NORMAL AND DEFECTIVE
COLOUR VISION

NORMAL AND DEFECTIVE COLOUR VISION

Edited by

J. D. MOLLON

University of Cambridge

J. POKORNY

University of Chicago

and

K. KNOBLAUCH

University of Lyon

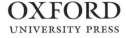

OXFORD
UNIVERSITY PRESS

Great Clarendon Street, Oxford OX2 6DP

Oxford University Press is a department of the University of Oxford.
It furthers the University's objective of excellence in research, scholarship,
and education by publishing worldwide in

Oxford New York

Auckland Bangkok Buenos Aires Cape Town Chennai
Dar es Salaam Delhi Hong Kong Istanbul Karachi Kolkata
Kuala Lumpur Madrid Melbourne Mexico City Mumbai Nairobi
São Paulo Shanghai Taipei Tokyo Toronto

Oxford is a registered trade mark of Oxford University Press
in the UK and in certain other countries

Published in the United States
by Oxford University Press Inc., New York

British Library Cataloging in Publication Data
(Data available)

Library of Congress Cataloging in Publication Data
(Data available)

ISBN 0 19 852530 3

10 9 8 7 6 5 4 3 2 1

Typeset by Newgen Imaging Systems (P) Ltd., Chennai, India
Printed in Great Britain
on acid-free paper by
Biddles Ltd, Guildford and King's Lynn

PREFACE

Those who study colour vision are drawn from many different disciplines, including physics, physiology, ophthalmology, optometry, and experimental psychology. Their publications are correspondingly scattered among scores of journals. The International Colour Vision Society (ICVS) exists to bring together colour scientists from different fields. The papers collected in this volume are selected from those given at a symposium held by the Society in Cambridge to mark the bicentennial of the lecture in which Thomas Young first proposed the trichromatic theory of colour vision. His paper was published in the *Philosophical Transactions* of the Royal Society for 1802. Young's theory was later given a quantitative basis by James Clerk Maxwell, and so it was appropriate that the Cambridge symposium was held at Clerk Maxwell's first college, Peterhouse.

Colour vision is arguably the most delicate of all our senses. For we can detect changes of less than 0.1% in the relative rates at which photons are absorbed in different classes of retinal photoreceptor. But the delicacy of our colour sense means that it is also very vulnerable, readily affected by toxins and by ocular and systemic disease. So the reader will find in this volume not only a survey of normal colour vision but also an account of the alterations of colour perception that occur in pathological conditions, as well as a discussion of the clinical tests that may be used to examine them. Clinical papers have always been integral to the ICVS, which began life in 1971 as an association of European clinicians and visual scientists, who were brought together by the Belgian ophthalmologist, Guy Verriest (1927–1988).

Some 8% of men exhibit an inherited deficiency or anomaly of colour vision, and these many variant forms of perception were already of interest to colour theorists in Thomas Young's day. Young's contemporary, John Dalton, described his own colour blindness in his first scientific paper, and Young rightly guessed that Dalton was lacking one of three types of receptor present in the normal eye. Inherited colour deficiencies continue to enjoy a central place in colour theory, and many of the papers in the present volume are concerned primarily or in part with this topic. What is new, however, is that the genetic basis of inherited colour deficiencies is increasingly yielding to molecular analysis; and Thomas Young's greatest contribution to modern science – the Principle of Interference – has recently provided a tool for analysing the three-dimensional structure of the photopigment molecules, the molecules on which all vision depends. Molecular genetics has also revived interest in the evolution of colour vision, and the reader will find this field well represented in the present volume. An interest in evolution has led visual scientists to ask how well our colour vision is matched to the chromatic properties of the theatre in which we live. At the Cambridge meeting this question was the subject of the Verriest Lecture by Dr D. I. A. MacLeod, and the Editors are grateful to Dr. MacLeod for allowing them to print the text of his Lecture.

All the papers included in the present volume have been refereed before publication. The Editors thank the contributors and referees for their work in making this book possible; and we are also grateful to The Wellcome Trust, The Colour Group of Great Britain, and the University of Cambridge for financial assistance that made possible both the meeting and the publication of selected papers.

Those wishing to learn more about the International Colour Vision Society are invited to consult the Society's web page: http://orlab.optom.unsw.edu.au/ICVS. Membership enquiries may be directed to the Membership Secretary, Dr Anne Kurtenbach, Department of Pathophysiology of Vision and Neuro-Ophthalmology, University Eye Hospital, Schleichstrasse, 72076 Tübingen, Germany.

The Editors would like to dedicate this volume to the memory of Professor C. R. Cavonius, who died on January 20, 2003. Professor Cavonius was an honorary member of the International Colour Vision Society and an editor of several of its earlier publications.

J. Mollon, J. Pokorny, K. Knoblauch

CONTENTS

Introduction: Thomas Young and the trichromatic theory of colour vision *page xix*

J. D. Mollon

Section 1   Photoreceptors and their evolution

1   Electrons and X-rays reveal the structure of rhodopsin: a prototypical G protein-coupled receptor–Implications for colour vision *page 3*

Jonathan J. Ruprecht and Gebhard F. X. Schertler

2   Photopigment polymorphism in prosimians and the origins of primate trichromacy *page 14*

Gerald H. Jacobs and Jess F. Deegan II

3   Did primate trichromacy evolve for frugivory or folivory? *page 21*

P. Sumner and J. D. Mollon

4   Lack of S-opsin expression in the brush-tailed porcupine (*Atherurus africanus*) and other mammals. Is the evolutionary persistence of S-cones a paradox? *page 31*

P. Ahnelt, K. Moutairou, M. Glösmann, and A. Kübber-Heiss

5   The arrangement of L and M cones in human and a primate retina *page 39*

J. K. Bowmaker, J. W. L. Parry, and J. D. Mollon

6   Comparison of human and monkey pigment gene promoters to evaluate DNA sequences proposed to govern L : M cone ratio *page 51*

C. McMahon, J. Neitz, and M. Neitz

Section 2   Retinal processes

7   Structure of receptive field centers of midget retinal ganglion cells *page 63*

Barry B. Lee

8   The neural circuit providing input to midget ganglion cells *page 71*

David W. Marshak

9   Coding of position of achromatic and chromatic edges by retinal ganglion cells *page 79*

Hao Sun, Barry B. Lee, and Lukas Rüttiger

Section 3   Spatial and temporal aspects of colour perception

10   Psychophysical correlates of parvo- and magnocellular function *page 91*
      Vivianne C. Smith and Joel Pokorny

11   Spatial contrast sensitivity for pulsed- and steady-pedestal stimuli *page 108*
      Anna Leonova, Joel Pokorny, and Vivianne C. Smith

12   Chromatic assimilation: evidence for a neural mechanism *page 114*
      Steven K. Shevell and Dingcai Cao

13   Reaction times to stimuli in isoluminant colour space *page 122*
      D. J. McKeefry, N. R. A. Parry, and I. J. Murray

14   Integration times reveal mechanisms responding to isoluminant chromatic
      gratings: a two-centre visual evoked potential study *page 130*
      A. G. Robson, J. J. Kulikowski, M. Korostenskaja, M. M. Neveu, C. R. Hogg,
      and G. E. Holder

15   Temporal frequency and contrast adaptation *page 138*
      Arthur G. Shapiro, S. Mary Hood, and J. D. Mollon

16   Contribution of achromatic and chromatic contrast signals to
      Fechner–Benham subjective colours *page 145*
      J. Le Rohellec, H. Brettel, and F. Viénot

17   Sensitivity to movement of configurations of achromatic and chromatic
      points in amblyopic patients *page 154*
      M. L. F. de Mattiello, M. Maneiro, and S. Buglione

18   Convergence as a function of chromatic contrast: a possible contributor to
      depth perception? *page 160*
      Galina V. Paramei and Wolfgang Jaschinski

Section 4   Rods and colour vision

19   The influence of rods on color naming during dark adaptation *page 173*
      Janice L. Nerger, Vicki J. Volbrecht, and Kristin A. Haase

20   Stimulus duration affects rod influence on hue perception *page 179*
      Steven L. Buck and Roger Knight

Section 5   Natural scenes and colour constancy

21   The Verriest Lecture: Colour discrimination, colour constancy and natural
      scene statistics *page 189*
      Donald I. A. MacLeod

22   Tritanopic colour constancy under daylight changes? *page 218*
      David H. Foster, Kinjiro Amano, and Sérgio M. C. Nascimento

23   Red–green colour deficiency and colour constancy under
     orthogonal-daylight changes *page 225*
     Kinjiro Amano, David H. Foster, and Sérgio M. C. Nascimento

24   Calculating appearances in complex and simple images *page 231*
     John J. McCann

25   The effect of global contrast distribution on colour appearance *page 239*
     K. Wolf and A. C. Hurlbert

Section 6   Colour spaces and their variation

26   Schopenhauer's "parts of daylight" in the light of modern
     colorimetry *page 251*
     Jan J. Koenderink

27   Representing an observer's matches in an alien colour space *page 267*
     Kenneth Knoblauch

28   Macular pigment: nature's notch filter *page 273*
     J. D. Moreland and S. Westland

29   How to find a tritan line *page 279*
     H. E. Smithson, P. Sumner, and J. D. Mollon

30   Some properties of the physiological colour system *page 288*
     C. von Campenhausen, and J. Schramme

Section 7   Inherited colour deficiency: molecular genetics

31   Genotypic variation in multi-gene dichromats *page 299*
     S. S. Deeb, W. Jagla, H. Jägle, T. Hayashi, and L. T. Sharpe

32   Hybrid pigment genes, dichromacy, and anomalous trichromacy *page 307*
     Wolfgang Jagla, Tanja Breitsprecher, Itala Kucsera, Gyula Kovacs, Bernd
     Wissinger, Samir S. Deeb, and Lindsay T. Sharpe

33   Middle wavelength sensitive photopigment gene expression is absent in
     deuteranomalous colour vision *page 318*
     Maureen Neitz, Kathryn Bollinger, and Jay Neitz

Section 8   Inherited colour deficiency: psychophysics and tests

34   Preliminary norms for the Cambridge colour test *page 331*
     D. F. Ventura, L. C. L. Silveira, A. R. Rodrigues, J. M. de Souza, M. Gualtieri,
     D. Bonci, and M. F. Costa

35   Evaluation of "Colour vision testing made easy" *page 340*
     Stephen J. Dain

36   Survey of the colour vision demands in fire-fighting   *page 347*
     Stephen J. Dain and Laura E. Hughes

37   Lantern colour vision tests: one light or two?   *page 354*
     Jeffery K. Hovis

38   Extreme anomalous trichromatism   *page 364*
     Jennifer Birch

39   Colour naming, colour categories, and central colour-coding in a case of
     X-linked incomplete achromatopsia   *page 370*
     J. B. Nolan, M. A. Crognale, and M. A. Webster

Section 9   Acquired deficiencies of colour vision

40   Effects of retinal detachment on S and M cone function in an animal model
     page 381
     Gerald H. Jacobs, Jack B. Calderone, Tsutomu Sakai,
     Geoffrey P. Lewis, and Steven K. Fisher

41   Colour vision in central serous chorioretinopathy   *page 389*
     Maija Mäntyjärvi and Tarja Maaranen

42   Early vision loss in diabetic patients assessed by the Cambridge Colour Test
     page 395
     D. F. Ventura, M. F. Costa, M. Gualtieri, M. Nishi, M. Bernick,
     D. Bonci, and J. M. de Souza

43   Colour-vision disturbances in patients with arterial hypertension   *page 404*
     Anke Schröder, Carl Erb, Stefan Falk, Gabriele Schwartze,
     Jörg Radermacher, and Rolf Winter

44   Visual dysfunction following mercury exposure by breathing mercury
     vapour or by eating mercury-contaminated food   *page 409*
     Luiz Carlos L. Silveira, Enira Terezinha B. Damin,
     Maria da Conceição N. Pinheiro, Anderson R. Rodrigues,
     Ana Laura A. Moura, Maria Izabel T. Côrtes, and Guilherme A. Mello

Index   *page 419*

CONTRIBUTORS

P. Ahnelt
Department of Physiology,
Medical School, University of Vienna,
Austria

Kinjiro Amano
Visual and Computational Neuroscience
Group,
Department of Optometry and
Neuroscience,
University of Manchester Institute of
Science and Technology,
Manchester, M60 1QD, UK

M. Bernick
Departamento de Psicologia
Experimental,
Nucleo de Neurosciencias e
Comportamento,
Instituto de Psicologia, Universidade de
Säo Paulo, Brasil

Jennifer Birch
Applied Vision Research Laboratory
City University, London EC1V OHB, UK

Kathryn Bollinger
Department of Ophthalmology
Medical College of Wisconsin
8701 Watertown Plank Rd.
Milwaukee, WI 53226, USA

D. Bonci
Departamento de Psicologia
Experimental,
Nucleo de Neurosciencias e
Comportamento,
Instituto de Psicologia, Universidade de
Säo Paulo, Brasil

J. K. Bowmaker
Department of Visual Science,
Institute of Ophthalmology
University College London, London
EC1V 9EL, UK

Tanja Breistsprecher
Department of Neuro-Ophthalmology
University Eye Clinic, D72076,
Tübingen, Germany

H. Brettel
CNRS URA 820, Ecole National
Superieur des Telecommunications,
Départment de Traitement du
Signal et de L'Image, 46 rue
Barrault, 75013, Paris, France

Steven L. Buck
Department of Psychology
University of Washington
Seattle WA 98155-1525, USA

S. Buglione
Laboratorio de Investigaciones Visuales
University of Buenos Aires, Argentina

Jack B. Calderone
Department of Psychology and
Neuroscience Research Institute
University of California
Santa Barbara, California, USA

C. von Campenhausen
Institut für Zoologie, Johannes
Gutenberg - Universität
Saarstr. 21, 55099 Mainz, Germany

Dingcai Cao
Visual Science Laboratories
The University of Chicago
940 East 57th St., Chicago, IL 60637, USA

Maria Izabel T. Côrtes
Departamento de Fisiologia,
Universidade Federal do Para 66075-900
Belém, Pará, Brasil

M. F. Costa
Departamento de Psicologia
Experimental,
Nucleo de Neurosciencias e
Comportamento,
Instituto de Psicologia, Universidade de
Säo Paulo, Brasil

M. A. Crognale
Department of Psychology,
University of Nevada,
Reno, NY 89557, USA

Stephen J. Dain
School of Optometry and Vision Science
University of New South Wales
Sydney NSW 2052 Australia

Enira Terezinha B. Damin
Departamento de Fisiologia,
Universidade Federal do Para 66075-900
Belém, Pará, Brasil

S. S. Deeb
Departments of Medicine and Genome
Sciences
University of Washington, Seattle
WA 98195, USA

Jess F. Deegan II
Department of Psychology,
California State University, Bakersfield,
USA

Carl Erb
Medizinische Hochschule Hannover,
Department of Ophthalmology
Carl-Neuberg-Str. 1, 30625, Hannover,
Germany

Stefan Falk
Medizinische Hochschule Hannover,
Department of Ophthalmology,
Carl-Neuberg-Str.1, 30625,
Hannover, Germany

Steven K. Fisher
Department of Psychology and
Neuroscience Research Institute
University of California
Santa Barbara, California, USA

David H. Foster
Visual and Computational Neuroscience
Group,
Department of Optometry and
Neuroscience,
University of Manchester Institute of
Science and Technology,
Manchester, M60 1QD, UK

M. Glösmann
Department of Physiology,
Medical School
University of Vienna, Austria

M. Gualtieri
Departamento de Psicologia
Experimental,
Nucleo de Neurosciencias e
Comportamento,
Instituto de Psicologia, Universidade de
Säo Paulo, Brasil

Kristin A. Haase
Department of Psychology, Behavioral
Neuroscience Program,
Colorado State University
Fort Collins, CO, USA

T. Hayashi
Departments of Medicine and Genome
Sciences
University of Washington, Seattle WA
98195, USA

C. R. Hogg
Department of Electrophysiology
Moorfields Eye Hospital
City Road, London, EC1V 2PD, UK

G. E. Holder
Department of Electrophysiology
Moorfields Eye Hospital
City Road, London, EC1V 2PD, UK

S. Mary Hood
Department of Experimental Psychology
Cambridge University, Cambridge,
CB2 3EB, UK

Jeffery K. Hovis
School of Optometry
University of Waterloo
Waterloo, ON N2L 3G4, Canada

Laura E. Hughes
School of Optometry and Vision Science,
University of New South Wales,
Sydney, NSW 2052, Australia

A. C. Hurlbert
Henry Wellcome Building,
School of Biology, Framlington Place,
Newcastle upon Tyne, NE2 4HH, UK

Gerald H. Jacobs
Neuroscience Research Institute &
Department of Psychology,
University of California, Santa Barbara,
CA 93106, USA

W. Jagla
Department of Neuro-Ophthalmology,
University Eye Clinic, D72076
Tübingen, Germany

H. Jägle
Department of Neuro-Ophthalmology,
University Eye Clinic, D72076
Tübingen, Germany

Wolfgang Jaschinski
Institute for Occupational Psychology at
the University of Dortmund,
Ardeystrasse 67, D-44139 Dortmund
Germany

Roger Knight
Department of Psychology
University of Washington
Seattle WA 98155-1525, USA

Kenneth Knoblauch
INSERM Unité 371
Cerveau et Vision
18 avenue du Doyen Lépine
69675 Bron Cedex, France

Jan J. Koenderink
Universiteit Utrecht
Faculteit Natuur- en Sterrenkunde,
Princetonplein 5,
3584 cc Utrecht, Postbus 80000,
The Netherlands

M. Korostenskaja
Visual Sciences Laboratory
Department of Optometry and
Neuroscience
UMIST, Manchester, UK

Gyula Kovacs
COLORYTE HUNGARY Inc.,
Budapest, H-1121, Hungary

A. Kübber-Heiss
Department of Pathology and Forensic
Medicine,
Veterinary University, Vienna, Austria

Itala Kucsra
COLORYTE HUNGARY Inc., Budapest,
H-1121, Hungary

J. J. Kulikowski
Visual Sciences Laboratory
Department of Optometry and
Neuroscience,
UMIST, Manchester, UK

Barry B. Lee
SUNY College of Optometry, New York,
NY, 10036, USA and
Max Plank Institute for Biophysical
Chemistry
Göttingen, Germany

Anna Leonova
Visual Science Laboratories
The University of Chicago
940 East 57th St., Chicago, IL 60637

J. Le Rohellec
Muséum National d'Histoire Naturelle
Laboratoire de Photobiologie,
43 rue Cuvier, 75005 Paris, France

Geoffrey P. Lewis
Neuroscience Research Institute
University of California
Santa Barbara, California, USA

Tarja Maaranen
Department of Ophthalmology
University of Kuopio and University
Hospital of Kuopio
Kuopio, Finland

Donald I. A. MacLeod
Psychology Department
UCSD, La Jolla, CA 92093, USA

Marta Maneiro
Laboratorio de Investigaciones Visuales
University of Buenos Aires, Argentina

Maija Mäntyjärvi
Department of Ophthalmology
University of Kuopio and University
Hospital of Kuopio
Kuopio, Finland

David W. Marshak
Department of Neurobiology and
Anatomy,
University of Texas Medical School
Houston, Texas, 77225, USA

María L. F. de Mattiello
Laboratorio de Investigaciones Visuales
University of Buenos Aires, Argentina

John J. McCann
McCann Imaging, Belmont MA 02478
USA

D. J. McKeefry
Department of Optometry
University of Bradford
Bradford, UK

C. McMahon
Department of Cell Biology,
Neurobiology, and Anatomy
Medical College of Wisconsin
8701 Watertown Plank Rd.
Milwaukee, WI 53226, USA

Guilherme A. Mello
Departamento de Fisiologia,
Universidade Federal do Para 66075-900
Belém, Pará, Brasil

J. D. Mollon
Department of Experimental Psychology
Cambridge University, Downing St.,
Cambridge, CB2 3EB, UK

J. D. Moreland
MacKay Institute of Communication &
Neuroscience,
Keele University, UK

Ana Laura A. Moura
Departamento de Fisiologia,
Universidade Federal do Para 66075-900
Belém, Pará, Brasil

K. Moutairou
Département de Biochimie et de Biologie
Cellulaire
Université Nationale du Benin
BP 525 Cotonou, Rep Benin

I. J. Murray
Visual Sciences Laboratory
Department of Optometry and
Neuroscience
UMIST, Manchester, UK

Sérgio M. C. Nascimento
Departamento de Física
Campus de Gualtar
Universidade do Minho
4710-057 Braga, Portugal

J. Neitz
Department of Cell Biology,
Neurobiology, and Anatomy
Medical College of Wisconsin
8701 Watertown Plank Rd.
Milwaukee, WI 53226, USA

M. Neitz
Department of Ophthalmology,
Medical College of Wisconsin
8701 Watertown Plank Rd.
Milwaukee, WI 53226, USA

Janice L. Nerger
Department of Psychology,
Behavioural Neuroscience Program,

Colorado State University
Fort Collins, CO, USA

M. Neveu
Department of Electrophysiology
Moorfields Eye Hospital
City Road, London, EC1V 2PD, UK

M. Nishi
Departamento de Psicologia
Experimental,
Nucleo de Neurosciencias e
Comportamento,
Instituto de Psicologia, Universidade de
Säo Paulo, Brasil

J. B. Nolan
Department of Psychology,
University of Nevada,
Reno NV 89557, USA and
Department of Psychology
Southwestern University
Winfield, KS 67156, USA

Galina V. Paramei
Institute for Occupational Psychology at
the University of Dortmund
Ardeystrasse 67, D-44139 Dortmund,
Germany

J. W. L. Parry
Department of Visual Science,
Institute of Ophthalmology
University College London, London
ECIV 9EL, Uk

N. R. A. Parry
Vision Science Centre, Manchester Royal
Eye Hospital, UK

Maria da Conceiçao N. Pinheiro
Núcleo de Medicina Tropical,
Universidade Federal do Para 66075-900
Belém, Pará, Brasil

Joel Pokorny
Visual Science Laboratories
The University of Chicago
940 East 57th St., Chicago, IL 60637, USA

Jorg Rädermacher
Medizinische Hochschule Hannover
Department of Nephrology
Carl-Neuberg-Str.
Hannover, Germany

A. G. Robson
Department of Electrophysiology,
Moorfields Eye Hospital, City Road,
London, ECIV 2PD, UK and
Visual Sciences Laboratory
Department of Optometry and
Neuroscience
UMIST, Manchester, UK

Anderson R. Rodrigues
Departmento de Fisiologia
Universidade Federal do Pará, 66075-900
Belém, Pará, Brasil

Jonathan J. Ruprecht
MRC Laboratory of Molecular Biology
Hills Road, Cambridge, CB2 2QH, UK

Lukas Rüttiger
Max Planck Institute for Biophysical
Chemistry, Göttingen, Germany

Tsutomu Sakai
Department of Ophthalmology
Jikei University School of Medicine
Tokyo, Japan

Gebhard F. X. Schertler
MRC Laboratory of Molecular Biology
Hills Road, Cambridge, CB2 2QH, UK

J. Schramme
Institut für Zoologie, Johannes

Gutenberg - Universität
Saarstr. 21, 55099 Mainz, Germany

Anke Schröder
Medizinische Hochschule Hannover,
Department of Ophthalmology
Carl-Neuberg-Str. 1, 30625, Hannover,
Germany

Gabriele Schwartz
Medizinische Hochschule Hannover,
Department of Ophthalmology
Carl-Neuberg-Str. 1, 30625, Hannover,
Germany

Arthur G. Shapiro
Department of Psychology
Bucknell University
Lewisburg, PA 17837, USA

L. T. Sharpe
Department of Neuro-Ophthalmology,
University Eye Clinic, D72076,
Tübingen, Germany and
Department of Psychology, University of
Newcastle
NE1 7RU Newcastle-upon-Tyne, UK

Steven K. Shevell
Departments of Psychology and
Ophthalmology, and Visual Science
Visual Science Laboratories,
The University of Chicago,
940 East 57th St., Chicago, IL 60637, USA

Luiz Carlos L. Silveira
Departmento de Fisiologia and
Núcleo de Medicina Tropical
Universidade Federal do Pará, 66075-900
Belém, Pará, Brasil

Vivianne C. Smith
Visual Science Laboratories
The University of Chicago
940 East 57th St., Chicago, IL 60637, USA

H. E. Smithson
Department of Experimental Psychology
Cambridge University, Downing St.,
Cambridge, CB2 3EB, UK

J. M. de Souza
Departamento de Psicologia
Experimental,
Nucleo de Neurosciencias e
Comportamento,
Instituto de Psicologia, Universidade de
Säo Paulo, Brasil

P. Sumner
Department of Experimental Psychology,
Cambridge University, Cambridge,
CB2 3EB, UK and
Neuroscience and Psychological
Medicine,
Imperial College School of Medicine,
London, W6 8RP, UK

Hao Sun
SUNY State College of Optometry
New York, NY, 10036, USA

D. F. Ventura
Departamento de Psicologia
Experimental,
Nucleo de Neurosciencias e
Comportamento,
Instituto de Psicologia, Universidade de
Säo Paulo, Brasil

F. Viénot
Muséum National d'Histoire Naturelle
Laboratoire de Photobiologie, 43 rue
Cuvier, 75005 Paris, France

Vicki J. Volbrecht
Department of Psychology
Behavioural Neuroscience Program,
Colorado State University,
Fort Collins, CO, USA

M. A. Webster
Department of Psychology,
University of Nevada,
Reno, NY 89557, USA

S. Westland
Colour Imaging Institute,
University of Derby, UK

Rolf Winter
Medizinische Hochschule Hannover,
Department of Ophthalmology
Carl-Neuberg-Str. 1, 30625, Hannover,
Germany

Bernd Wissinger
Departments of Medicine and Genome
Sciences
University of Washington, Seattle
WA 98195, USA

K. Wolf
Henry Wellcome Building,
School of Biology,
Framlington Place,
Newcastle upon Tyne, NE2 4HN, UK

INTRODUCTION: THOMAS YOUNG AND THE TRICHROMATIC THEORY OF COLOUR VISION

J. D. MOLLON

As this paper contains nothing which deserves the name, either of experiment or discovery, and as it is in fact destitute of every species of merit, we should have allowed it to pass among the multitude of those articles which must always find admittance into the collections of a Society, which is pledged to publish two or three volumes every year...

These critical words came from a distinguished pen, that of Henry Brougham (1778–1868), later Baron Brougham and Vaux. While still a teenager, Brougham had published optical and mathematical papers in the *Philosophical Transactions* of the Royal Society; and he was later to become Lord Chancellor, the chief law officer of the United Kingdom. He is remembered as a campaigner for abolition of the slave trade, as the counsel for Queen Caroline in the divorce proceedings against her, and as the co-founder of University College London. But in the history of optics he is also remembered for the essay whose opening lines are quoted above (Brougham 1803).

The object of Brougham's scorn was a Bakerian Lecture delivered in two parts to the Royal Society of London on November 12 and 19, 1801, and published in the *Philosophical Transactions* for 1802. It was in this Lecture that Thomas Young developed the wave theory of light, introduced the generalized Principle of Interference, and proposed the trichromatic theory of colour vision in its recognizably modern form.

Born at Milverton in Somerset in 1773, Thomas Young was the eldest son of a banker and mercer. The family were Quakers. Young could read by the age of two—if we believe his own account—and had read twice through the bible by the age of four (Peacock 1855). At the age of 17, he read Newton's *Principia* and *Opticks*, but—by the standard of Henry Brougham—he was relatively old when he published his first scientific paper. This paper, on the mechanism of visual accommodation, appeared in the *Philosophical Transactions* when Young was 20 (Young 1793) and secured his election to the Royal Society the following year. His uncle, Richard Brocklesby, was a prosperous London physician and intended Young as his successor. Young began his studies at St. Bartholomew's Hospital in London, and then moved to Edinburgh for the academic year 1794–5. It was here that

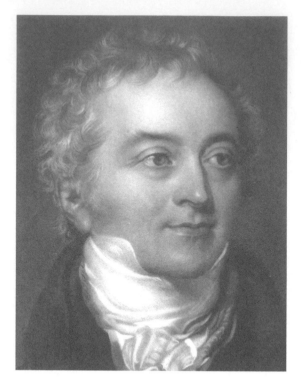

Figure i.1 Thomas Young (1773–1829).

he first crossed the path of Henry Brougham, for it is known that they both attended one of Joseph Black's last courses of chemical lectures (Cantor 1971).

The origins of the trichromatic theory

Young spent the academic year 1795–6 at the Georg-August University of Göttingen, which lay within the Hannoverian realms of George III. It was in Göttingen that Young probably first gave detailed thought to the nature of colour, as a result of contact with the physicist and aphorist, G. C. Lichtenberg. Although Young found most of the Göttingen professors rather distant and formal, he mentions in a letter to his uncle that 'Arnemann, in whose house I live, and Lichtenberg the lecturer on Natural Philosophy, are the most sociable' (Peacock 1855). Lichtenberg was an anglophile and a Fellow of the Royal Society, and brief entries in his diaries do record visits by Young ('Dr. Young bey mir') (Lee 2001). We know from Young's own account that he attended Lichtenberg's lectures on physics at 2.00 o'clock each afternoon (see Figure i.2). And we know from a transcript of Lichtenberg's lectures, taken down by a student and later published (Gamauf 1811), that Lichtenberg discussed in some detail the colour triangle of Tobias Mayer, the Göttingen astronomer. Mayer had died in 1762 and Lichtenberg had taken on the task of editing

" At 8, I attend Spittler's course on the History of the Principal States of Europe, exclusive of Germany.
    " At 9, Arnemann on Materia Medica.
    " At 10, Richter on Acute Diseases.
    " At 11, Twice a week, private lessons from Blessman, the
        academical dancing-master.
    " At 12, I dine at Ruhlander's table d'hôte.
    " At 1, Twice a week, lessons on the Clavichord from Forkel ;
        and twice a week at home, from Fiorillo on Drawing.
    " At 2, Lichtenberg on Physics.
    " At 3, I ride in the academical manège, under the instruc-
        tions of Ayrer, four times a week.
    " At 4, Stromeyer on Diseases.
    " At 5, Blumenbach on Natural History.
    " At 6, Twice Blessmen with other pupils, and twice Forkel.
    " Spittler, Arnemann and Blumenbach, follow, in lecturing,
their own compendiums, and Lichtenberg makes use of Erxle-
ben's. I mean to study regularly beforehand."

Figure i.2 Thomas Young's own account of his working day as a student in Göttingen in the academical year 1795–6. Reproduced from Peacock (1855).

his unpublished papers, which included the essay *On the Relationship of Colours* (Forbes 1971; Mayer 1775). Mayer had supposed that there were only three primary colours—red, yellow and blue—and that all other colours could be produced by mixing the primaries. The three primaries formed the apices of his colour-mixing triangle, and along each side there were twelve discriminably different mixtures.

Yet Newton's prismatic experiments had suggested that the physical variable underlying hue was a continuous one. In his lectures, Lichtenberg himself took a conventionally Newtonian position when discussing the dispersion of white light by a prism, but he also discussed the extensive eighteenth-century evidence that all colours could be constructed by mixing three 'primary' colours. The trichromacy of colour mixture had in fact been widely discussed before Mayer (e.g. Anonymous 1708; Castel 1740; Le Blon 1725) It was this accumulated evidence for trichromacy that led many commentators to suppose the Newton was wrong and that there were three physically distinct types of light. They were misled by a category error: they supposed that the trichromacy of colour mixture was a property of physics (Mollon 2003).

What most colour theorists lacked in the eighteenth century was the concept of a tuned transducer, that is, a retinal resonator responding to only part of the visible spectrum. Rather it was assumed, by Newton and by many subsequent writers, that the vibrations occasioned in the retina by rays of light were conveyed unchanged along the optic nerve to the sensorium, where they aroused sensations of hue. Without the concept of a tuned retinal transducer, it was not obvious that trichromacy was a property of our visual system rather than a fact of physics. An intermediate stage of understanding is represented by the shadowy figure of George Palmer (1740–95). A London dealer in coloured glass, Palmer was both a physical and a physiological trichromatist: he postulated three types of 'particle' or 'fibre' in the retina and three corresponding kinds of light (Mollon 1993; Palmer 1777). Colour blindness arose, said Palmer, when one or two of the three types of 'molecule' was constitutionally inactive or constitutionally over-active. His explanation of colour blindness first appeared in a scientific magazine edited by Lichtenberg's brother (Voigt 1781).

In summary, as the eighteenth century closed, there was accumulated evidence for the trichromacy of colour mixture, but this evidence seemed to be at odds with the Newtonian theory of light. It was to be Thomas Young who released colour science from the category error that held it back. And it was almost certainly in Göttingen in 1795–6 that he was first exposed to the issues in detail.

Acoustics and the principle of interference

It was not, however, the theory of light that primarily occupied Thomas Young in the period that immediately followed his return from Germany to Emmanuel College in Cambridge. He was to come to colour theory by an indirect route. In order to graduate as Doctor of Physic in Göttingen, he submitted a dissertation on the preservative powers of the human body, but he was also required to deliver a lecture on some topic relevant to medical studies. He chose to lecture on the human voice and a fragment of this lecture was printed at the end of his dissertation. He included a proposed universal alphabet of forty-seven letters, which were designed to express, by their combination, every sound that could be produced by the human vocal organs and thus any human language. Wanting to develop this work, he soon realized that he was limited by his understanding of the nature of sound. He gives an account in a later pamphlet defending his optical papers against the criticisms published by Brougham in the *Edinburgh Review*:

> 'When I began the outline of an essay on the human voice, I found myself at a loss for a perfect conception of what sound was, and during the three years that I passed at Emmanuel College, Cambridge, I collected all the information relating to it that I could procure from books, and I made a variety of original experiments on sounds of all kinds, and on the motions of fluids in general. In the course of these enquiries, I learned to my surprise, how much further our neighbours on the continent were advanced in the investigation of the motions of sounding bodies and of elastic fluids, than any of our countrymen; and in making some experiments on the production of sounds I was so forcibly impressed with the resemblance of the phenomena that I saw, to those of the colours of thin plates, with which I was already acquainted, that I began to suspect the existence of a closer analogy between them than I could before have easily believed.' (Young 1804)

The reason that Young did not start immediately in medical practice in 1797 was that new rules of the Royal College of Physicians required him to spend two consecutive years at one university (Gurney 1831). So this is how he came to enter Emmanuel College, Cambridge, as a Fellow-Commoner, that is, a gentleman entitled to dine with the Fellows although still *in statu pupillari*. One of his contemporaries at the college recorded that he was known in Emmanuel as 'Phaenomenon Young' and wrote:

> '...his room had all the appearance of belonging to an idle man. I once found him blowing smoke through long tubes, and I afterwards saw a representation of the effect in the Transactions of the Royal Society to illustrate one of his papers upon sound; but he was not in the habit of making experiments.' (Peacock 1855)

The paper referred to in this passage must be Young's 'Outlines of experiments and inquiries respecting sound and light', published in the *Philosophical Transactions* for 1800. In this paper he applies the principle of interference to acoustics but does not yet generalize it to optics. He devotes most of the text to acoustics but in §10 he does suggest an analogy between the colours of thin plates and the resonance of organ pipes. He does not yet have the critical insight—that the colours of thin plates are the product of constructive and destructive interference—for it is only in the following section of the paper ('Of the coalescence of musical sounds') that he uses the yet-unnamed principle of interference to explain the beating that is heard when two tones are of very similar but not identical frequency.

The *Parlour Book* of Emmanuel College records a wager dated 14 March 1799 between Young and Pemberton that 'Young will produce a pamphlet or paper on sound more satisfactory than anything that has already appeared, before he takes his Bachelor's degree' (Figure i.3). An Audit of Wagers in the *Parlour Book* for 1802 records that Young was held to have lost the bet.

Yet the Principle of Interference was to prove perhaps the single most important concept in the physics of the subsequent two centuries. According to college tradition at Emmanuel, Young first observed interference patterns in the ripples produced by a pair of swans on the rectangular pond in the college paddock (Bendall *et al.* 1999). It is a pleasant legend, but I have not found any nineteenth-century reference to it. However, in defending his theory of light against Brougham's criticisms, Young does certainly use a lake as his model:

> 'Suppose a number of equal waves of water to move upon the surface of a stagnant lake, with a certain constant velocity, and to enter a narrow channel leading out of the lake. Suppose then another similar cause to have excited another equal series of waves, which arrive at the same channel, with the same velocity, and at the same time as the first. Neither series of waves will destroy the other, but their effects will be combined: if they enter the channel in such a manner that the elevations of one series coincide with those of the other, they must together produce a series of greater joint elevations; but if the elevations of one series are so situated as to correspond to the depressions of the other, they must exactly fill up those depressions, and the surface of the water must remain smooth; at least I can discover no alternative, either from theory or from experiment.' (Young 1804)

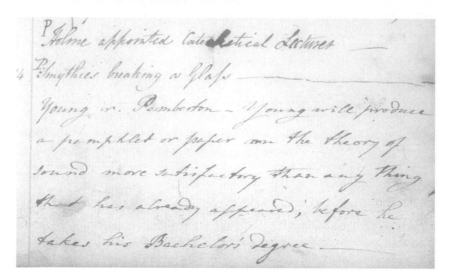

Figure i.3 A wager between Young and Pemberton recorded in the Parlour Book of Emmanuel College, Cambridge. The preceding entries record an appointment celebrated and a clumsiness fined.

The Bakerian Lecture of 1801

By Young's own account, it was not until May, 1801 that he realized that interference could be used to explain the colours of thin plates—the colours of soap bubbles and oil films, and the coloured rings observed by Newton when a convex lens was pressed against a glass plate (Newton 1730). Young set out the hypothesis in the Bakerian Lecture that was to draw Brougham's attack. The lecture was read in two parts to the Royal Society, on 12 and 19 November 1801, and published the following spring (Young 1802a). He supposed that light consisted of waves in an all pervading ether. Different wavelengths corresponded to different hues, the shortest wavelengths appearing violet, the longest red. In his initial model of 1802, the undulations were longitudinal—along the line of the ray—rather than transverse, as Fresnel was later to show them to be.

Young proposed that the colours of thin films depended on constructive and destructive interference between light reflected at the first surface and light reflected at the second: when the peak of one wave coincides with the trough of another, the two will cancel, but when the path length of the second ray is such that the peaks coincide for a given wavelength, then the hue corresponding to that wavelength will be seen (Young 1802a).

The principle of interference, in its generalized form, was first actually published in the *Syllabus* for the Royal Institution Lectures that Young gave in the winter of 1801–2 (Young 1802c). There he writes (page 117):

> 'But the general law, by which all these appearances are governed, may be very easily deduced from the interference of two coincident undulations, which either cooperate, or destroy each other, in the same manner as two musical notes produce an alternate intension and remission, in the beating of an imperfect unison.'

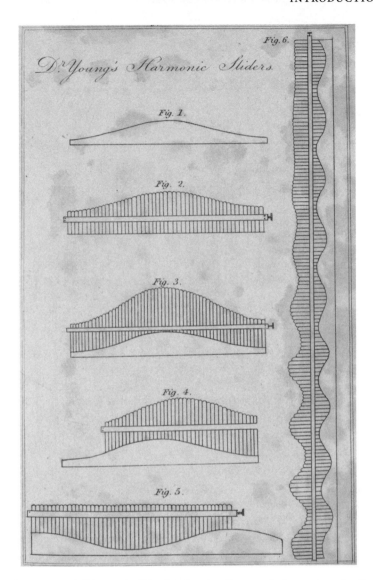

Figure i.4 Thomas Young's 'Harmonic sliders', designed to illustrate the interaction of optical or acoustic waves. A set of sliding rods of varying length (Fig. 2 in the diagram) can be placed on a shaped board representing a second wave (Fig. 1 in the diagram). In different phases (Figures 3–5 in the diagram), the two waveforms constructively or destructively interfere. Figure 6 in the diagram illustrates beating.

To illustrate the concept to his audience at the Royal Institution, Young developed the apparatus shown in Figure i.4: one of two component waves is formed by sliders of different length, the second by a shaped board. The former can be placed in different positions on the latter, to represent different phases (Young 1802b).

Colours.	Length of an Undulation in parts of an Inch, in Air.	Number of Undulations in an Inch.	Number of Undulations in a Second.	Wavelength nm
Extreme -	.0000266	37640	463 millions of millions	
Red - -	.0000256	39180	482	650
Intermediate	.0000246	40720	501	
Orange - -	.0000240	41610	512	609
Intermediate	.0000235	42510	523	
Yellow -	.0000227	44000	542	576
Intermediate	.0000219	45600	561 $(= 2^{48}$ nearly$)$	
Green - -	.0000211	47460	584	536
Intermediate	.0000203	49320	607	
Blue - -	.0000196	51110	629	497
Intermediate	.0000189	52910	652	
Indigo - -	.0000185	54070	665	469
Intermediate	.0000181	55240	680	
Violet - -	.0000174	57490	707	444
Extreme - -	.0000167	59750	735	

Figure i.5 Young's estimates of the wavelengths and frequencies corresponding to particular hues (Young, 1802a). Values of wavelength in nanometers are added to the right.

By applying his interference hypothesis to Newton's measurements of the colours of thin films, Young was able to map particular hues to the underlying physical variable. Figure i.5 shows his table of the wavelengths that correspond to given colours (Young 1802a). On the right, I have re-expressed Young's values in nanometers. They closely resemble modern estimates. A good test of their accuracy is the value that Young gives for yellow, since this is the part of the spectrum where hue changes rapidly with wavelength and where therefore a physical error would easily reveal itself. His value converts to 576 nm and this is within a nanometer of modern estimates of the wavelength that appears neither reddish nor greenish to an average eye in a neutral state of adaptation (Ayama *et al.* 1987). His estimates for orange, green and violet are similarly close to modern ones. But what makes the accuracy so impressive is that Thomas Young was using not his own measurements but rather those made by Newton in the seventeenth century.

The value given in Figure i.5 for blue (497 nm) is a longer wavelength than would be given today for the blue that is neither reddish nor greenish. However, Newton's 'blew' was embedded in a spectrum that also included indigo. 'Blew' may have been close to cyan, resembling the primary colour term *golyboi* in modern Russian.

The trichromatic theory

In the broader domain of science, Young's Bakerian Lecture is most important for the principle of interference, for the explanation of the colours of thin films, and for the first quantification of the visible spectrum. Visual scientists, however, most often cite the Lecture for its statement of the trichromatic theory of vision. Having grasped that the physical variable corresponding to hue was wavelength and very unlikely to be anything other than a continuous variable, Young saw that the results of colour mixing must be determined by the physiology of the human visual system, by the presence in the retina of a limited number of types of resonator. Yet he introduces the theory only briefly, and as an aside:

'Now, as it is almost impossible to conceive each sensitive point of the retina to contain an infinite number of particles, each capable of vibrating in perfect unison with every possible undulation, it becomes necessary to suppose the number limited, for instance, to the three principal colours, red, yellow, and blue, of which the undulations are related in magnitude nearly as the numbers 8, 7, and 6; and that each of the particles is capable of being put in motion less or more forcibly, by undulations differing less or more from a perfect unison; for instance, the undulations of green light being nearly in the ratio of 6 1/2, will affect equally the particles in unison with yellow and blue, and produce the same effect as a light composed of those two species: and each sensitive filament of the nerve may consist of three portions, one for each principal colour...' (Young 1802a)

Notice that in this first account, Young does not refer explicitly to the trichromacy of colour mixture, and he remains hesitant about the number of types of resonator. His uncertainty at this period (1801–2) is clear from the manuscript notes of his Royal Institution Lectures (University College London Archives, *Ms. Add. 13./14, 13./15*): at one point he offers red, yellow and blue as the primitive colours, but at another point he derives all colours from '4 simple colours', red, green, blue and violet. And neither in the manuscript notes nor in the printed *Syllabus* does he clearly explain to his audience what he means by 'simple' or 'primitive' colours.

In his later account of 'Chromatics', written for *Encyclopaedia Britannica* (Young 1817), the trichromatic theory takes on a more sophisticated form. Young assumes the three distinct 'sensations' to be red, green and violet. The rays occupying intermediate places in the Newtonian spectrum excite mixed sensations. Thus monochromatic yellow light excites both the red and green sensations, while monochromatic blue light excites both the violet and the green sensations. By 'sensation' he means here the excitation of his 'sympathetic fibres' or resonators. So he explains that 'mixed excitations' of the fibres— whether produced by monochromatic lights or mixtures—may produce 'a simple idea only', as when excitation of the green and violet fibres leads to the sensation of a pure blue. This is a critical insight. Young realized that the peak sensitivities of the receptors do not necessarily correspond to the hues that are phenomenologically the purest. This insight was not always shared by those who later adopted his theory.

There is a second way in which Young's version of the trichromatic theory was more advanced than that of his successors. For he allowed that the perceived colour of a patch in a complex scene depends not just on the relative excitations of the three types of fibre in the part of the retina illuminated by that patch. It depends also on the context, on the spectral distributions of surfaces in the surrounding field. Already in his *Syllabus* of 1802 he recognizes the existence of colour constancy, the approximate stability of our perception of surface colour when we view a given surface in illuminants of different colour.

> 'Other causes, probably connected with some general laws of sensation, produce the imaginary colours of shadows, which have been elegantly investigated and explained by Count Rumford. When a general colour prevails over the whole field of vision, excepting a part comparatively small, the apparent colour of that part is nearly the same as if the light falling on the whole field had been white, and the rays of the prevalent colour only had been intercepted at one particular part, the other rays being suffered to proceed.' (Young 1802c).

Young was not sympathetic, however, to the phenomenological approach of his contemporary, Goethe. Young's editor saw fit to suppress Young's review of the *Farbenlehre* from his collected works. A short quotation will give a feel for Young's style—and for his opinion :

> 'Our attention has been less directed to this work of Mr. von Goethe, by the hopes of acquiring from it anything like information, than by a curiosity to contemplate a striking example of the perversion of the human faculties, in an individual who has obtained enough of popularity among his countrymen, by his literary productions, to inspire him with a full confidence in his own powers, and who seems to have wasted those powers for the space of twenty years, by forcing them into a direction, in which he had originally mistaken his way, for want of profiting by the assistance of a judicious guide.' (Young 1814).

'. . .but he was not in the habit of making experiments'

Thomas Young published no original experiments on colour mixing or on the perception of colour. Although he did enter into the spirit of the Royal Institution and devised demonstrations to illustrate his lectures (*v.* Figure i.6), and although the two-slit experiment described in his published *Lectures* has proved one of the most influential experiments in modern physics, he was not at heart a committed experimentalist. His lifelong friend and first biographer, Hudson Gurney, records:

> 'In the winters of 1790 and 1791, having prepared himself by previous reading, he attended the lectures of Dr Higgins in chemistry, and began to make some simple experiments of his own on a small scale. But he was afterwards accustomed to say, that at no period of his life was he particularly fond of repeating experiments, or even of very frequently attempting to originate new ones; considering that, however necessary to the advancement of science, they demanded a great sacrifice of time, and that when the fact was once established, that time was better employed in considering the purposes to which it might be applied, or the principles which it might tend to elucidate.'

Similarly, his second biographer, George Peacock, quotes Young as saying: 'acute suggestion was...always more in the line of my ambition than experimental illustration' (Peacock 1855). Later in life, Young opposed any addition to the fund that Wollaston

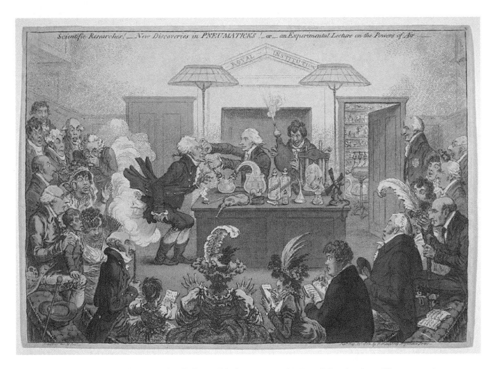

Figure i.6 A satire by Gillray on the fashionable lectures at the Royal Institution. The engraving was published in May 1802 and almost certainly depicts Thomas Young as lecturer (centre). Young is experimenting on Sir J. C. Hippisley, applying gas to his mouth. To the right of Young, holding the bellows, is Humphry Davy, and standing on the right is Count Rumford.

had left to the Royal Society for the support of experimental science, declaring: 'For my part, it is my pride and pleasure, as far as I am able, to supersede the necessity of experiments, and more especially of expensive ones' (Mayer 1875). The criticisms of Young by Henry Brougham (see above) were taken by nineteenth-century commentators to be inspired purely by personal bitterness (Tyndall 1892)—in the *British Magazine* for 1800 Young had scathingly criticized a mathematical paper by 'a young gentleman of Edinburgh' (Brougham)—but in fact Brougham was also expressing the preference for inductive science and critical experiment that was favoured in the Scottish methodological tradition (Cantor 1971). To be fair to Young, it has to be allowed that the Bakerian lecture of 1801 contains one imaginative set of measurements (on the colours produced by striated surfaces); but for the most part it is theoretical, and in particular it postulates a luminiferous ether, an unobservable that members of the Scottish school could not accept.

The trichromatic theory is a good example of the 'acute suggestion' that Young saw as his role. He never attempted to place the theory on a quantitative basis. In his *Lectures* he describes demonstrations in which colours are mixed on rotating discs, but such demonstrations were already antique in 1802. Young's contribution was to release colour science from the category error that had held back the understanding of physical optics in the eighteenth century. He realized that the trichromacy of colour mixture did not mean that there were only three physical kinds of light. Rather it meant that colours were represented by just three variables somewhere in our visual apparatus. James Clerk Maxwell was later to write:

> 'So far as I know, Thomas Young was the first who, starting from the well known fact that there are three primary colours, sought for the explanation of this fact, not in the nature of light, but in the constitution of man.' (Maxwell 1871).

The trichromatic theory after 200 years

It was Clerk Maxwell who first attempted to estimate quantitatively the spectral sensitivities of Young's retinal resonators, by identifying the sets of colours in the trichromat's colour space that were confused by a dichromat (Maxwell 1855). Yet general agreement on the spectral sensitivities, and even the number, of the receptors did not come until the second half of the Twentieth Century, when estimates by Maxwell's method were found to be consistent with direct measurements by reflection densitometry of the fundus of the eye, by microspectrophotometry of individual receptors, and by electrical records from isolated receptors sucked into a micropipette.

Today, it is known that there are four classes of photoreceptor in the normal retina: the rods, which subserve our vision at low light levels, and three kinds of cone, which subserve colour vision as well as the other functions of daytime vision. The rods are most sensitive near 500 nm, a wavelength that appears blue green. The peak sensitivities of the cones lie in the violet, the green, and the yellow-green regions of the spectrum (Figure i.7), and the three types are referred to as short-wave, medium-wave and long-wave respectively. The long- and middle-wave cones are more numerous than the short-wave cones (see Chapter 5).

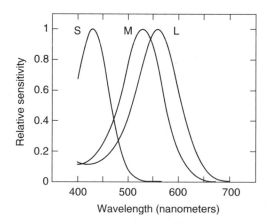

Figure i.7 Sensitivities of the three types of cone receptor in the normal eye. S= 'short-wave', M= 'middle-wave', L='long-wave'.

Each of the four classes of photoreceptor obeys the *Principle of Univariance* (Baylor *et al.* 1987; Rushton 1972): although the stimulus may vary in its radiance and in its wavelength, the response of the photoreceptor varies on only one dimension—the difference in electrical potential between the inside and the outside of the cell. Once an individual photon has been absorbed, all information about its wavelength—its electromagnetic frequency—is lost. What does vary with wavelength is the *probability* of a given photon being absorbed, and spectral sensitivity curves, such as those of Figure i.7, reflect this changing probability.

Each class of photoreceptor gains its characteristic light sensitivity from the photopigment molecules embedded in the enfolded membrane of the cell. Each photopigment is a member of the extended family of G-protein coupled receptors and has a heptahelical structure: the 'opsin', or protein part of the molecule, consists of seven helices, running between the inside and the outside of the cell membrane; and these form a splayed palisade that surrounds the chromophore, 11-*cis*-retinal (see Chapter 1). Variations in the amino acid sequence of the opsin lead to variations in the wavelength of peak sensitivity of the molecule. The short-wave cone opsin is encoded by a gene on chromosome 7, whereas the long- and middle-wave opsins are encoded by genes on the q arm of the X-chromosome (Nathans *et al.* 1986). Most of the common types of inherited colour deficiency are associated with alterations of this cluster of genes at Xq28 (see Chapters 31–33). The gene for the short-wave pigment is ancient and antedates the mammals, whereas the long- and middle-wave photopigments are thought to have diverged during the evolution of the primates, as the result of the duplication of an ancestral gene on the X-chromosome. The ecological factors that drove this divergence are the subject of current debate (see Mollon (2002) and Chapter 3).

The univariance of photoreceptors means that any individual cone, or individual class of cone, is colour blind. The long-wave cones, for example, will give the same signal to lights from any part of the visible spectrum, provided only that the radiances of the lights are adjusted to give the same rates of photon absorption in this class of cones. To find out what colour is present, the visual system must compare the rates at which photons are absorbed in different classes of cone. This is achieved already within the retina, by particular types of ganglion cell that draw inputs of different sign—excitatory or inhibitory—from different classes of cone. Such 'chromatically opponent' cells are typically excited by one part of the spectrum and inhibited by another (see Chapters 7–9).

There are several types of chromatically opponent cell in the retina, distinct in the signals they carry, in their morphology, and in their central projections. At least two minority types of cell oppose the short-wave cone signal to some combination of the signals of the other receptors (Dacey *et al.* 2003), and these ganglion cells project to the koniocellular layers of the lateral geniculate nucleus. The more numerous midget ganglion cells draw opposed inputs from the long- and middle-wave receptors; and these ganglion cells project to the parvocellular laminae of the lateral geniculate nucleus.

For much of its history, the trichromatic theory had the disadvantage of being tied to a simple form of Müller's 'Doctrine of Specific Nerve Energies': there were three types of receptor, these directly excited three types of nerve, and the latter secreted red, green, or blue sensations at some central site. When chromatically opponent cells were first reported in the primate visual system (De Valois 1965), it became the fashion to identify them with the red-green and yellow-blue antagonistic mechanisms postulated by Hering (1878) and to declare that the Young-Helmholtz theory held at the level of the receptors while the Opponent Process Theory held at a post-receptoral level. In fact, the chromatically opponent channels of the early visual system do not correspond in a simple way to the red-green and yellow-blue axes of phenomenological colour space: for example, at the wavelength of unique blue (c. 480 nm), the blue that looks neither reddish nor greenish, a neural channel that extracts the ratio of middle- and long-wave cone signals will not be in equilibrium but will be strongly polarized in the +M direction (Mollon & Estévez 1988). To this day, we do not understand how to incorporate phenomenological observations into our mechanistic theory of colour vision; but the trichromatic theory itself has been released from the ancient demand that it should account for how colours look.

References

Anonymous (1708). *Traité de la Peinture en mignature.* La Haye, van Dole.

Ayama, M., Nakatsue, T. & Kaiser, P. K. (1987). Constant hue loci of unique and binary balanced hues at 10, 100, and 100 Td. *Journal of the Optical Society of America* **4A**, 1136–44.

Baylor, D. A., Nunn, B. J. & Schnapf, J. L. (1987). Spectral sensitivity of cones of the monkey *Macaca fascicularis. Journal of Physiology* **390**, 145–60.

Bendall, S., Brooke, C. & Collinson, P. (1999). *A history of Emmanuel College,Cambridge.* Woodbridge: Boydell Press.

Brougham, L. (1803). The Bakerian Lecture on the Theory of Light and Colours. By Thomas Young M.D. F.R.S. Professor of Natural Philosophy of the Royal Institution. *The Edinburgh Review or Critical Journal* **1**, 450–56.

Cantor, G. N. (1971). Henry Brougham and the Scottish methodological tradition. *Studies in the History and Philosophy of Science* **2**, 69–89.

Castel, P. (1740). *L'Optique des Couleurs.* Paris, Briasson.

Dacey, D. M., Peterson, B. B., Robinson, F. R. & Gamlin, P. D. (2003). Fireworks in the primate retina: in vitro photodynamics links dendritic morphology, physiology and connectivity of diverse cell types in the retinogeniculate pathway. *Neuron* **37**, 15–27.

De Valois, R. L. (1965). Analysis and coding of color vision in the primate visual system. *Cold Spring Harbor Symposia on Quantitative Biology* **30**, 567–79.

Forbes, E. G. (1971). *Tobias Mayer's Opera Inedita.* London, Macmillan.

Gamauf, G. (1811). *Lichtenberg über Luft und Licht nach seinen Vorlesungen herausgegeben. Erinnerungen aus Lichtenbergs Vorlesungen über Erxlebens Anfangsgründe der Naturlehre.* Vienna & Trieste, Geistinger.

Gurney, H. (1831). *Memoir of the life of Thomas Young, M.D., F.R.S.* London, John & Arthur Arch.

Hering, E. (1878). *Zur Lehre vom Lichtsinne. Sechs Mittheilungen an die Kaiserliche Akademie der Wissenschaften in Wien.* Wien: Carl Gerlold's Sohn.

Le Blon, J. C. (1725). *Coloritto; or the Harmony of Colouring in Painting: Reduced to Mechanical Practice under Easy Precepts, and Infallible Rules.* London, W. and J. Innys.

Lee, B. B. (2001). Colour science in Göttingen in the 18th Century. *Color Research and Application* **26**, S25–S31.

Maxwell, J. C. (1855). Experiments on Colour, as perceived by the Eye, with remarks on Colour-blindness. *Transactions of the Royal Society of Edinburgh* **21**, 275–98.

Maxwell, J. C. (1871). On colour vision. *Proceedings of the Royal Institution of London*, 260–71.

Mayer, A. M. (1875). The history of Young's discovery of his theory of colours. *American Journal of Science* **9**, 251.

Mayer, T. (1775). *Opera Inedita.* Göttingen: J. C. Dieterich.

Mollon, J. D. (1993). George Palmer (1740–1795). *The Dictionary of National Biography.* C. S. Nicholls. Oxford, Oxford University Press: pp. 509–10.

Mollon, J. D. (2002). When the rainbow resembles the tricolour of France: The two subsystems of colour vision. *Rétine, cerveau et vision.* Y. Chisten, M. Doly and M.-T. Droy-Lefaix. Marseille, Solal: pp. 3–17.

Mollon, J. D. (2003). The origins of modern color science. *The Science of Color.* S. Shevell. Washington, Optical Society of America.

Mollon, J. D. & **Estévez, O.** (1988). Tyndall's paradox of hue discrimination. *Journal of the Optical Society of America* **5A**, 151–59.

Nathans, J., Thomas, D. & **Hogness, D. S.** (1986). Molecular genetics of human color vision: The genes encoding blue, green, and red pigments. *Science* **232**, 193–202.

Newton, I. (1730). *Opticks, or a Treatise of the Reflections, Refractions, Inflections & Colours of Light.* London, Wm. Innys.

Palmer, G. (1777). *Theory of colours and vision.* London, S. Leacroft.

Peacock, G. (1855). *Life of Thomas Young MD, FRS.* London, John Murray.

Rushton, W. A. H. (1972). Pigments and signals in colour vision. *Journal of Physiology* **220**, 1–31P.

Tyndall, J. (1892). *New Fragments.* New York, Appleton.

Voigt, J. H. (1781). Des herrn Giros von Gentilly Muthmassungen über die Gesichtsfehler bey Untersuchung der Farben. *Magazin für das Neueste aus der Physik und Naturgeschichte (Gotha)* **1**, 57–61.

Young, T. (1793). Observations on Vision. *Philosophical Transactions of the Royal Society* **83**, 169–81.

Young, T. (1802a). The Bakerian Lecture. On the Theory of Light and Colours. *Philosophical Transactions of the Royal Society of London* **92**, 12–48.

Young, T. (1802b). Harmonic sliders. *Journals of the Royal Institution*, 261–4.

Young, T. (1802c). *A syllabus of a course of lectures on natural and experimental philosophy.* London, Royal Institution.

Young, T. (1804). *Reply to the animadversions of the Edinburgh reviewers on some papers published in the Philosophical Transactions.* London, Longman & Co.

Young, T. (1814). Zur Farbenlehre. On the Doctrine of Colours. By Goethe. *Quarterly Review* **10**, 427–41.

Young, T. (1817). Chromatics. *Supplement to the Encyclopaedia Britannica.* 3, 141–63.

PHOTORECEPTORS AND THEIR EVOLUTION

ELECTRONS AND X-RAYS REVEAL THE STRUCTURE OF RHODOPSIN: A PROTOTYPICAL G PROTEIN-COUPLED RECEPTOR–IMPLICATIONS FOR COLOUR VISION

JONATHAN J. RUPRECHT AND GEBHARD F. X. SCHERTLER

Introduction

A fundamental aim in vision research is to elucidate the factors that subtly modify the absorption maxima of the visual pigments—the G protein-coupled receptors (GPCRs) responsible for transducing visual stimuli. Humans have four visual pigments (Nathans 1999), found in the two classes of retinal cells responsible for light detection: rod cells for dim-light detection, and cones for colour vision. Human rod cells contain rhodopsin, which has an absorption maximum (λ_{max}) at ~500 nm, and plays little role in colour vision. Rhodopsin is important for vision in dim light, and is currently the most intensively studied visual pigment. Human cone cells contain a blue or short-wavelength pigment (λ_{max}~425 nm), a green or middle-wavelength pigment (λ_{max}~530 nm) and a red or long-wavelength pigment (λ_{max}~560 nm) (Nathans 1989, 1999; Oprian *et al.* 1991; Merbs and Nathans 1992).

Despite their different absorption maxima, the visual pigments contain the same chromophore, 11-*cis*-retinal, which is attached by a Schiff base linkage to the ε-amino group of a lysine residue in transmembrane helix VII. In organic solvents, the protonated Schiff base of 11-*cis*-retinal has a λ_{max} at 440 nm (Kochendoerfer *et al.* 1999). The visual pigments confine 11-*cis*-retinal within a binding pocket, where specific amino acids cause environmental perturbations that shift λ_{max}—this is called the opsin shift (Nakanishi *et al.* 1980). The opsin shift, or spectral tuning, is also used to refer to the differences in λ_{max} among the visual pigments. Several chromophore–protein interactions have been described that might be responsible for this effect (Kochendoerfer *et al.* 1999; Nathans 1999). Weakening the interaction of the positively charged protonated Schiff base with its negatively charged counterion or hydrogen-bonding partners could promote delocalization of the positive charge throughout the π electron system of the chromophore, resulting in a red-shift of λ_{max} (Baasov et al. 1987; Blatz et al. 1972; Nathans 1999). Modifying the dipolar environment of the conjugated chromophore backbone by the placement of charged (Asenjo et al. 1994; Honig et al. 1976; Kropf and Hubbard 1958; Neitz et al. 1991) or polarizable (Blatz and Mohler 1975; Irving et al. 1970) groups close to the polyene chain of the chromophore would be expected to shift λ_{max}. Finally, planarization of the polyene chain caused by the protein environment could alter λ_{max} (Blatz and Liebman 1973).

Several studies have identified amino acid groups in the cone pigments that may be responsible for spectral tuning. Recent crystal structures of bovine rhodopsin allow us to reinterpret the results of some of these studies. This article will review the structural work that has been carried out on rhodopsin, with a view towards spectral tuning.

Structural studies of rhodopsin

Several properties of rhodopsin make it an ideal candidate for structural studies. Rhodopsin is present at very high concentrations in the outer segment membranes of retinal rod cells, where it comprises over 80 per cent of the protein (Papermaster and Dreyer 1974). In contrast, the cone cell pigments are much less abundant, and show low expression in mammalian cells (e.g. Lin et al. 1998). Rhodopsin is one of the most stable and detergent-tolerant GPCRs known. The abundance and stability of rhodopsin mean that it can be isolated relatively simply from retinas, in large enough quantities for crystallization trials. To date, rhodopsin is the only GPCR to have been crystallized in 2D or in 3D.

Cryo-electron microscopy (cryo-EM) studies

The first evidence for the arrangement of rhodopsin's seven transmembrane α-helices came from a 9 Å projection structure of bovine rhodopsin (Schertler et al. 1993). This revealed an elongated arc-shaped feature, predicted to be three-tilted α-helices, and four well-resolved peaks of density, corresponding to α-helices oriented nearly perpendicular to the membrane. Structural constraints obtained from a comparison of GPCR sequences were used to allocate helices to the 9-Å projection map (Baldwin 1993). A low-resolution 3D structure of bovine rhodopsin (Unger and Schertler 1995) and projection structures of frog rhodopsin in two different crystal forms (Schertler and Hargrave 1995) confirmed the position of the three least tilted helices (IV, VI, and VII), while helix V showed a more elongated density, indicating that it was tilted or bent. Helices I, II, and III were not resolved. It became apparent that the maps of rhodopsin differed from those of bacteriorhodopsin, an extensively studied seven transmembrane helix light-driven proton pump from salt-loving archaebacteria (Schertler and Hargrave 1995; Schertler 1998). Significantly, this revealed that bacteriorhodopsin, whose atomic model had been published in 1990 (Henderson et al. 1990), would not provide a suitable model for GPCR structure.

Extraction of frog cell membranes with Tween 80 resulted in the formation of well-ordered 2D crystals, allowing a 3D map to be calculated with a resolution of 7.5 Å in the membrane plane and 16.5 Å normal to it (Unger *et al.* 1997). All seven of the trans-membrane α-helices were resolved in this map, and the molecule was shown to have a three-layered structure, with helix IV being separated from helices VI and VII by helices II and III. The helices were shown to be close-packed towards the intracellular side, opening towards the extracellular side where a cavity for retinal binding is formed by helices III, IV, V, VI, and VII. Reconstitution experiments have led to the production of improved 2D crystals of bovine rhodopsin, allowing a 5-Å resolution projection map to be calculated, and for the first time, electron diffraction patterns could be recorded (Krebs *et al.* 1998).

A 3D structure of squid (*Loligo forbesi*) rhodopsin has now been obtained (Davies *et al.* 2001). This follows on from the publication of an 8-Å projection structure of squid rhodopsin (Davies *et al.* 1996). Squid rhodopsin differs from vertebrate rhodopsin by interacting with different target molecules (G_q and phospholipase C rather than trans-ducin and cGMP phosphodiesterase), and by having a unique C-terminal extension. However, the projection structure of squid rhodopsin is clearly similar to that of bovine and frog rhodopsin, despite squid rhodopsin showing only 35 per cent sequence identity with mammalian rhodopsins (50 per cent overall homology with conservative substi-tutions). Docking the atomic structure of bovine rhodopsin into the 3D squid density map has shown that the helix packing and extracellular plug structure are conserved. This supports the conservation in structure of rhodopsin from phylogenetically distant organisms. The structure indicates that the C-terminal helix VIII, which lies transverse to the membrane, may make the lattice contacts that drive the formation of the ordered lattice found in cephalopod photoreceptor membranes.

A model based on the EM data and an extensive sequence comparison of GPCRs, which provided additional structural constraints, was constructed. This produced the first detailed α-carbon template for the seven transmembrane helices of GPCRs (Baldwin *et al.* 1997).

X-ray diffraction studies

Recently, the X-ray structure of rhodopsin has been obtained from a P4$_1$ crystal form (Palczewski *et al.* 2000; reviewed in Teller *et al.* 2001 and in Menon *et al.* 2001). In our laboratory, we have obtained P3$_1$ crystals, and have determined the structure of rhodopsin in this crystal form by molecular replacement, to a resolution better than 3.2 Å (Edwards *et al.*, Li *et al.*, in preparation). The two X-ray structures superimpose well, particularly in the transmembrane region. The X-ray structures have confirmed the arrangement of transmembrane helices revealed by EM, but are at higher, isotropic, resolutions, providing a tremendous amount of information about rhodopsin's struc-ture. For the first time, the palmitoylation and oligosaccharide modifications, and the molecular architecture of the retinal-binding pocket, have been revealed. An important finding has been that the C-terminus forms a short helix (helix VIII), which lies parallel to the membrane plane. This helix lies where an additional density feature was found in the frog rhodopsin 3D EM map (Unger *et al.* 1997). X-ray diffraction studies of heavy-atom labelled 2D crystals of bovine rhodopsin have provided the first direct proof that this density is part of helix VIII (Mielke *et al.* 2002). Another important finding has been the structure of the extracellular loops, which associate together to form a "plug". The second extracellular loop folds into the transmembrane region of the molecule, so that β-strand 4 actually forms part of the retinal-binding pocket (Fig. 1.1(b)). The rest of the discussion in this article, and the figures shown, will describe the B chain in the asymmetric unit of the rhodopsin structure produced by our laboratory.

Mechanism of the opsin shift in rhodopsin

A weaker electrostatic interaction between the counterion (Glu113) and the protonated Schiff base due to greater separation is thought to explain most of the opsin shift in rhodopsin compared to an 11-*cis*-retinal protonated Schiff base in organic solvents (Lin *et al.* 1998; Livnah and Sheves 1993). However, theoretical molecular orbital calculations indicate that second-order interactions (e.g. dipole–dipole and dipole–induced dipole) play an important role by subtly altering the orientation of groups in the retinal-binding pocket (Kusnetzow *et al.* 2001). It appears that this opsin shift cannot be adequately explained by considering individual residues alone.

Spectral tuning in the middle- and long-wavelength cone pigments

Nathans and colleagues published the first sequences of the human cone pigments in 1986 (Nathans *et al.* 1986). This work revealed that the middle- and long-wavelength opsins

---

Figure 1.1 See also colour plate section. Views of an atomic model of bovine rhodopsin. Helices are labelled: I is helix I etc. The 11-*cis*-retinal chromophore is in green, and the counterion (Glu113) is in cyan. (a) Atomic model of rhodopsin viewed from the extracellular side of the membrane. Extracellular and cytoplasmic loops have been removed from this view, to allow the retinal-binding pocket to be viewed more easily. Residues implicated in a red-shift are shown in red, and are labelled (Ala164, Phe261, and Ala269—Chan *et al.* 1992; His100, Ile214, Ile217, and Phe293—Asenjo *et al.* 1994). (b): Side view of the retinal-binding pocket, with the extracellular surface at the top of the figure. Helix VI to the C terminus has been removed to expose the retinal-binding site. The β-sheet regions contributing to part of the extracellular "plug" are shown in yellow. β3 and β4 are in the second extracellular loop. The residues Glu181 and Gln184 are shown in red. The corresponding residues in the red and green cone pigments are thought to form a chloride ion-binding site, which red-shifts these visual pigments compared to rhodopsin (Wang *et al.* 1993). (c): Atomic model of rhodopsin viewed from the extracellular side of the membrane. Extracellular and cytoplasmic loops have been removed from this view, to allow the retinal-binding pocket to be viewed more easily. Residues whose mutation results in a blue-shift in the "blue-rhodopsin" mutant are shown in blue, and are labelled (Met86, Gly90, Ala117, Glu122, Ala124, Trp265, Ala292, Ala295, and Ala299—Lin *et al.* 1998). These images were created in Swiss-Pdb viewer, and rendered in POV-Ray (Guex and Peitsch 1997).

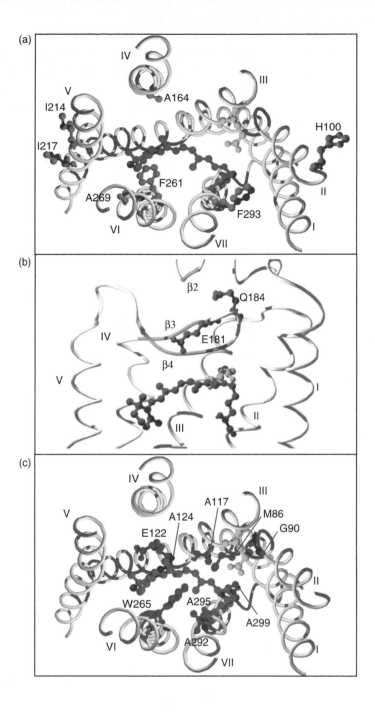

(a)

IV

V

I214

I217

A164

III

H100

F261

A269

F261

F293

VI

VII

I

II

(b)

β2

Q184

β3

E181

IV

β4

V

III

II

I

(c)

IV

III

A117

M86

V

A124

G90

E122

W265

A295

A299

A292

VI

VII

I

II

differ only in 15 amino acids. Furthermore, only seven of these were non-homologous substitutions lying within predicted transmembrane regions, which were therefore likely to affect chromophore–protein interactions. In an elegant analysis of the nucleotide sequences of eight primate photopigment genes, Neitz and colleagues identified three key amino acid residues (at positions 180, 277, and 285 in the cone pigments) that accounted for the variation in the λ_{max} of the primate cone pigments (Neitz *et al.* 1991; reviewed in Mollon 1991). In each case, replacement of a non-polar amino acid with a hydroxyl-bearing amino acid at these positions produced a red-shift. The authors hypothesized that these three amino acid substitutions were responsible for the difference in λ_{max} between the human red and green visual pigments.

Sakmar and colleagues tested this hypothesis by mutating the three equivalent residues in rhodopsin (Ala164, Phe261, and Ala269) and evaluating the effects on the spectral properties of the mutant pigments (Chan *et al.* 1992). Non-polar residues normally present in rhodopsin and the green visual pigments were mutated to hydroxyl-bearing residues normally present in the red visual pigment. Two of the substitutions (Phe261Tyr and Ala269Thr) caused significant red-shifts in λ_{max}, while Ala164Ser caused only a slight red-shift. Combinations of substitutions were found to cause approximately additive red-shifts. Resonance Raman spectroscopy has revealed that the Schiff-base vibrational structures of the human red and green visual pigments are identical (Kochendoerfer *et al.* 1999). This indicates that the shift in λ_{max} between red and green visual pigments is due to electrostatic interactions of residues with the ground and excited electronic states of the chromophore. Mainly non-polar residues surround the 11-*cis*-retinal in the green pigment—a possible exception is a glutamate (the equivalent residue in rhodopsin is Met86, see Fig. 1.1(c)), and shielding by water molecules was proposed to weaken any interaction between this residue and the chromophore. However, the crystal structures reveal that the equivalent residue in rhodopsin lies further from the chromophore, 8–9 Å from the protonated Schiff base, compared to 5 Å in the earlier models (Kochendoerfer *et al.* 1999). Using a model of the red visual pigment, based on existing models of rhodopsin, Sakmar and colleagues concluded that Ser164, Tyr261, and Thr269 (rhodopsin numbering) in the red pigment were ideally positioned to stabilize the excited-state charge distribution of the chromophore, thus producing the red-shift. In the excited-state, a significant proportion of the positive charge of the protonated Schiff base is thought to be delocalized into the chromophore chain towards the cyclohexenyl ring (Honig *et al.* 1976). The crystal structures of rhodopsin provide us with a better model of the retinal-binding pocket (Fig. 1.1(a)). The chromophore position in the crystal structure is different from that in the model used by Sakmar—the cyclohexenyl ring lies almost perpendicular to the membrane, rather than parallel to it. The location of individual amino acid residues is also different. Ala164 in rhodopsin lies in transmembrane helix IV, quite far from the chromophore, and does not directly contribute to the retinal-binding pocket (Fig. 1.1(a)). This supports the finding that the Ala164Ser mutant shows only a slight red-shift (Chan *et al.* 1992). Ala269 lies on transmembrane

helix VI, about $4\,\text{Å}$ away from the C_{17} atom of the retinal, and plays a role in con-
straining the position of the cyclohexenyl ring (Fig. 1.1(a)). Mutation of this residue to
threonine would bring a hydroxyl group close to the cyclohexenyl ring. As suggested
by Sakmar and colleagues, Thr269 could interact preferentially with the excited-state
charge distribution, thus producing a red-shift (Kochendoerfer et al. 1999). Phe261, on
transmembrane helix VI, points right into the retinal-binding pocket, and pairs with
Gly121 to form one boundary of the retinal-binding pocket (Fig. 1.1(a)). Phe261 lies
underneath the cyclohexenyl ring, towards the cytoplasmic surface. Mutation of this
residue to tyrosine would place a hydroxyl group very close to the cyclohexenyl ring, in
position to stabilize the excited-state of the chromophore, producing the red-shift, as
suggested by Sakmar (Kochendoerfer et al. 1999). Since Phe261 and Ala269 both form
parts of the retinal-binding pocket, mutations of these amino acids may cause rearrange-
ments of other parts of the retinal-binding pocket. This may account for the fact that the
Phe261Tyr/Ala269Thr double mutant caused a red-shift greater than either mutation
alone, but was not additive (Chan et al. 1992).

An extensive mutagenesis study carried out by Oprian et al. has revealed that the
spectral differences between the green and red pigments is due to seven amino acids
alone (Asenjo et al. 1994). This work is consistent with Chan et al. (1992) in that
amino acids at positions 180, 277, and 285 determined a major portion of the spectral
shift. However, amino acids at positions 116, 230, 233, and 309 also played a role. The
equivalent residues in rhodopsin (His100, Ile214, Ile217, and Phe293) lie quite far from
the binding pocket: His100 lies at the extracellular end of helix II; Ile214, and Ile217 lie in
helix V, and Phe293 lies in the middle of helix VII (Fig. 1.1(a)). It thus appears likely that
these residues alter λ_{max} via an indirect effect on the retinal-binding pocket, for example
mutation of the residues equivalent to Ile214 and Ile217 could alter the tilt of helix V.

This work has elucidated key residues responsible for the opsin shift between
red and green visual pigments. The opsin shift between these pigments and the
rhodopsins and short-wavelength pigments has also been addressed. Mutagenesis of
the human red and green colour vision pigments has identified His197 and Lys200 as
forming a chloride ion-binding site, with His197 having the dominant contribution
(Wang et al. 1993). Cl^--binding produces a large red-shift in the λ_{max}. Furthermore,
His197 and Lys200 are conserved in all long-wavelength cone pigments, but are absent
in all rhodopsins and short-wavelength cone pigments. It therefore appears that His197
and Lys200 are responsible for the red-shift of the green and red pigments compared to
rhodopsin and the short-wavelength cone pigments. The equivalent residue of His197
in rhodopsin is Glu181. This residue lies in the long extracellular loop 2, which is fol-
ded into the core of the membrane-embedded region of the protein (Fig. 1.1(b)). The
carboxylic acid side chain of Glu181 points towards the centre of the polyene chain of
the chromophore, and it has been proposed that Glu181 may influence the delocalized
electron density of the chromophore so that photoisomerization occurs exclusively at
the C_{11}–C_{12} bond (Menon et al. 2001). The equivalent His197 in the green and red cone
pigments may thus be ideally located for spectral tuning.

Spectral tuning in short-wavelength pigments

Spectral tuning within the short-wavelength pigments is less well-defined than in the medium- and long-wavelength pigments. However, a site-directed mutagenesis study of bovine rhodopsin has identified nine positions where simultaneous substitution with the respective residues from the human blue cone sequence can account for about 80 per cent of the opsin shift between rhodopsin and the human blue cone pigment (Lin *et al.* 1998). The substitutions required to create the "blue-rhodopsin" mutant lie on helix II (Met86Leu and Gly90Ser), helix III (Ala117Gly, Glu122Leu, and Ala124Thr), helix VI (Trp265Tyr) and helix VII (Ala292Ser, Ala295Ser, and Ala299Cys). The Trp265Tyr mutant showed the largest single opsin shift out of the single substitutions examined. Resonance Raman spectroscopy has helped to elucidate possible mechanisms for this opsin shift (Lin *et al.* 1998). The authors conclude that Ser90, Ser292, Ser295, and Cys299 do not blue-shift the λ_{max} by either directly or indirectly altering the hydrogen bonding of the Schiff base nitrogen or its electrostatic interaction with the protein. Instead, the blue-shift is due to through-space electrostatic interactions of the added dipole groups with the chromophore. This conclusion is supported by the crystal structure—residue 292 is the only one that directly forms part of the retinal-binding pocket, and whilst the residues lie close to the chromophore, they are from 5 to 9 Å away from the Schiff base (Fig. 1.1(c)). The blue-shift caused by Trp265Tyr mutation is also attributed to a through-space electrostatic effect on the chromophore, decreasing polarizability close to the cyclohexenyl ring. Trp265 directly forms part of the retinal-binding pocket in rhodopsin. It lies about 6 Å from the cyclohexenyl ring, with the plane of the tryptophan ring lying almost parallel to the cyclohexenyl ring, supporting the conclusion (Fig. 1.1(c)). The combination of these effects is thought to cause a blue-shift to about 460 nm. The blue-shift below 440 nm requires two additional mutations on helix III (Ala117Gly and Glu122Leu), which appear to act synergistically with the mutations on helices II, VI, and VII. Resonance Raman spectroscopy (Lin *et al.* 1998; Kochendoerfer *et al.* 1999) indicates that this synergistic effect is due to local structural reorganization of the retinal-binding pocket. This reorganization is thought to reposition or reorient the Glu113 counterion (which also lies on helix III), or surrounding water, thus allowing better solvation of the protonated Schiff base, and allowing the counterion to move closer to the Schiff base. This would stabilize the positive charge near the protonated Schiff base, lowering the ground-state energy and blue-shifting λ_{max}. Since Glu122 and Ala117 directly form part of the retinal-binding pocket (Fig. 1.1(c)), mutation of these residues may indeed cause its reorganization.

Recent theoretical molecular orbital calculations on a model of the violet cone opsin ($\lambda_{max} = 425$ nm) using the $P4_1$ rhodopsin structure (Palczewski *et al.* 2000) as a template have indicated that the loss of the Glu122–His211 pair, which are sufficiently close together to form a salt bridge, can account for ~75 per cent of the blue-shift compared to rhodopsin (Kusnetsow *et al.* 2001). Although this calculation assumes a Glu(−) His(+) charge, it is significant that the Glu122–His211 pair is also absent from the human blue cone pigment. Furthermore, the Glu122Leu mutation used by Lin *et al.* (1998) would disrupt this potential salt bridge.

Conclusions

Extensive mutagenesis studies, coupled with spectroscopy, have identified key amino acid residues responsible for the opsin shift, and have identified possible mechanisms. Stabilization of the excited-state charge distribution of the chromophore by hydroxyl-bearing residues around the cyclohexenyl ring produces a red-shift. Stabilization of the ground-state charge distribution by residues around the chromophore, coupled with reorganization of the retinal-binding pocket to move the counterion closer to the protonated Schiff base, or to better solvate the protonated Schiff base, results in a blue-shift. Theoretical calculations highlight the importance of considering the entire binding site, especially secondary interactions among the residues, to fully explain opsin shifts. The rhodopsin crystal structures support the findings of earlier studies, and help to explain the key role played by certain residues. These structures provide for the first time an ideal basis for developing improved models of the structures of the cone pigments, and for further theoretical calculations on the mechanism of spectral tuning. Furthermore, the structure of the retinal-binding pocket will enable us to design specific mutations to test proposed mechanisms for opsin shifts.

References

Asenjo, A. B., Rim, J., & Oprian, D. D. (1994). Molecular determinants of human red/green color discrimination. *Neuron*, *12*, 1131–38.

Baasov, T., Friedman, N., & Sheves, M. (1987). Factors affecting the C=N stretching in protonated retinal Schiff base: a model study for bacteriorhodopsin and visual pigments. *Biochemistry*, *26*, 3210–17.

Baldwin, J. M. (1993). The probable arrangement of the helices in G protein-coupled receptors. *EMBO J.*, *12*, 1693–703.

Baldwin, J. M., Schertler, G. F. X. & Unger, V. M. (1997). An alpha-carbon template for the transmembrane helices in the rhodopsin family of G-protein-coupled receptors. *J. Mol. Biol.*, *272*, 144–64.

Blatz, P. E. & Liebman, P. A. (1973). Wavelength regulation in visual pigments. *Exp. Eye Res.*, *17*, 573–80.

Blatz, P. E. & Mohler, J. H. (1975). Effect of selected anions and solvents on the electron absorption, nuclear magnetic resonance, and infrared spectra of the *N*-retinylidene-*n*-butylammonium cation. *Biochemistry*, *14*, 2304–09.

Blatz, P. E., Mohler, J. H., & Navangul, H. V. (1972). Anion-induced wavelength regulation of absorption maxima of Schiff bases of retinal. *Biochemistry*, *11*, 848–55.

Chan, T., Lee, M., & Sakmar, T. P. (1992). Introduction of hydroxyl-bearing amino acids causes bathochromic spectral shifts in rhodopsin. Amino acid substitutions responsible for red-green color pigment spectral tuning. *J. Biol. Chem.*, *267*, 9478–80.

Davies, A., Gowen, B. E., Krebs, A. M., Schertler, G. F. X., & Saibil, H. R. (2001). Three-dimensional Structure of an Invertebrate Rhodopsin and Basis for Ordered Alignment in the Photoreceptor Membrane. *J. Mol. Biol.*, *314*, 455–63.

Davies, A., Schertler, G. F. X., Gowan, B. E., & Saibil, H. R. (1996). Projection structure of an invertebrate rhodopsin. *J. Struct. Biol.*, *117*, 36–44.

Edwards, P., Li, J., Burghammer, M., McDowell, J., Villa, C., Hargrave, P. A., & Schertler, G. F. X. (2002). Crystals of native and modified bovine Rhodopsins and their heavy atom derivatives. *J. Mol. Biol.*, submitted.

Guex, N. & Peitsch, M. C. (1997). SWISS-MODEL and the Swiss-PdbViewer: An environment for comparative protein modeling. *Electrophoresis*, *18*, 2714–23.

Henderson, R., Baldwin, J. M., Ceska, T. A., Zemlin, F., Beckmann, E., & Downing, K. H. (1990). Model for the structure of bacteriorhodopsin based on high-resolution electron cryo-microscopy. *J. Mol. Biol.*, *213*, 899–929.

Honig, B., Greenberg, A. D., Dinur, U., & Ebrey, T. G. (1976). Visual-pigment spectra: implications of the protonation of the retinal Schiff base. *Biochemistry*, *15*, 4593–9.

Irving, C. S., Byers, G. W., & Leermakers, P. A. (1970). Spectroscopic model for the visual pigments. Influence of microenvironmental polarizability. *Biochemistry*, *9*, 858–64.

Kochendoerfer, G. G., Lin, S. W., Sakmar, T. P., & Mathies, R. A. (1999). How color visual pigments are tuned. *Trends Biochem. Sci.*, *24*, 300–5.

Krebs, A., Villa, C., Edwards, P. C., & Schertler, G. F. (1998). Characterisation of an improved two-dimensional p22$_1$2$_1$ crystal from bovine rhodopsin. *J. Mol. Biol.*, *282*, 991–1003.

Kropf, A. & Hubbard, R. (1958). The Mechanism of Bleaching Rhodopsin. *Ann. New York Acad. Sci.*, *74*, 266–80.

Kusnetzow, A., Dukkipati, A., Babu, K. R., Singh, D., Vought, B. W., Knox, B. E., & Birge, R. R. (2001). The photobleaching sequence of a short-wavelength visual pigment. *Biochemistry*, *40*, 7832–44.

Lin, S. W., Kochendoerfer, G. G., Carroll, K. S., Wang, D., Mathies, R. A., & Sakmar, T. P. (1998). Mechanisms of spectral tuning in blue cone visual pigments. Visible and raman spectroscopy of blue-shifted rhodopsin mutants. *J. Biol. Chem.*, *273*, 24583–91.

Livnah, N. & Sheves, M. (1993). Model Compounds Can Mimic Spectroscopic Properties of Bovine Rhodopsin. *J. Am. Chem. Soc.*, *115*, 351–3.

Menon, S. T., Han, M., & Sakmar, T. P. (2001). Rhodopsin: structural basis of molecular physiology. *Physiol. Rev.*, *81*, 1659–88.

Merbs, S. L. & Nathans, J. (1992). Absorption spectra of human cone pigments. *Nature*, *356*, 433–5.

Mielke, T., Villa, C., Edwards, P. C., Schertler, G. F. X., & Heyn, M. P. (2002). X-ray diffraction of heavy-atom labelled two-dimensional crystals of rhodopsin identifies the position of cysteine 140 in helix 3 and cysteine 316 in helix 8. *J. Mol. Biol.*, *316*, 693–709.

Mollon, J. (1991). G protein-coupled receptors. Hue and the heptahelicals. *Nature*, *351*, 696–7.

Nakanishi, K., Balogh-Nair, V., Arnaboldi, M., Tsujimoto, K., & Honig, B. (1980). An External Point-Charge Model for Bacteriorhodopsin To Account for Its Purple Color. *J. Am. Chem. Soc.*, *102*, 7945–47.

Nathans, J. (1989). The genes for color vision. *Sci. Am.*, *260*, 42–9.

Nathans, J. (1999). The evolution and physiology of human color vision: insights from molecular genetic studies of visual pigments. *Neuron*, *24*, 299–312.

Nathans, J., Thomas, D., & Hogness, D. S. (1986). Molecular genetics of human color vision: the genes encoding blue, green, and red pigments. *Science*, *232*, 193–202.

Neitz, M., Neitz, J., & Jacobs, G. H. (1991). Spectral tuning of pigments underlying red-green color vision. *Science*, *252*, 971–4.

Oprian, D. D., Asenjo, A. B., Lee, N., & Pelletier, S. L. (1991). Design, chemical synthesis, and expression of genes for the three human color vision pigments. *Biochemistry*, *30*, 11367–72.

Palczewski, K., Kumasaka, T., Hori, T., Behnke, C. A., Motoshima, H., Fox, B. A., Le Trong, I., Teller, D. C., Okada, T., Stenkamp, R. E., Yamamoto, M., & Miyano, M. (2000). Crystal structure of rhodopsin: A G protein-coupled receptor. *Science*, *289*, 739–45.

Papermaster, D. S. & Dreyer, W. J. (1974). Rhodopsin content in the outer segment membranes of bovine and frog retinal rods. *Biochemistry*, *13*, 2438–44.

Schertler, G. F. (1998). Structure of rhodopsin. *Eye*, *12*, 504–10.

Schertler, G. F. X. & Hargrave, P. A. (1995). Projection structure of frog rhodopsin in two crystal forms. *Proc. Natl. Acad. Sci. USA*, *92*, 11578–82.

Schertler, G. F. X., Villa, C., & Henderson, R. (1993). Projection Structure of Rhodopsin. *Nature*, *362*, 770–2.

Teller, D. C., Okada, T., Behnke, C. A., Palczewski, K., & Stenkamp, R. E. (2001). Advances in determination of a high-resolution three-dimensional structure of rhodopsin, a model of G-protein-coupled receptors (GPCRs). *Biochemistry*, *40*, 7761–72.

Unger, V. M., Hargrave, P. A., Baldwin, J. M., & Schertler, G. F. X. (1997). Arrangement of rhodopsin transmembrane alpha-helices. *Nature*, *389*, 203–6.

Unger, V. M. & Schertler, G. F. X. (1995). Low resolution structure of bovine rhodopsin determined by electron cryo-microscopy. *Biophys. J.*, *68*, 1776–86.

Wang, Z., Asenjo, A. B., & Oprian, D. D. (1993). Identification of the Cl^--binding site in the human red and green color vision pigments. *Biochemistry*, *32*, 2125–30.

CHAPTER 2

PHOTOPIGMENT POLYMORPHISM IN PROSIMIANS AND THE ORIGINS OF PRIMATE TRICHROMACY

GERALD H. JACOBS AND JESS F. DEEGAN II

Introduction

It is generally believed that among mammals only primates have evolved the biological machinery required for trichromatic color vision. Anthropoid primates achieve their trichromacy in either of two ways (for reviews see Jacobs 1996, 1998). Catarrhine monkeys, apes, and people have multiple X-chromosome opsin genes that specify spectrally distinct middle-wavelength sensitive (M) and long-wavelength sensitive (L) cone pigments, which in conjunction with an autosomal gene yielding short-wavelength sensitive (S) cone pigment provide the pigment basis for trichromacy. In distinction, most platyrrhine monkeys are polymorphic at a single X-chromosome opsin gene site. This polymorphism permits heterozygous females to produce two types of M and L cone pigments and, with an S-cone opsin of autosomal origin, become trichromatic. A limitation of this arrangement is that homozygous females and all males are obligatory dichromats and these species thus can encompass a variable number of color vision phenotypes. There has been reason to believe that members of the eight primate families classified as Prosimians had neither of these arrangements. Rather, earlier examinations of three species suggested that they were similar to most non-primate mammals in having only a single X-chromosome opsin gene without any polymorphic variation (Jacobs and Deegan II 1993; Deegan II and Jacobs 1996).

The implication that was drawn from the above sketch is that among primates only anthropoids are trichromatic. However, a recent genetic analysis strongly implies that cone photopigment arrangements in prosimians may be more varied than the earlier results indicated. Specifically, screening of M/L opsin genes obtained from twenty prosimian species revealed the presence of polymorphic variation in three species (Tan and Li 1999). Each of these three had two different M/L opsin genes thus predicting polymorphic color vision similar to that seen in platyrrhine monkeys. Because this result has important implications for prosimian color vision as well as for the evolution of primate color vision, we have searched for direct evidence of photopigment polymorphism in prosimi-ans and report here confirming observations made on individuals from one species of diurnal prosimian, *Varecia variegata variegata*—the black and white ruffed lemur. There was as well a specific motivation for examining this particular prosimian, because it is one of those species where the genetic analysis detected no polymorphism in examina-tion of genes from a total of five animals (Tan and Li 1999). This seemed intriguing to us because opsin gene polymorphism was found in the red ruffed lemur (*Varecia variegata rubra*), an animal usually classified as differing from the black and white ruffed lemur only at the sub-species level (Rowe 1996).

Methods

We used a noninvasive electrophysiological technique, electroretinogram (ERG) flicker photometry, to measure spectral sensitivity in prosimians. Both the apparatus and the procedure for making measurements of this kind have been fully described (Jacobs *et al.* 1996*a*; Jacobs and Deegan II 1997). In brief, the fundamental component of the ERG response to high-frequency (31.25 Hz) flickering light was recorded from a bipolar contact-lens electrode placed on the eye of a sedated subject. The stimuli were presented in Maxwellian view through a dilated pupil in the form of a circular field subtending 57 deg. The recordings were made with ambient illumination set to photopic levels. Flicker photometric equations were obtained between an achromatic reference light (3.3 log td) and monochromatic test lights that were successively varied in 10 nm steps from 450 to 650 nm. Spectral sensitivity functions were subsequently derived from the photometric equations.

Recordings were obtained from three adult (one male, two female) black and white ruffed lemurs (*Varecia variegata variegata*) during the course of routine physical exam-inations conducted at the Santa Ana Zoo, Santa Ana, California. Animals were initially anesthetized with isoflurane (5 per cent) delivered through a mask. They were sub-sequently intubated and maintained on 1.5–2.0 per cent isoflurane throughout the recording session.

Results

Under these stringent photopic test conditions large and reliable ERG signals were recor-ded from each of the three subjects implying that the retinas of black and white ruffed lemurs, like those of other diurnal prosimians (Peichl *et al.* 2001), contain a signific-ant cone population. Complete spectral sensitivity functions were measured twice for each animal and these values were averaged. The deviations between the two separ-ately determined equations at each test wavelength typically did not exceed 0.04 log unit. Each of the three lemurs had a distinctly different spectral sensitivity function. Those obtained from the two animals shown at the top of Fig. 2.1 were closely fitted by

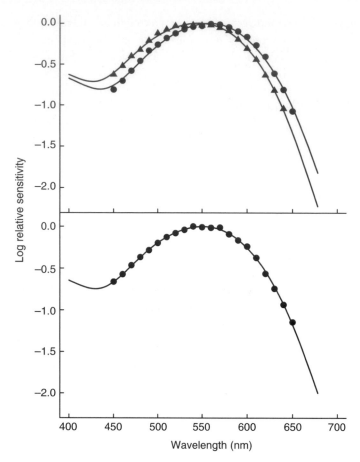

Figure 2.1 Spectral sensitivity functions for three black and white ruffed lemurs. The data points are averaged ERG flicker photometric equation values. These values were corrected for pre-retinal absorption using lens absorption measurements appropriate for another similarly sized, diurnal primate, the macaque monkey (Jacobs and Deegan II 1997). The solid lines are best fits to standard photopigment absorption curves. The curves for the two animals at the top have peak values of 546.3 nm (triangles, the male subject) and 558.4 nm (circles, a female), respectively. The function for the third animal (bottom) has been best fitted by linearly summing these same two curves in the relative proportions 60.7 per cent and 39.3 per cent.

standard photopigment absorption curves (Govardovskii *et al.* 2000) having respective peak values of 546.3 and 558.4 nm. The third animal (Fig. 2.1, bottom) had a spectral sensitivity function somewhat broader than that predicted by the absorption spectrum of a single type of photopigment. It could, however, be very tightly fit (continuous line) by a linear summation of the two absorption functions of the first two subjects, that is, a combination of absorption spectra having respective peak values of 546 and 558 nm.

Discussion

It has been clearly established that spectra measured with ERG flicker photometry provide valid photopigment indices and thus the results of Fig. 2.1 show that each of the three animals had a different complement of M/L cone pigments. The picture that emerges from these recording experiments is in line with what would be expected from the earlier survey of prosimian M/L cone opsin genes. In that survey, individual diurnal prosimians were found to have M/L opsin genes that differed in structure in a fashion that predicts they would yield pigments with different spectral absorption properties and, additionally, some females of these species were found to have copies of both of the genes (Tan and Li 1999). From examination of the amino acids inferred to be present at each of the five locations in the cone opsins believed crucial for spectral tuning (positions 180, 229, 233, 277, and 285), the genetic analysis predicts prosimian M/L cone pigments having spectral peaks of about 543 nm and 558 nm. These values are close to those established by our *in vivo* measurements and thus the present experiment provides strong validation of the genetic results. The peaks we found for the M/L pigments of black and white ruffed lemurs (546, 558 nm) are also virtually identical (545, 558 nm) to those recently measured in another polymorphic prosimian, Coquerel's sifaka (*Propithecus verreauxi coquereli*) (Jacobs *et al.* 2002).

Tan and Li (1999) failed to detect polymorphic M/L opsin gene variation in the five black and white ruffed lemurs they studied while, somewhat surprisingly, we found different phenotypes in each of the three animals examined. That difference in outcome probably reflects nothing other than an example of the role that chance plays in cases where one is limited to studying small numbers of animals drawn from polymorphic species. In any case, it seems clear that these very closely related species of ruffed lemur (*Varecia variegata variegata* and *Varecia variegata rubra*) share in common an M/L cone pigment polymorphism.

The pigment polymorphism seen in black and white ruffed lemurs in turn predicts variations in color vision. Two of the animals should be dichromatic, each with distinctly different color vision characteristics, while the third (a female) has the photopigment basis for trichromacy. Emergence of trichromatic color vision depends, of course, on having both three types of cone pigment and an appropriately organized visual system. Structural examinations of prosimian visual systems show that they share many features in common with anthropoid visual systems (Casagrande and Kaas 1994) and, specifically, there is evidence that prosimian retinas have P-type ganglion cells of the sort known to support M/L opponency and thus serve as a critical neural link to trichromacy in anthropoids (Yamada *et al.* 1998). Direct tests of color vision would obviously be a useful addition to this story, but in their absence it seems reasonable to suppose that these diurnal lemurs have a color vision polymorphism that allows the presence of both dichromatic and trichromatic individuals. Since there is only a single opsin gene locus this predicts that all of the males and some females will be dichromatic. The incidence of trichromatic females among these lemurs will depend on the relative frequencies of

Table 2.1 Distribution of cone pigment polymorphism among prosimians

Family	Number of species	Circadian behavior	M/L cone polymorphism
Tarsiidae	5	Nocturnal	No
Loridae	6	Nocturnal	No
Galagonidae	12	Nocturnal	No
Cheirogaleidae	9	Nocturnal	?*
Megaladapidae	7	Nocturnal	Unknown
Lemuridae	10	Diurnal/cathemeral/ crepuscular	Variable
Indridae	6	Diurnal	Yes
Dauentoniidae	1	Nocturnal	No

*A member of this group, the greater dwarf lemur, was originally claimed to be poly-morphic (Tan and Li 1999). This conclusion is now less certain because of possible errors in the identification of the species of the animals from which the genetic samples were obtained (Y. Tan 2001, personal communication).

the two M/L opsin genes in the population, but in any case it cannot exceed 50 per cent unless additional undiscovered M/L pigments exist in the population.

With the recent evidence that prosimians have cone opsin gene and photopigment polymorphisms it seems clear the idea that only anthropoid primates can be trichromatic was mistaken. At the same time, it is equally clear that the number of prosimians potentially enjoying trichromacy may be limited. Table 2.1 summarizes the evidence so far gathered. While it should be emphasized that there are many prosimian species whose photopigment status is unknown, so far representatives from only two of the eight families in this group are certainly known to have the pigments required for trichromacy. Table 2.1 also contains summary statements about the nominal activity patterns of these prosimians. Most prosimians are nocturnal and it is evident from Table 2.1 that only animals from diurnal species are so far known to have M/L cone polymorphism. Prosimians from the family Lemuridae are of particular interest in this regard since this group contains animals that vary in activity patterns from strongly diurnal to crepuscular to cathemeral (Rowe 1996). It will be interesting to learn if photopigment polymorphism, and thus the potential for color vision variation, is distributed across this family in accord with nominal activity pattern.

Primitive primates have traditionally been considered to have been nocturnal (Martin 1990), and the argument has been advanced that diurnality appeared following the divergence of strepsirrhines and haplorhines, possibly only after the latter group had additionally split into tarsier and anthropoid clades (Ross 2000). Based on their finding of cone opsin polymorphism in prosimians, Tan and Li (1999) made a counter proposal, that the common ancestors of strepsirrhines and tarsiers may have been diurnal and trichromatic. Evidence against this idea comes from a reconstruction of activity patterns in fossil primates and an analysis of the evolution of several features of the visual system by Heesy and Ross 2001. They analyzed estimated orbit size/body size ratios from skull fragments of fossil adapiformes (the sister taxon to modern strepsirrhines) and these, by comparison to the ratios in modern primates, supported the idea that the basal condition of strepsirrhines was nocturnal and that diurnality has arisen sporadically in just a few lines of prosimians. The evidence from extant and fossile haplorhines suggested that the omomyiformes (the Eocene fossil group most closely related to tarsiers and anthropoids) were also nocturnal, diurnality arising later in the stem lineage of anthropoids. Additionally, by calculating the most parsimonious interpretations of the activity patterns and color vision of ancestral primates based on current knowledge of these traits in extant primates, they robustly reconstructed nocturnality and dichromacy as primitive traits for primates. If they are right, diurnality evolved in the stem lineage of the anthropoids and, sporadically, in a few of the lines to modern prosimians. Table 2.1 would suggest that it is only in those diurnal lines that cone pigment polymorphism has emerged as an adaptive trait.

Whether M/L cone pigment polymorphism preceded the acquisition of routine trichromacy in catarrhine primates or not is unknown. The fact that such polymorphism did precede the evolution of universal trichromacy in the only platyrrhine genus (*Alouatta*) to achieve that status suggests that it may be the usual progression to the acquisition of two separate M and L cone opsin genes (Jacobs *et al.* 1996*b*; Kainz *et al.* 1998; Dulai *et al.* 1999). That latter step has apparently not been achieved in any of the lines to modern prosimians. Nevertheless, the appearance of very similar photopigment polymorphism in prosimians and platyrrhines suggests that the basic organizational pattern of the primate retina provides a very fertile ground in which opsin gene polymorphisms can opportunistically take root and yield trichromatic color vision.

Acknowledgements

We thank L. Boldrick and C. Sweet for their cooperation and assistance and an anonymous referee for helpful comments. This research was supported by a grant from the National Eye Institute (EY02052).

References

Casagrande, V. A. & Kaas, J. H. (1994). The afferent, intrinsic, and efferent connections of primary visual cortex in primates. In A. Peters & K. S. Rockland (Eds.), *Primary Visual Cortex in Primates* (Vol. 10, pp. 201–59). New York: Plenum Press.

Deegan II, J. F. & Jacobs, G. H. (1996). Spectral sensitivity and photopigments of a nocturnal prosimian, the bush baby (*Otolemur crassicaudatus*). *American Journal of Primatology, 40*, 55–66.

Dulai, K. S., von Dornum, M., Mollon, J. D., & Hunt, D. M. (1999). The evolution of trichromatic color vision by opsin gene duplication in New World and Old World primates. *Genome Research*, *9*, 629–38.

Govardovskii, V. I., Fyhrquist, N., Reuter, T., Kuzmin, D. G., & Donner, K. (2000). In search of the visual pigment template. *Visual Neuroscience*, *17*, 509–28.

Heesy, C. P., & Ross, C. F. (2001). Evolution of activity patterns and chromatic vision in primates: Morphometrics, genetics and cladistics. *Journal of Human Evolution*, *40*, 111–49.

Jacobs, G. H. (1996). Primate photopigments and primate color vision. *Proceedings of the National Academy of Sciences USA*, *93*, 577–81.

Jacobs, G. H. (1998). A perspective on color vision in platyrrhine monkeys. *Vision Research*, *38*, 3307–13.

Jacobs, G. H. & Deegan II, J. F. (1993). Photopigments underlying color vision in ringtail lemurs (*Lemur catta*) and brown lemurs (*Eulemur fulvus*). *American Journal of Primatology*, *30*, 243–56.

Jacobs, G. H. & Deegan II, J. F. (1997). Spectral sensitivity of macaque monkeys measured with ERG flicker photometry. *Visual Neuroscience*, *14*, 921–8.

Jacobs, G. H., Deegan II, J. F., Tan, Y., & Li, W.-H. (2002). Opsin gene and photopigment polymorphism in a prosimian primate. *Vision Research*, *42*, 11–18.

Jacobs, G. H., Neitz, J., & Krogh, K. (1996a). Electroretinogram flicker photometry and its applications. *Journal of the Optical Society of America A*, *13*, 641–8.

Jacobs, G. H., Neitz, M., Deegan, J. F., & Neitz, J. (1996b). Trichromatic colour vision in New World monkeys. *Nature*, *382*, 156–8.

Kainz, P. M., Neitz, J., & Neitz, M. (1998). Recent evolution of uniform trichromacy in a New World monkey. *Vision Research*, *38*, 3315–20.

Martin, R. D. (1990). *Primate Origins and Evolution*. Princeton: Princeton University Press.

Peichl, L., Rakotondraparany, F., & Kappeler, P. (2001). Photoreceptor types and distributions in nocturnal and diurnal Malagasy primates. *Investigative Ophthalmology and Visual Science*, *42*, S48.

Ross, C. F. (2000). Into the light: The origin of Anthropoidea. *Annual Review of Anthropology*, *29*, 147–94.

Rowe, N. (1996). *The Pictorial Guide to the Living Primates*. East Hampton, New York: Pogonias Press.

Tan, Y. & Li, W.-H. (1999). Trichromatic vision in prosimians. *Nature*, *402*, 36.

Yamada, E. S., Marshak, D. W., Silveira, L. C. L., & Casagrande, V. A. (1998). Morphology of P and M retinal ganglion cells of the bush baby. *Vision Research*, *38*, 3345–52.

CHAPTER 3

DID PRIMATE TRICHROMACY EVOLVE FOR FRUGIVORY OR FOLIVORY?

P. SUMNER AND J. D. MOLLON

Introduction

Primate colour vision

Most mammals have two types of cone photopigment, short-wave-sensitive (S) and long-wave-sensitive (L); and a dichromatic colour sense is provided by a comparison of the signals from the different cones in which these two pigments reside (Jacobs 1993). Most platyrrhine primates (New World monkeys), and probably some lemuriformes of Madagascar, exhibit sex-linked polymorphic colour vision: some females are trichromatic, having two different L photopigments with peak sensitivity (λ_{max}) in the range 536–564 nm (in addition to their S pigment, λ_{max} 430 nm), whereas other females and all males possess only one L photopigment, and are therefore dichromatic (Bowmaker et al. 1987; Jacobs and Blakeslee 1984; Jacobs et al. 1981; Mollon et al. 1984; Tan and Li 1999; Jacobs and Deegan, Chapter 2). All catarrhines (Old World monkeys and apes) and one genus of platyrrhines, *Alouatta*, have developed uniform trichromacy, such that all individuals possess two L pigments with λ_{max} values at about 530 and 560 nm, the former of which is normally referred to as a middle-wave (M) pigment (Bowmaker et al. 1991; Dulai et al. 1994; Dulai et al. 1999; Hunt et al. 1998; Jacobs and Deegan 1999; Jacobs et al. 1996; Kainz et al. 1998).

Whether the primates possess one or two types of L pigment, a comparison of the signal from L cones and S cones is mediated by a small population of bistratified ganglion cells, which project to the koniocellular layers of the Lateral Geniculate Nucleus and constitute a neural channel that is thought to remain largely separate from other visual pathways (Dacey and Lee 1994; Hendry and Reid 2000; Martin et al. 1997). In primates with two types of L cone (often called M and L), a separate comparison of the signals from these two types is mediated by the parvocellular system (which is present in all primates and is thought to subserve the resolution of spatial detail). Together these S/L and L/M subsystems create trichromacy.

The uniform trichromacy of *Alouatta* is known to have arisen separately from that of catarrhines, perhaps from a polymorphic arrangement similar to that seen in other platyrrhines. The polymorphic state may be ancestral to all primates, anteceding the catarrhine uniform trichromacy also. Alternatively, the polymorphism of platyrrhines, the polymorphism of Malagasy strepsirhines, and the uniform trichromacy of catarrhines, may all have arisen separately from a dichromatic ancestor. Regan et al. (2001) review this debate.

The advantage of trichromacy?

What was the selective advantage of the extra, L/M, subsystem of colour vision? The main hypothesis has been that the advantage lay in finding fruit amongst foliage (Allen 1879; Mollon 1989; Osorio and Vorobyev 1996; Polyak 1957). Primary evidence in support of this frugivory hypothesis has come from Regan et al. (1998, 2001), who measured (1) the spectral properties of the fruit in the diets of three platyrrhine species in French Guiana, (2) the spectral properties of the leaves that form the natural background against which these fruit must be found, and (3) the various illumination conditions of the forest environment. By modelling the signal-to-noise ratios for detecting fruit against foliage for all possible pairs of L pigment sensitivities, they found that the photopigments of *Alouatta seniculus* and of the trichromatic individuals of *Ateles paniscus* and *Cebus apella* are well optimized for detecting the fruit in the monkeys' diets against the natural background of forest leaves.

It has further been proposed that fruit signals and primate colour vision have co-evolved (Polyak 1957). For a recent discussion, see Regan et al. (2001). However, the relative advantages of different fruit colours to the plants, and the question of whether or not the plants' evolution has been affected by primate colour vision, do not directly impinge on our primary concern here—the selective advantage of trichromacy to the primates.

Lucas et al. (1998) have suggested an alternative hypothesis: that the advantage of trichromatic vision lay in the detection of red or reddish/brown colouration in the edible young leaves of some tropical plants. This folivory hypotheses has been compared to the frugivory theory by Sumner and Mollon (2000a). We used methods similar to those of Regan et al. (1998, 2001), but applied them to six catarrhine species in an African forest (Kibale, Uganda). We found that the L/M subsystem provides an advantage for detecting both fruits and young leaves amongst mature foliage, and furthermore, that the spectral positions of the primates' pigments are optimized for both tasks. We concluded that finding any of these food items may have been an important selective advantage in the original development, and in the subsequent maintenance and tuning, of primate trichromacy.

However, Dominy and Lucas (2001) have concluded, from similar spectral data also collected in Kibale, that "leaf consumption [has] unique value in maintaining tri-chromacy in catarrhines," that "the fruit-feeding hypothesis for trichromacy in higher primates is unconvincing," and that "full trichromatic vision evolved originally for leaf foraging in higher primates." Note that they make conclusions about both the original selective advantage and the advantage that maintains trichromacy today, factors which need not be the same. In addition, there are at least three "original" events to consider: the establishment of the polymorphic situation, perhaps more than once, the establishment of uniform trichromacy in *Alouatta*, and the establishment of uniform trichromacy in catarrhines. The most important selective advantage may have been different for each of these cases, just as the relative importance of folivory and frugivory in maintaining polymorphism or uniform trichromacy may differ between different species today.

We examine below how Dominy and Lucas, using data similar to ours, reached different conclusions and why we believe that the evidence cannot support their claims.

Evidence and arguments for the folivory and frugivory hypotheses

The spectroradiometric evidence

Dominy and Lucas' derived their conclusions both from their primary evidence, and from secondary arguments. We consider first their primary arguments, which may be summarized as follows:

(1) Leaves that primates select have higher than average ratios of protein to toughness (their Fig. 2).

(2) This ratio is correlated with the leaves' signal in the L/M colour subsystem (calculated as $L/(L + M)$, where L and M are the quantum catches of the L and M cones).

(3) $L/(L+M)$ is better than luminance at discriminating consumed from mature leaves.

(4) The pre-existing colour signal (calculated as $S/(L + M)$) cannot discriminate between consumed leaves and mature leaves, but can discriminate between fruit and mature leaves because the average of the fruit's $S/(L + M)$ values is lower than that of mature leaves (their Fig. 3), and thus the L/M channel is unnecessary for finding fruit, but necessary for finding edible leaves.

(5) While the fruit diets of different primates differ in their chromaticity distributions, the leaf diets of the different primates do not, possibly explaining why all primates with uniform trichromacy have very similar λ_{max} values for their M and L cones (close to 530 and 560 nm, see Introduction, this chapter).

Dominy and Lucas supported points (1) and (2) with important new data. These arguments, however, while consistent with the folivory hypothesis, do not elevate it above the frugivory hypothesis because similar points can be made for fruit: Dominy and Lucas do not report the physicochemical characteristics of the fruit they measured, but primates tend to select ripe fruit, which have higher than average nutrient content (e.g. Simmen and Sabatier 1996; Wrangham *et al.* 1993) and lower than average hardness or toughness. For example, we found that for most species of consumed fruit in Kibale, the force required to puncture the skin of samples of different maturity (our measure of ripeness) was inversely related to their $L/(L + M)$ chromaticity values (Sumner and Mollon 2000*b*).

Likewise, point (3), that edible and mature leaves can better be discriminated by their $L/(L + M)$ chromaticity values than by luminance, is indeed consistent with the folivory hypothesis (and replicates our findings, e.g. figure 11A of Sumner and Mollon 2000a), but it is not inconsistent with the frugivory hypothesis, because fruits too can be better detected amongst mature leaves by their $L/(L + M)$ chromaticity values than by luminance (e.g. Sumner and Mollon 2000a, pp. 1973–4). Dominy and Lucas do not report how they calculated that "the red–green colour channel was a far better discriminant," and do not give the equivalent results for the fruits they measured. We suggest that a comparison of the mean signal-to-noise ratios may be appropriate. For our data collected in Kibale, the signal-to-noise ratio for detecting edible leaves against mature leaves (measured in the canopy in cloudy conditions) was about seven times higher using $L/(L + M)$ than luminance ($L + M$ or simply L for a dichromat), and for detecting ripe fruits against mature leaves it was about 14 times higher (the exact values depend on the relative sampling of different species and of different stages of maturity, on the type of illumination (sunlight, blue sky or cloudy) and on the exact λ_{max} of the dichromat's L cone)[1].

The main pillar of Dominy and Lucas' proposal that trichromacy evolved for folivory was argument (4), that frugivores do not need the additional "red–green" ($L/(L + M)$) colour channel, because the fruit was discriminable from mature leaves by the dichromat's existing "blue–yellow" ($S/(L + M)$) channel. However, they showed only that the distributions of the $S/(L + M)$ signal for fruit and foliage have statistically distinguishable means (their Fig. 3). This is to confound (a) the discriminability of two overlapping statistical distributions and (b) the discriminability of individual elements drawn from those distributions. To be camouflaged, a class of objects does not have to display the whole range of visual appearances found in their surroundings, they need only appear like a subsection of their surroundings. To be detected, therefore, a target must lie outside

---

1   Although the chromaticity and luminance distributions in figure 1 of Dominy and Lucas (2001) are similar to our data, the exact values on each axis are different. Dominy and Lucas do not give the details of how they calculated S, M, and L, or luminance, and nor do they tell us how they defined the boundary of their "domain of mature foliage (outlined in green)" in their figure 1. The differences in $L/(L + M)$ and $S/(L + M)$ probably arose from different normalization of the S, M, and L sensitivity curves (i.e. different assumptions about relative sensitivity of the cone classes) (D. Osorio, personal communication; P. Lucas, personal communication). This would affect the values, but not the form of the results, because, for example, a change in the relative sensitivity of L and M must affect equally all samples with equal $L/(L + M)$ values. Since no arguments are made from the absolute values of the results, all conclusions will be unaffected. The luminance axis may not be so easily dismissed: although labelled "luminance," the legend states that it is "a proportion of reflectance from a compacted barium-sulphate powder standard" (i.e. mean reflectance), but does not say what sensitivity function (e.g. $V\lambda$ or $L + M$) this has been weighted by, or even whether one was used at all. It seems unlikely that a weighting factor for the primates' sensitivity was omitted, but some of the reflectance values plotted by Dominy and Lucas in their figure 1b are curiously low (values below 2 per cent would normally appear black to a human observer).

the distractor distribution, not simply away from the mean. The important thing to a primate observer is whether a *particular* chromaticity is more likely to be a fruit or a leaf, regardless of what chromaticities other leaves and other fruits may have. If targets are much rarer than distractors (as in the case of fruit in the forest), when any particular chromaticity that might be a target or distractor is observed from a distance, it will most likely be a distractor. This argument is effectively taking a Bayesian approach of prior probability. The "frequency" axis of Dominy and Lucas' figure 3 gives, we assume, simply the number of samples they collected of each category. If the plots were scaled to reflect the total number of fruit and leaves that might be in a primate's visual field as it scans the canopy, then at nearly every $S/(L+M)$ chromaticity value the number of fruits would be dwarfed by the number of leaves (see Fig. 3.1). Even if some fruit were detectable by a dichromat using S/L, as long as the L/M channel provided an added advantage, it would still be selected for (this is the same argument as put forward above for luminance—that although some edible leaves and fruit have higher luminance than mature leaves, the L/M channel is a "better discriminant").

Where diets of primates are concerned, any argument that relies crucially on the exact statistics of samples will be insecure, because samples from different studies will vary. For example, although the mean $S/(L+M)$ values for the edible leaves and fruit differed in Dominy and Lucas' study, in our data they do not. Dominy and Lucas' samples of

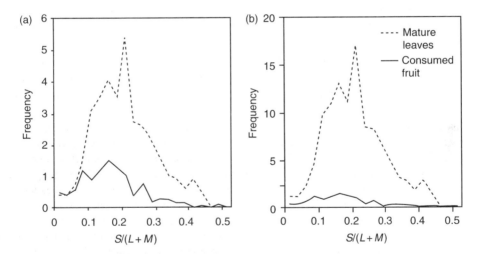

Figure 3.1 (a) Distribution of $S/(L+M)$ chromaticity values for the consumed fruits and mature leaves in figure 3.3A of Dominy and Lucas (2001). The "frequency" axis corresponds to the total number of samples measured, and thus the relative scaling of fruit and leaves is somewhat arbitrary. The ratio of leaves to fruit in the field of view of a primate searching for fruit, while difficult to estimate exactly, would probably range from 100 : 1 to much higher ratios. (b) Replots of the data of (a) with a very conservative ratio of 10 : 1 for the total number of mature leaves and fruit. At every value of $S/(L+M)$ chromaticity, the mature leaves outnumber the fruits, and thus any given chromaticity in the $S/(L+M)$ colour system is more likely to represent a distractor than a target.

these eaten items may be more representative because their fieldwork extended over a longer period (8 months vs 4 months). However, in the case of the mature foliage, we do claim to have made measurements that are more representative of the distribution viewed by a primate in the canopy. Dominy and Lucas measured the chromaticities only of collected samples, and these do not fully represent the distribution of signals in the forest. We additionally made measurements of leaves *in situ* in the canopy, and these display an extended range of S/L chromaticity values compared to our measurements of collected samples (especially when viewed from below), owing to light transmitted though the blade in the canopy as well as reflected light (see Sumner and Mollon 2000*a*, pp. 1971–3 and Regan *et al.* 2001, pp. 249–51). *In situ* the range of luminances is also extended, owing to differing angles of leaf blade and local shadows. When measurements of collected samples are compared, it appears that some fruits and edible leaves lie outside the mature leaf distribution on the luminance and S/L axes, and thus would be detectable by dichromats. But when the distribution of foliage *in situ* is considered, the food items do not lie outside the foliage distribution in S/L, and very few do in luminance, and thus the dichromatic primate could not reliably spot the fruit or young leaves on the basis of their colour, and would find it very difficult on the basis of luminance (especially for fruit, which tend to grow more in the shadows of the mature leaves than do the young leaves). On the other hand, in the phylogenetically newer, L/M channel of the trichromat, even the *in situ* foliage produces only a very limited distribution of signals, and most targets lie outside this distribution. Therefore, in the natural forest environment, the advantage of trichromacy for finding both fruit and leaves is larger than estimated from collected samples alone.[2]

It is clear that the L/M ("red–green") channel offers an advantage for finding both fruits and young leaves. There are other useful cues too, such as shape, position, smell, touch, or sound (e.g. alerting from birds) (Dominy *et al.* 2001), but their existence would not stop trichromacy being selected for if it gave a primate a competitive edge. Since all the arguments raised above apply to both frugivory and folivory, how might we distinguish between the theories? In the absence of other constraints, we might expect the L/M channel to be optimized for the task that most influenced its evolution. Following the modelling procedure developed by Regan and Mollon (Regan *et al.* 1998, 2001), we have calculated signal-to-noise ratios for detecting target food items amongst foliage for all possible combinations of M and L cone spectral sensitivities (Sumner and Mollon 2001). We did this separately for the fruit and leaf diets of the six studied primates in Kibale and we found that in all cases the maximum signal-to-noise ratios were yielded by a pair of pigments very close to those that the primates actually possess: about 530

---

2   Dominy and Lucas cite Sumner and Mollon (2000*b*) to support their claim that "although the red–green colour channel can help a group to identify such fruits at long range, the yellow–blue channel can often do this too." However in that paper we discussed the separate task of discriminating ripe fruit from unripe fruit (at short range), not the task of detecting fruit amongst foliage.

and 560 nm. The two sets of targets, edible leaves and fruit, produce virtually identical results because it is not the exact spectral properties of the targets themselves, but rather the properties of the mature foliage background that determine which spectral positions are optimal: the pair of λ_{max} values that yield maximum signal-to-noise is determined chiefly by minimising the variance of the chromaticities of mature leaves (Sumner and Mollon 2000*a*). This may explain why all extant trichromatic primates have similar photopigment tuning despite varied diets (cf point (5) of Dominy and Lucas' argument above). It also means that spectroradiometric data cannot tell us whether the most important things to detect amongst foliage were fruit, young leaves, or something else altogether, such as conspecifics or other animals.

Secondary arguments

Since spectroradiometric data cannot decide the folivory–frugivory debate, we might turn to other evidence. The primate species that are polymorphic for colour vision (most platyrrhines and at least some lemuroids; see Introduction of this chapter) offer the opportunity for directly testing whether trichromatic individuals are more successful than dichromatic conspecifics in foraging for fruit or for young leaves in the forest. However, since a study of this kind has not yet been published, let us briefly assess some of the secondary arguments.

Dominy and Lucas point out ecological differences between the diets and habitats of those primates exhibiting uniform trichromacy (Old World monkeys and apes, plus *Alouatta*) and those exhibiting polymorphic vision. The folivory hypothesis is supported by the fact that young leaves tend to be a more important food resource (in terms of both overall quantity consumed and reliance on it in times of fruit shortage) to catarrhines and *Alouatta* than to many platyrrhines, and that there seem to be more reddish young leaves in Africa and Asia than in South America (see Dominy and Lucas 2001; Dominy 2002). In the case of the folivorous colobines, which eat very little ripe fruit, leaf-finding is probably more important than fruit-finding in maintaining their trichromacy today, but this need not be true of when it originally evolved. It is believed that the specialized leaf-eating of colobines is a derived characteristic and that the ancestral catarrhine, being small, ate much more fruit than leaves (Martin 1990). Dominy and Lucas mention also that fruit may be found using other pre-ingestive cues, such as smell and texture. It could equally be argued that young edible leaves are a much less sporadic resource in the forest than fruit and can be found by their likely position at the ends of twigs.

Dominy and Lucas further argue that because 'basically dichromatic' platyrrhine species eat similar fruit to catarrhine primates and find it with 'no apparent difficulty', the idea that catarrhine trichromacy evolved for fruit-finding is implausible. However, firstly, no known diurnal platyrrhine is uniformly dichromatic. Secondly, no-one has reported that platyrrhines have difficulty finding young leaves: there are no published data on individual differences in fruit-finding or leaf-finding between trichromatic and dichromatic individuals. Thirdly, the use of a trait for a particular need in one population might easily occur without the invention or use of that trait in another population with a similar need: in the latter population there may be other means of solving the problem, there may be reasons for not wanting the trait, or the necessary step of invention may simply not have occurred.

If the initial genetic event needed to create uniform trichromacy from the polymorphic state has simply never occurred in the lineages of extant polymorphic primates, then comparisons of the diets and habitats of uniformly trichromatic and polymophic species are in fact not relevant. In order for a polymorphic species to become uniformly trichromatic, there needs to be an unequal cross-over at mieosis, so creating an X chromosome with two different viable middle/long-wave photopigment genes. This X chromosome then needs to be spread and maintained in the population. Why has this happened only in catarrhines and separately in *Alouatta*, but not in any other primate lineages despite the advantages in finding fruit and young leaves that should benefit all species? There are three possible types of reason: (1) As mentioned above, the required genetic event, followed by fertilization of the egg and survival of the embryo, may have occurred only in catarrhines and *Alouatta* and the polymorphism in other species may have been maintained by 'pure heterozygous advantage' (Mollon *et al.* 1984). (2) The advantage of trichromacy to catarrhines and *Alouatta* may have been more than to other platyrrhines and lemuroids (e.g. because the latter eat fewer leaves, as Dominy and Lucas argue, or because their social behaviour enables dichromatic individuals to find food via trichromatic individuals, or because South American fruits can more easily be spotted by their lightness or found using other pre-ingestive cues). (3) There may be advantages in being dichromatic, or in having a polymorphic group with dichromacy and different types of trichromacy all present. The latter possibility is discussed in detail by Mollon *et al.* (1984) and Regan *et al.* (2001).

Conclusions

The spectroradiometric evidence is consistent with both the folivory and frugivory hypotheses, and tests of intraspecific differences in foraging success between dichromatic and trichromatic individuals are yet to be reported. Therefore, there is at present no primary evidence that distinguishes between the theories. Secondary arguments can be made in favour of each theory, but our tentative conclusions would be that leaf-finding was probably important (as well as fruit-finding) in the spread of uniform trichromacy in *Alouatta*, and may now be the most important factor maintaining trichromacy in highly folivorous catarrhine species. In other species there is probably a range in the relative importance of frugivory and folivory in maintaining trichromacy, depending on diet, on fruiting and leafing cycles of the habitat, and on other uses of trichromacy such as discriminating the colours of pelage. Since ancestral primates are believed to have relied much more on fruit than leaves, fruit-finding was probably the most important factor in the original emergence of uniform trichromacy in Old World primates, and probably also in the emergence of the polymorphic states in South American monkeys and in lemurs.

Acknowledgement

We thank Dr Benedict Regan for comments.

References

Allen, G. (1879). The Colour-Sense: Its Origin and Development. London: Trubner & Co.

Bowmaker, J. K., Astell, S., Hunt, D. M., & Mollon, J. D. (1991). Photosensitive and photostable pigments in the retinae of Old World monkeys. *Journal of Experimental Biology* **156**, 1–19.

Bowmaker, J. K., Jacobs, G. H., & Mollon, J. D. (1987). Polymorphism of photopigments in the squirrel monkey: a sixth phenotype. *Proceedings of the Royal Society of London B* **231**, 383–90.

Dacey, D. M. & Lee, B. B. (1994). The 'blue on' opponent pathway in primate retina originates from a distinct bistratified ganglion cell type. *Nature* **367**, 731–5.

Dominy, N. J. (2002). Incidence of red leaves in the rain forest of Kibale National Park, Uganda: shade-tolerators and light-demanders compared. *African Journal of Ecology* **40**, 94–6.

Dominy, N. J., & Lucas, P. W. (2001). Ecological importance of trichromatic vision to primates. *Nature* **410**, 363–6.

Dominy, N. J., Lucas, P. W., Osorio, D., & Yamashita, N. (2001). The sensory ecology of primate food perception. *Evolutionary Anthropology* **10**, 171–86.

Dulai, K. S., Bowmaker, J. K., Mollon, J. D., & Hunt, D. M. (1994). Sequence divergence, polymorphism and evolution of middle-wave and long-wave visual pigment genes of great apes and Old World monkeys. *Vision Research* **34**, 2483–91.

Dulai, K. S., von Dornum, M., Mollon, J. D., & Hunt, D. M. (1999). The evolution of trichromatic color vision by opsin gene duplication in New World and Old World primates. *Genome Research* **9**, 629–38.

Hendry, S. H. C. & Reid, R. C. (2000). The koniocellular pathway in primate vision. *Annual Reviews in Neuroscience* **23**, 127–53.

Hunt, D. M., Dulai, K. S., Cowing, J. A., Julliot, C., Mollon, J. D., Bowmaker, J. K., Li, W.-H., & Hewett-Emmett, D. (1998). Molecular evolution of trichromacy in primates. *Vision Research* **38**, 3299–306.

Jacobs, G. H. (1993). The distribution and nature of colour vision among the mammals. *Biological Reviews* **68**, 413–71.

Jacobs, G. H. & Blakeslee, B. (1984). Individual variations in color vision among squirrel monkeys (*Saimiri sciureus*) of different geographical origins. *Journal of Comparative Psychology* **98**, 347–57.

Jacobs, G. H., Bowmaker, J. K., & Mollon, J. D. (1981). Behavioural and microspectrophotometric measurements of colour vision in monkeys. *Nature* **292**, 541–3.

Jacobs, G. H. & Deegan, J. F. (1999). Uniformity of colour vision in Old World monkeys. *Proceedings of the Royal Society of London B* **266**, 2023–8.

Jacobs, G. H., Neitz, M., Deegan, J. F., & Neitz, J. (1996). Trichromatic colour vision in New World monkeys. *Nature* **382**, 156–8.

Kainz, P. M., Neitz, J., & Neitz, M. (1998). Recent evolution of uniform trichromacy in a New World monkey. *Vision Research* **38**, 3315–20.

Lucas, P. W., Darvell, B. W., Lee, P. K. D., Yuen, T. D. B., & Choong, M. F. (1998). Colour cues for leaf food selection by long-tailed macaques (*Macaca fascicularis*) with a new suggestion for the evolution of trichromatic colour vision. *Folia Primatologica* **69**, 139–52.

Martin, P. R., White, A. J. R., Goodchild, A. K., Wilder, H. D., & Sefton, A. E. (1997). Evidence that blue-on cells are part of the third geniculocortical pathway in primates. *European Journal of Neuroscience* **9**, 1536–41.

Martin, R. D. (1990). Primate Origins and Evolution. Princeton: Princeton University Press.

Mollon, J. D. (1989). "Tho she kneel'd in that Place where they grew . . . ." *Journal of Experimental Biology* **146**, 21–38.

Mollon, J. D., Bowmaker, J. K., & Jacobs, G. H. (1984). Variations of colour vision in a New World primate can be explained by polymorphism of retinal photopigments. *Proceedings of the Royal Society of London B* **222**, 373–99.

Osorio, D. & Vorobyev, M. (1996). Colour vision as an adaptation to frugivory in primates. *Proceedings of the Royal Society of London B* **263**, 593–99.

Polyak, S. (1957). The Vertebrate Visual System. Chicago: University of Chicago Press.

Regan, B. C., Julliot, C., Simmen, B., Viénot, F., Charles-Dominique, P., & Mollon, J. D. (1998). Frugivory and colour vision in *Alouatta seniculus*, a trichromatic platyrrhine monkey. *Vision Research* **38**, 3321–7.

Regan, B. C., Julliot, C., Simmen, B., Viénot, F., Charles-Dominique, P., & Mollon, J. D. (2001). Fruits, foliage and the evolution of the primate colour-sense. *Philosophical Transactions of the Royal Society of London B* **356**, 229–83.

Simmen, B. & Sabatier, D. (1996). Diets of some French Guianan primates: food composition and food choices. *International Journal of Primatology* **17**, 661–93.

Sumner, P. & Mollon, J. D. (2000*a*). Catarrhine photopigments are optimised for detecting targets against a foliage background. *Journal of Experimental Biology* **203**, 1963–86.

Sumner, P. & Mollon, J. D. (2000*b*). Chromaticity as a signal of ripeness in fruits taken by primates. *Journal of Experimental Biology* **203**, 1987–2000.

Tan, Y. & Li, W.-H. (1999). Trichromatic vision in prosimians. *Nature* **402**, 36.

Wrangham, R. W., Conklin, N. L., Etot, G., Obua, J., Hunt, K. D., Hauser, M. D., & Clark, A. P. (1993). The value of figs to chimpanzees. *International Journal of Primatology* **14**, 243–56.

CHAPTER 4

LACK OF S-OPSIN EXPRESSION IN THE BRUSH-TAILED PORCUPINE (*ATHERURUS AFRICANUS*) AND OTHER MAMMALS. IS THE EVOLUTIONARY PERSISTENCE OF S-CONES A PARADOX?

P. AHNELT, K. MOUTAIROU, M. GLÖSMANN, AND A. KÜBBER-HEISS

Introduction

Rodents are a heterogeneous order, comprising near half of present day placental mammals (DeBry and Sagel 2001). Recent studies on the photoreceptor layers reveal a surprising variance of photoreceptor topographies (reviews in Ahnelt and Kolb 2000; Szél *et al.* 2000). Extending our knowledge on further rodent families may reveal common trends of adaptive specializations under varying lifestyles and may point to phylogenetic constraints on mammalian retinal design. The porcupines represent a rodent family with very distinct characteristics, in particular, varying sets of defensive spines. They are relatively large herbivores with mostly nocturnal activity patterns.

   The present study gives a description of the photoreceptor layer of the African brush-tailed porcupine (*Atherurus africanus*) and surveys the occurrence of secondary short wavelength cone (pigment) sensitivity loss. This loss is a seemingly frequent event in recent placental mammalian evolution, and it contrasts with the long persistence of the S-cone system in the early Mesozoic mammals. The loss may point to changing roles of the short-wavelength-sensitive (SWS) system during different stages of mammalian evolution.

Materials and methods

Five Brush Tailed African Porcupines (ca. 3 kg) were captured in Benin from the wild according to CITES regulations and sacrificed. Eyes were removed and fixed in P-buffered 4 per cent paraformaldehyde, some after removal of lens and cornea for 1 day, and were transferred to 1 per cent P-buffered PF for transport. After pre-incubation in 10 per cent bovine serum albumin (BSA) and 3 per cent normal goat serum (NGS) overnight, they were incubated for 24 h in the primary antibodies JH 455 1 : 30 000 or JH492 1 : 20 000, (kindly provided by J. Nathans, Johns Hopkins University). After Biotin/Extravidin–Peroxidase incubation, DAB was used for visualization. Retinas were transferred in 95 per cent glycerol on to glass slides for inspection. Cell densities were sampled using counting frames on a Hamamatsu camera/Macintosh computer system and then mapped using *DeltaGraph* (*SPSS*) and *Canvas* (*Deneba*) software.

Results and discussion

Lack of S-opsin expression in Atherurus

Rods dominate the *Atherurus* photoreceptor cell layer and reach densities of ca. $400\,000/mm^2$ in superior retina (Fig. 4.1(a)). An immuno-histochemical study on the opsin topographies in the retina of the brush-tailed porcupine by labeling of wholemounts and sections with opsin antibodies (JH455, JH492) reveals a sparse population (ca. $2000/mm^2$) of presumptive middle-to-long wavelength sensitive (M/L-) cones (Fig. 4.1(b)). The density in the superior retina is relatively higher (maximum of ca. $3600/mm^2$) but still yields cone proportions <1 per cent. JH455 fails to detect S-opsins in all regions.

Convergent trend to S-cone deficiency

These observations indicate that at least one species in an additional rodent family has evolved towards secondary monochromacy. Data from various mammalian orders including rodents, whales, carnivores, primates, and pholidotes (review in: Ahnelt and Kolb 2000) now indicate a multiple and independent trend towards abandonment of functional S-cones (See Table 4.1). In the species studied so far, S-cone pigment deficiency appears associated with nocturnal or aquatic lifestyles. This link is not strict however since there are S-cones in nocturnal species (e.g. Tarsius (Hendrickson *et al.* 2000)) and in the semi-aquatic hippopotamus (Peichl *et al.* 2001) and the manatee (Ahnelt *et al.* in preparation).

So far SWS-deficiencies have been tracked to actual opsin defects of the opsin gene in a few instances only: human tritanopes (Weitz *et al.* 1992), owl monkey and bushbaby (Jacobs *et al.* 1996) and the dolphin (Fasick *et al.* 1998). The defects have different loci including deletions and insertions and it seems likely that further alterations will be detected in other species.

Of course negative findings could be limited by the sensitivity of current methods of detection. For murid rodents and rabbits, variable thresholds of different antibodies have led to differences in topographic mappings and evaluation of the extent of opsin-coexpression. In the mouse and the rabbit for example, the use of M-opsin antibodies with different affinities has led to different interpretations of the extent of opsin coex-pression. While monoclonal COS-1 antibody failed to stain cone outer segments in

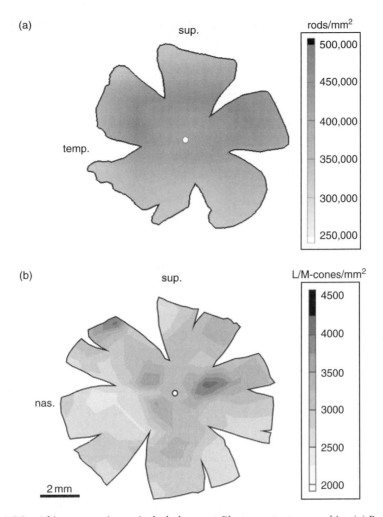

Figure 4.1 West African porcupine, retinal wholemount. Photoreceptor topographies. (a) Rod density. (b) M/L-cone density. See text for details.

the ventral retina (Szél *et al.* 1994; Röhlich *et al.* 1994), labelling with polyclonal anti-sera revealed the presence of M-opsin over the entire retina with gradients of M-opsin expression diminishing from dorsal to ventral (Glösmann and Ahnelt 1998; Hack and Peichl 1999; Pflug 1999; Applebury *et al.* 2000; Ng *et al.* 2001). There is evidence that available S-opsin markers also have different affinities. In the mouse lemur, monoclonal OS-2 antibody gives negative results, whereas polyclonal JH455 detects a population of S-cones (Dkhissi-Benyahya *et al.* 2001; Peichl *et al.* 2001). Interestingly, in the hedgehog, both monoclonal and polyclonal S opsin markers completely fail to label cone outer segments. However, a subset of bipolar cells is distinctly labeled by JH455 (Glösmann

Table 4.1 Current data on SWS-opsin deficiencies in mammals

Systematics	Common name	Reference
Rodents		
Muride		
Cricetomys	African giant rat	Peichl & Moutairou 1998; Szél *et al.* 1994, 1996
Mus pahari	Shrew mouse	
Apodemus microps		Szél *et al.* 1994
Apodemus flavicollis		Glösmann, unpublished
Spalax ehrenbergi	Mole rat	David-Gray *et al.* 2000
Myoxidae		
Glis glis	Dormouse	Glösmann, 2 specimens, unpublished
Hystricidae		
Atherurus	W. African porcupine	Ahnelt *et al.* 2001
Insectivores		
Erinaceids	European hedgehog	Glösmann 2001, Opsin in Bipolars?
Pholidota		
Manis tetradactyla	Scaled anteater	Ahnelt *et al.* 2001
Primates		
Galago,	Bushbaby	Wikler & Rakic 1990; Ahnelt & Kolb 2000 (single
Lori		sample); Wikler & Rakic 1990; Jacobs *et al.* 1996
Aotus	Owl monkey	
Carnivores		
Fissipediia		
Potos flavus	Kinkajou	Jacobs & Deegan 1992; Peichl & Pohl 2000
Procyon cancrivorus	Racoon	
Pinnipedia		
Phoca	Seals	Peichl and Moutairou 1998; Peichl *et al.* 1901
Cetaceans		
Both Odontoceti and	Dolphins	Fasick *et al.* 1998; Peichl *et al.* 2001
Mysticeti	Baleen whales	Levenson *et al.* 2000

et al. 2001). This result suggests that the lack of S opsin in cone photoreceptors can result from mechanisms different from S opsin gene defects.

In any case, these conditions imply a loss of functional SWS-cones with normal thresholds, a conversion to cone monochromacy. While these losses must have occurred in geologically recent time (<60 Mio years), they are elements of a stepwise reduction of spectral differentiation during mammalian evolution. SWS2 and RH2 opsins—present in fish and reptiles and therefore most likely also in synapsid mammalian ancestors—may have been lost during or before the first phase of mammalian evolution (<100 Mio years) from the early Jurassic to the late Cretaceous. During this period a SWS1 pigment was preserved together with rhodopsin and a LW-opsin.

We may assume that (except for some catastrophic events) environmental light conditions had a similar range in both phases of mammalian evolution. It then seems paradoxical that the SWS1-cone pigment (and thus the precondition for color vision) was maintained in those early (small nocturnal insectivore-like) mammals while many recent descendants apparently have remained competitive without it. In most vertebrates S-cones comprise a minor subpopulation allowing them to serve mainly for hue rather than spatial discrimination. Thus shifts in the functional roles of S-opsins and even disappearance may be under fewer selective constraints than apply to L-opsins and related pathways.

Consequently other non-visual functions may have been involved in SWS1-conservation:

Role as promoter

(a) For the mosaic organization of other retinal cell types (Wikler *et al.* 1996).

(b) For maintaining circuitries shared with/required for other pathways.

Role in non-visual tasks driven by light

(a) Sensor for (circa-dian, circa-lunar, circa-annual) biorhythm.

(b) Guiding fast vegetative responses such as pupillary reflexes (Lucas *et al.* 2001).

From UV to blue sensitivity

In this respect it is most notable that the present mammalian S-pigments originate from the class of SWS1-opsins, which in fish and reptiles are mostly positioned in the UV-range (Yokoyama 2000) whereas most modern mammals have "Blue" SWS1-opsins. The finding of UV-sensitivity in murid rodents could then indicate that murids have "back-mutated" their SWS1 opsins after their ancestors had shared a phase of blue sensitivity with the other mammals (Fig. 4.2(a)). Alternatively, the UV-SWS1 varieties were also present in all/most early mammals. Indeed the murine SWS1 opsin shares significant numbers of amino acid sites with UV-pigments of other vertebrates. Thus these rodents may have preserved primary conditions rather than undergone secondary shifts (Fig. 4.2(b)). The present blue range would then be a result from a single upward shift of ancestral UV-pigments and not vice-versa.

SWS-1 photopigments in early mammals could have been UV-sensitive, providing general information about the photic environment. Such capabilities, not requiring image representation, have been present in organisms since the beginning of life itself but until recently little attention had been directed to them in mammals. Now cryptochromes, which may relay information about light conditions to the suprachiasmatic nucleus (Selby *et al.* 2000), are being detected in non-photoreceptoral retinal neurons.

UV-SWS1 opsins serving as (non-visual) complementary light detectors might have been of selective relevance originally. In descendants with photopic or arhythmic lifestyles they supported dichromatic color discrimination by shifting towards longer (blue) wavelengths. Finally, for certain modern groups specialized to specific environments

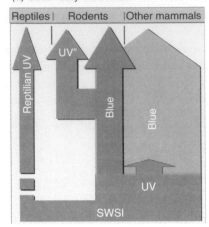
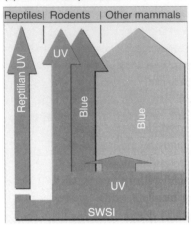

Figure 4.2 Possible scenarios for the origins of rodent UV-sensitive pigments within the evolutionary history of mammalian SWS-opsin family. (a) Secondary regression after general conversion to blue sensitivity in early mammals. (b) UV-sensitivity persisted unchanged in some rodents besides the trend towards longer wavelengths in other mammals.

these "blue-ified" opsins apparently have become dispensable. It should be expected that these losses be buffered by the continuing presence of non-photoreceptoral pigments, cryptochromes, and possibly also "displaced-expression"-opsins (Glösmann *et al.* 2001).

References

Ahnelt, P. K. & **Kolb, H.** (2000). The mammalian photoreceptor mosaic-adaptive design. *Progress in Retinal and Eye Research, 19,* 711–77.

Applebury, M. L., Antoch, M. P., Baxter, L. C., Chun, L. L., Falk, J. D., Farhangfar, F., Kage, K., Krzystolik, M. G., Lyass, L. A., & **Robbins, J. T.** (2000). The murine cone photoreceptor: a single cone type expresses both S and M opsins with retinal spatial patterning. *Neuron, 27,* 513–23.

David Gray, Z. K., Cooper, H. M., Janssen, J. W., Nevo, E., & **Foster, R. G.** (1999). Spectral tuning of a circadian photopigment in a subterranean 'blind' mammal (*Spalax ehrenbergi*). *FEBS-Letter, 461,* 343–7.

DeBry, R. W. & **Sagel, R. M.** (2001). Phylogeny of Rodentia (Mammalia) inferred from the nuclear-encoded gene IRBP. *Molecular Phylogeny and Evolution, 19,* 290–301.

Dkhissi Benyahya, O., Szél, A., Degrip, W. J., & **Cooper, H. M.** (2001). Short and mid-wavelength cone distribution in a nocturnal Strepsirrhine primate (*Microcebus murinus*). *Journal of Comparative Neurology, 438,* 490–504.

Fasick J. I., Cronin T. W., Hunt, D. M., & **Robinson, P. R.** (1998). The visual pigments of the bottlenose dolphin (*Tursiops truncatus*). *Visual Neuroscience, 15,* 643–51.

Glösmann, M. & **Ahnelt, P. K.** (1998). Coexpression of M- and S-opsin extends over the entire inferior mouse retina. *Investigative Ophthalmology & Visual Science, 39* (Suppl.), 1059 (Abstract).

Glösmann, M., Harlfinger, P. J., & Ahnelt, P. K. (2001). S-opsin-like immunoreactivity is localized to bipolar cells but not cone photoreceptors in the European hedgehog. *Investigative Ophthalmology & Visual Science, 42* (Suppl.), 362 (Abstract).

Hack, I. & Peichl, L. (1999). Horizontal cells of the rabbit retina are non-selectively connected to the cones. *European Journal of Neuroscience, 11,* 2261–74.

Hendrickson, A., *et al.* (2000). Nocturnal Tarsier retina has both short and medium-wavelength cones in an unusual topography. *Journal of Comparative Neurology, 424,* 718–30.

Jacobs, G. H. & Deegan, J.F. (1992). Cone photopigments in nocturnal and diurnal procyonids. *Journal of Comparative Physiology A, 171,* 351–8.

Jacobs, G. H., Neitz, M., & Neitz, J. (1996). Mutations in S-cone pigment genes and the absence of colour vision in two species of nocturnal primate. *Proceedings Royal Society London B, Biological Sciences, 263,* 705–10.

Levenson, D. H., Dizon, A., & Ponganis P. J. (2000). Identification of loss-of-function mutations within the short-wavelength sensitive cone opsin genes of baleen and odontocete cetaceans. *Investigative Ophthalmology & Visual Science, 41* (Suppl.), 610 (Abstract).

Lucas, R. J., Douglas, R. H., & Foster, R. G. (2001). Characterization of an ocular photopigment capable of driving pupillary constriction in mice. *Nature Neuroscience, 4,* 621–6.

Ng, L., Hurley, J. B., Dierks, B., Srinivas, M., Salto, C., Vennstrom, B., Reh, T. A., & Forrest, D. (2001). A thyroid hormone receptor that is required for the development of green cone photoreceptors. *Nature Genetics, 27,* 94–8.

Peichl, L. & Moutairou, K. (1998). Absence of short-wavelength sensitive cones in the retinae of seals (Carnivora) and African giant rats (Rodentia). *European Journal of Neuroscience, 10,* 2586–94.

Peichl, L. & Pohl, B. (2000). Cone types and cone/rod ratios in the crab-eating racoon and coati (Procyonidae). *Investigative Ophthalmology & Visual Science, 41,* S495.

Peichl L., Behrmann, G., & Kröger, R. H. (2001). For whales and seals the ocean is not blue: a visual pigment loss in marine mammals. *European Journal of Neuroscience, 13,* 1520–8.

Pflug, R. & Reitsamer, H. (1999). Topographic variation of cone interactions in spectral sensitivities determined from small field ERGs of rabbit retina. *Investigative Ophthalmology & Visual Science, 40* (Suppl.), 238 (Abstract).

Selby, C. P., Thompson, C., Schmitz, T. M., Van Gelder, R. N., & Sancar, A. (2000). Functional redundancy of cryptochromes and classical photoreceptors for nonvisual ocular photoreception in mice. *Proceedings of the National Academy of Science USA, 97,* 14697–702.

Szél, A., Csorba, G., Caffe, A. R., Szél, G., Röhlich, P., & van Veen, T. (1994). Different patterns of retinal cone topography in two genera of rodents, *Mus* and *Apodemus. Cell Tissue Research, 276,* 143–50.

Szél, A., Röhlich, P., Caffe, A. R., & van Veen, T. (1996). Distribution of cone photoreceptors in the mammalian retina. *Microscopy Research Techniques,* 35, 445–62.

Szél, A., Lukáts, A., Fekete, T., Szepessy Z., & Röhlich, P. (2000). Photoreceptor distribution in the retinas of subprimate mammals. *Journal of the Optical Society of America A,* 568–79.

Weitz, C. J., Miyake, Y., Shinzato, K., Montag, E., Zrenner, E., Went, L. N., & Nathans, J. (1992). Human tritanopia associated with two amino acid substitutions in the blue-sensitive opsin. *American Journal of Human Genetics, 50*, 498–507.

Wikler, K. C. & Rakic, P. (1990). Distribution of photoreceptor subtypes in the retina of diurnal and nocturnal primates. *Journal of Neuroscience, 10*, 3390–401.

Wikler, K. C., Szél, A., & Jacobsen, A. L. (1996). Positional information and opsin identity in retinal cones. *Journal of Comparative Neurology*, 374, 96–107.

Yokoyama, S. (2000). Molecular evolution of vertebrate visual pigments. *Progress in Retinal and Eye Research, 19*, 385–419.

CHAPTER 5

THE ARRANGEMENT OF L AND M CONES IN HUMAN AND A PRIMATE RETINA

J. K. BOWMAKER, J. W. L. PARRY, AND J. D. MOLLON

Introduction

The relative numerosities and the spatial arrangement of the long-wave (L) and middle-wave (M) cones in the human and primate retina have long been debated. This topographical organization of cones is fundamental to our understanding of visual sensitivity and of colour vision. To date, owing to the very similar structure of the L and M opsins (Nathans *et al.* 1986), it has not been possible to label the two spectral classes of cone independently, and thus indirect methods have had to be employed. In humans, psychophysical estimates (Vos and Walraven 1971; Cicerone and Nerger 1989; Pokorny *et al.* 1991) suggested a preponderance of L cones, with an average L : M cone ratio close to 2 : 1, but with considerable variation between individuals, the estimated ratios ranging from about 0.3 : 1 to 3 : 1 (Rushton and Baker 1964). More recent findings, including ERG measurements (Carroll *et al.* 2000; Dobkins *et al.* 2000), suggest a similar average ratio and confirm the individual variability, with ratios as high as 12 : 1. Adaptive optics have made possible the direct imaging of the photoreceptor mosaic for spatially localized retinal densitometry and have allowed the L : M ratio to be estimated by differential bleaching (Roorda and Williams 1999; Brainard *et al.* 2000; Roorda *et al.* 2001). For two individuals this method gave ratios of 1.2 : 1 and 3.8 : 1. The distribution of L and M cones appeared random.

Estimates of the L : M cone ratio have also been made from the levels of mRNA, either in whole retina or in regionally located pieces of retina. In human retinae the ratio appears to increase from central retina to periphery, with a ratio in the fovea of about 1.3 : 1 rising to between 3.5 : 1 and 5 : 1 in the mid periphery (Yamaguchi *et al.* 1997; Hagstrom *et al.* 1998, 2000). There was considerable variation between individuals. The suggestion that the relative number of L cones increases towards the periphery (Hagstrom *et al.* 1998) implies that the cone-rich rim of the retina at the *ora serrata* may be dominated by L cones.

In the human retina a stochastic process is thought to determine which form of long- or middle-wave opsin will be expressed in a given cone. The L and M opsin genes are located on the X-chromosome in a tandem array, with one L opsin gene followed by two (or more) M opsin genes (Nathans *et al.* 1986). A locus control region (LCR), upstream of the first opsin gene, is thought to bend back to interact with a promoter region at the beginning of one of the opsin genes (Wang *et al.* 1992, 1999). Only the gene that is coupled to the LCR is favoured for expression. The probability of a given gene being expressed may depend on (i) the exact sequence of the promoter region and (ii) the distance of the gene from the LCR (Winderickx *et al.* 1992). In human females, the system of random X-chromosome inactivation is superposed on the stochastic choice of opsin gene within the expressed chromosome; and thus there is the possibility of more than two types of long-/middle-wave cone within a given retina (Mollon and Jordan 1988).

The organization of the L and M gene array in nonhuman Old World primates is similar to that in humans (Dulai *et al.* 1994, 1999), though normally there is only a single copy of the M gene (Onishi *et al.* 1999). Thus it might be expected that the arrangement of cones within Old World primates would be identical to that in humans. However, spectral sensitivities determined by flicker ERG for chimpanzees (Jacobs *et al.* 1996) suggested a ratio of about 1.3 : 1, somewhat lower than in humans. A lower ratio has also been reported for catarrhine monkeys from direct microspectrophotometric measurements (Bowmaker *et al.* 1991; Mollon and Bowmaker 1992), from flicker ERG (Jacobs and Deegan 1997), from red–green equiluminance matches for magnocellular units (Dobkins *et al.* 2000) and from L and M cone inputs to H1 horizontal cells (Dacey *et al.* 2000). Spatially localized retinal densitometry gave a ratio of 1.4 : 1 in an individual macaque (Roorda *et al.* 2001). Estimates of the L : M cone ratio made from mRNA levels (Deeb *et al.* 2000) yielded a value for macaques of about 1.6 : 1, lower than the value for humans of 4 : 1.

By contrast, in the case of most platyrrhine primates, such as marmosets, there is only a single opsin gene on the X-chromosome, but this locus is polymorphic in many species of New World monkey. In females heterozygous at the single locus, the random process of X-chromosome inactivation will ensure that only one or other opsin allele is expressed in a given cone (Mollon *et al.* 1984). Thus, in a trichromatic female, if X-chromosome inactivation is strictly random, the ratio of the two classes of cone in the red/green spectral region should be close to unity.

We have addressed the question of the numerosity of L and M cones in the human fovea directly by microspectrophotometry of individual cones, in a similar manner to that used previously for talapoin monkeys (Mollon and Bowmaker 1992). However, in the case of *post mortem* human tissue, where the photoreceptors are fully bleached, we have reconstituted the cone visual pigments with a synthetic retinaldehyde. We have also attempted to examine cones at the *ora serrata* and have analysed the foveal array of a trichromatic female New World monkey, *Callithrix jacchus jacchus*.

Methods

Tissue

Human retinal tissue was obtained from the eye bank of Moorfields Eye Hospital. For the successful preparation of foveal cone arrays, we have found that the tissue has to be less than 48–72 hours *post mortem* and from donors less than about 55–60 years old. From the eye cup, a small disc about 2 mm diameter centred in the macula was removed, along with a section of the *ora serrata* from the nasal region. In these preparations, the photoreceptors were fully bleached, since it was not possible at any stage *post mortem* for the eyes to be maintained in the dark. A dark-adapted retina from a female marmoset was obtained about 5 hours *post mortem*, by courtesy of Dr Martin Tovée of Newcastle University.

Reconstitution of visual pigments

We have developed a protocol for reconstituting visual pigments with synthetic retinaldehyde isomers, using the goldfish retina as a model system (Parry and Bowmaker 2000). Ideally, reconstitution would be carried out with 11-*cis* retinal, but because 11-*cis* retinal is not available commercially and because of the relatively large quantities necessary to reconstitute whole pieces of retina, we have used 9-*cis* retinal. The goldfish was chosen as a model system because it has, in addition to rods (λ_{max} 522), four spectral classes of cone extending throughout the spectrum with λ_{max} at about 380, 450, 535, and 620 nm. These pigments are all porphyropsins, based on vitamin A_2, and were reconstituted with both 11-*cis* retinal$_1$, to form rhodopsins, and 9-*cis* retinal$_1$, to form isorhodopsins (Knowles and Dartnall 1977). 11-*cis* retinal was a gift from Dr Rosalie Crouch and 9-*cis* was obtained commercially (Sigma).

Retinal tissue was incubated at 4 °C for about 3 hours, in a solution containing lipid vesicles incorporating retinal. Retinal and phosphatidylcholine were each dissolved in hexane and aliquotted together, then evaporated to dryness under argon and stored at −20 °C. Vesicles were formed by the addition of saline to an aliquot, vortexing for 10 min, then sonicating on ice for 3 min (Parry and Bowmaker 2000). The vesicles were present in excess to ensure complete reconstitution of visual pigments, but typically contained 60 μg 9-*cis* retinal and 1.5 mg phosphatidylcholine in 150 μl of saline.

Microspectrophotometry

After incubation, small pieces of retinal tissue were mounted on a cover slip and squashed under a second cover slip. Microspectrophotometric recordings were made in the conventional manner using a Liebman dual-beam microspectrophotometer (Liebman and Entine 1964; Mollon *et al.* 1984; Bowmaker *et al.* 1991). Spectra were recorded at 2-nm intervals from 750 to 350 nm and from 351 to 749 nm on the return scan. The outward and return scans were averaged. A baseline spectrum was measured for each cell, with both beams in an unoccupied area close to the cell, and this was subtracted from the

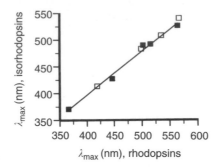

Figure 5.1 Correlation of λ_{max} of visual pigments based on 11-*cis* retinal (rhodopsins) and 9-*cis* retinal (isorhodopsins). Filled squares, the rod and four cone pigments from the goldfish (from Parry and Bowmaker 2000); open squares, the rod and three cone pigments from humans.

intracellular scan to derive the final spectrum. Two baseline scans were recorded for each cell and averaged. Cells were not routinely bleached, so as to avoid the possibility of low levels of bleaching in neighbouring cells in the array.

From the λ_{max} of the reconstituted goldfish pigments, it was possible to establish a linear relationship between the λ_{max} values of the rhodopsins and isorhodopsins (Parry and Bowmaker 2000). In the case of the human tissue, the L and M cone and rod pigments behave in an identical manner, exhibiting the same linear relationship (Fig. 5.1). The λ_{max} values of the L and M cones are displaced from about 565 and 535 nm to about 540 and 510 nm in the isorhodopsin form. Since we are interested only in whether an individual cone is L or M (or S), the precise λ_{max} is not important, but in all cases, a given cone could be assigned to either the L or the M class.

Results

Human tissue—foveal region

From two individuals, small patches of cone arrays from regions close to the fovea were successfully measured. In two further individuals, although clear arrays were not observed, sufficient cones in close proximity were recorded to estimate the ratio of L : M cones.

In a foveal array from a male (H24, aged 56) 44 cones were identified, one of which was an S cone (Fig. 5.2). Five additional cones, in close proximity to the array were also measured, together with eight rods. The cones were clearly divided into two classes with a ratio of L : M cones of 1.2 : 1. It was noticeable that the S cone did not disrupt the array and that two rods measured in the area of the array were in a slightly different focal plane of the preparation and did not fall within the array.

From a second individual (H25, a female aged 48) a less precise array was observed from which 37 cones were measured (Fig. 5.3). Again, one of these was an S cone and the other 36 fell into two distinct populations of L and M cones, with an L : M ratio of 2 : 1.

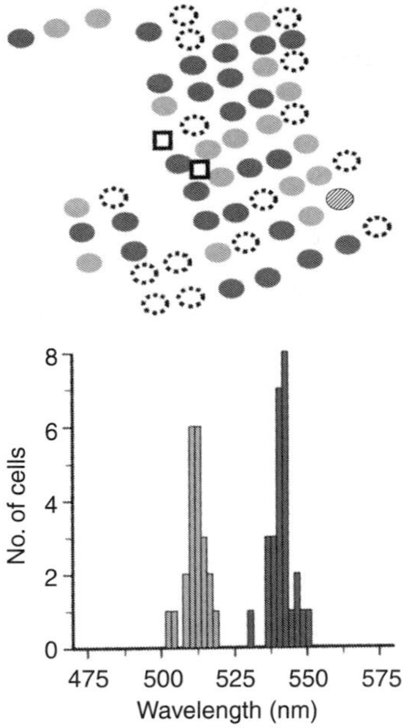

Figure 5.2 Foveal sample from a male (H24). Dark circles, L cones; light circles, M cones; ▨, S cone; dashed circles, cones not possible to measure; open squares, rods out of the plane of the cone array. Histograms of the distribution of the λ_{max} of individual L and M cones. The ratio of L : M cones is 1.2 : 1.

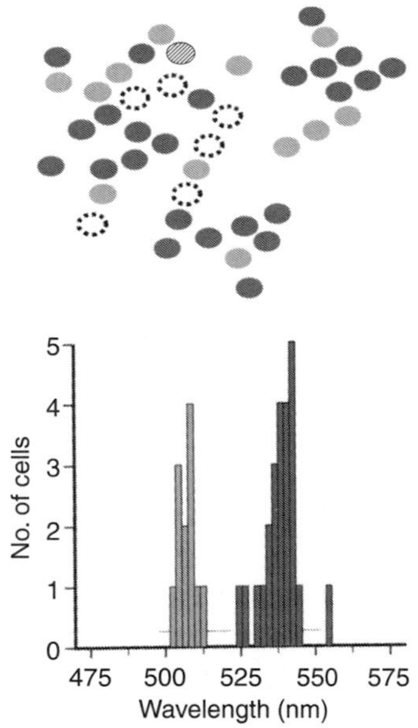

Figure 5.3 Foveal sample from a female (H25). Dark circles, L cones; light circles, M cones; ▨, S cone; dashed circles, cones not possible to measure. Histograms of the distribution of the λ_{max} of individual L and M cones. The ratio of L : M cones is 2.0 : 1.

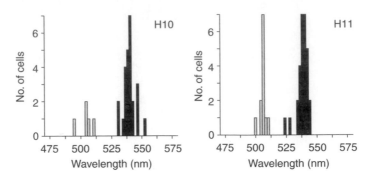

Figure 5.4 Histograms of the distribution of the λ_{max} of individual L (black bars) and M cones (grey bars) from two further males, H10 and H11. The ratio of L : M cones is 5.0 : 1 for H10 and 2.4 : 1 for H11.

The further two retinae were both from males (H10 aged 48 and H11 aged 45) and yielded a sufficiently large number of cones, though not in a clear array, to give ratios of L : M cones. In H10, 30 cones were recorded with an L : M ratio of 5 : 1, whereas in H11, 41 cones gave a distinctly different L : M ratio of 2.4 : 1 (Fig. 5.4).

Human tissue—ora serrata

Tissue from this region proved very difficult to record from, primarily because of excessive vitreous humour adhering to the retina. This proved almost impossible to remove and problems were further exacerbated by unavoidable contamination from pigment epithelium. Only in H24 were we able to make any significant measurements and here we recorded from only nine cones. Nevertheless, eight of the cones were L cones, which is suggestive of a considerably higher ratio of L : M cones than in the fovea.

Marmoset tissue

A relatively large parafoveal array was obtained from an individual female marmoset (Fig. 5.5). A total of 50 cones were recorded and these could be readily divided into two populations with the ratio of the longer to the shorter of 0.7 : 1.

Discussion

Human

The ratio of L : M cones in the four individuals ranged from 1.2 : 1 to 5.0 : 1 (Table 5.1). In total, from the four retinae, 156 L and M cones were identified with a mean ratio of 2.1 : 1. This figure agrees remarkably well with an overall ratio derived from microspectrophotometric data from twelve previous human eyes (some published (Dartnall *et al.* 1983*a, b*) and some not) that were obtained directly from enucleations and were not bleached. From these earlier twelve eyes, a total of 450 cones were measured, 303 L and 147 M, giving a ratio of 2.1 : 1. Although the numbers from any single retina were small,

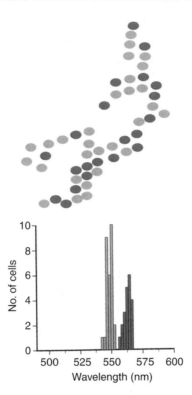

Figure 5.5 Foveal sample from a female marmoset (*Callithrix jacchus jacchus*). Dark circles: longer-wave cones; light circles: shorter-wave cones. Histograms of the distribution of the λ_{max} of individual cones. The ratio of the longer cones to the shorter is 0.7 : 1.

Table 5.1 Human foveal samples

Subject, age (years)	L : M cones	L : M ratio
H24 male, 56	27 : 22	1.23 : 1
H25 female, 48	24 : 12	2.00 : 1
H11 male, 45	29 : 12	2.42 : 1
H10 male, 48	25 : 5	5.00 : 1
Total	105 : 51	2.06 : 1

the individual ratios ranged from 0.9 : 1 to 4.3 : 1, a range not dissimilar from that of the four reconstituted retinae presented in this paper, 1.2 : 1 to 5.0 : 1.

These data strongly suggest that the ratio of L : M cones in the foveal region in humans varies between individuals from close to unity to at least as high as 5L : 1M. However, the average for the population is close to 2 : 1 (Table 5.1).

Although the size of the arrays was small, it is clear that the L and M cones do not form a systematic alternating array (e.g. Fig. 5.2), but appear to be randomly arranged with some indication of clumping. A χ^2 test in the array from H24 showed that the frequencies of three possible types of transition from cone to cone (L–L, M–M or L–M, in the direction of the long axis of the array), did not differ significantly from chance (χ^2 = 2.86, d.f. = 2), supporting a random distribution, but with a bias towards clumping or aggregation.

Comparison with other species

It is clear that in humans the relative proportion of L and M cones is on average about 2 : 1, but the ratio varies between individuals from about 1 : 1 to at least as high as 6 : 1, with some suggestion that the ratio may be even higher in extreme cases. This could be argued to reflect the order of L and M genes and their relative distances from the LCR in the gene array on the X chromosome. The first gene is usually an L gene and the first gene may be most likely to be coupled to the LCR (Winderickx *et al.* 1992; Yamaguchi *et al.* 1997). A weakness of this argument, however, is that the ratio of L to M cones appears to be lower in Old World monkeys and Apes, even though the arrangement of the gene array is thought to be similar across catarrhine primates (Dulai *et al.* 1994, 1999; Onishi *et al.* 1999). Data for Great Apes appears to be limited to the chimpanzee (*Pan troglodytes*), which has an estimated ratio of about 1.3 (Jacobs *et al.* 1996). Our direct microspectrophotometric studies of foveal tissue from ten talapoin monkeys (*Miopithecus talapoin*) gave an overall ratio of 0.9 : 1 (Mollon and Bowmaker 1992) from 545 cones. The individual ratios varied from 0.4 to 1.6. A similar collection of data from a total of 219 cones from macaque monkeys gave a ratio of 0.7 : 1 (unpublished). In addition, data from four baboons (*Papio papio*) (Bowmaker *et al.* 1991) gave a ratio from 120 cones of 0.7 : 1 with a range from 0.5 to 1.1, and individuals from five further catarrhine species gave a mean ratio of 1.2 from a total of 231 cones, with the individual ratios ranging from 0.8 to 2.5 (Bowmaker *et al.* 1991).

Estimates of the proportions of L and M cones in macaques, derived from analyses of the spectral luminosity function (Dobkins *et al.* 2000) were consistent with a cone ratio of 1 : 1; and a ratio of 1.4 : 1 was found from a large array of more than 900 cones in an individual macaque by spatially localized retinal densitometry made possible by adaptive optics (Roorda *et al.* 2001).

This apparent difference between humans and Old World monkeys is further supported by findings from analysis of mRNA in whole retinae (Deeb *et al.* 2000). The L : M ratio of mRNA from 26 monkeys, primarily *Macaca nemestrina*, ranged from 0.6 to 7.0 with a mean of about 1.6. This is markedly different from a similar analysis of mRNA from more than 50 human retinae where the range was from about 1–10 with a mode of 4 (Yamaguchi *et al.* 1997). These L : M ratios, somewhat higher than physiological estimates, may be a consequence of whole retinal extracts that will reflect the overall retinal ratio and not that of the foveal region (Neitz *et al.* 1996; Yamaguchi *et al.* 1997), but nonetheless, they reinforce the evidence for a difference between human and Old World monkeys.

Marmoset

In the case of the single female marmoset the two types of long-wave cone were in the ratio 0.7 : 1. This value does not differ significantly from 1.0 ($\chi^2 = 0.98$, d.f. $= 1$), the value that would be expected if X-chromosome inactivation were truly random and did not favour the maternal or the paternal chromosome. A ratio of unity similarly gave the simplest description of earlier data for another New World monkey, the squirrel monkey, *Saimiri sciureus* (Bowmaker *et al.* 1985).

A χ^2 analysis of transitions, similar to that performed on the array of H24, shows that the marmoset array does not depart significantly from chance ($\chi^2 = 4.21$, d.f. $= 2$). It is often held that X-chromosome inactivation occurs at an early embryonic stage, when the number of cells is small, and that the same chromosome remains inactivated in all the descendants of a given cell. The randomness observed in the marmoset photoreceptor matrix suggests either that the specificity of a cone is determined only at the last cell division or that a mixing of retinal cells is ensured by an active migration of cones during development.

Functional significance

What might be the functional significance of the individual variation in the ratio of L and M cones in humans? Traditionally, the ratio is held to affect the photopic luminous efficiency function, as measured by, say, flicker photometry (De Vries 1947); and indeed Rushton and Baker (1964) found an association between flicker photometric settings and reflection densitometric measurements of the proportions of L and M pigments in individual retinas. The relative numbers of L and M cones should not, however, affect Rayleigh equations: when subjects make a foveal colour match, they are thought to equate the quantum catches in the photopigments on the two sides of the stimulus field and so the equation ought to hold for each individual cone, whatever the numbers of a given type of cone. It has been proposed that settings of unique yellow reflect the ratio of L and M cones (Cicerone 1990), but differences in the expected direction are not found between female carriers of protan and deutan deficiencies, who are thought to have low numbers of L and M cones, respectively (Mollon and Jordan 1997; Miyahara *et al.* 1998).

A disproportion in the two types of cone should also affect the spatial properties of chromatic discrimination. Midget ganglion cells, which are thought to carry the L/M opponent signal, draw their centre input from a single cone. According to one hypothesis (Lennie *et al.* 1991), the antagonistic surround is drawn arbitrarily from both L and M cones in the neighbourhood. On this account, since a superabundance of one type of cone will produce homogeneous patches of mosaic, many midget ganglion cells would not be chromatically opponent. However, any ganglion cell drawing its centre input from the minority type of cone would be strongly opponent, since its surround would on average be purer than it would be in a more equilibrated retina. According to the hypothesis of Reid and Shapley (1992), the surround input is drawn specifically from cones of the type opposite to the cone that gives the centre input. On this account, a ganglion cell drawing its centre input from the superabundant class would have on average to seek its opponent input at a greater distance than would such a cell in an equilibrated retina, but the opposite would be true for a ganglion cell drawing its centre input from the minority type.

Acknowledgement

This work was supported by the Medical Research Council.

References

Bowmaker, J. K., Astell, S., Hunt, D. M., & Mollon, J. D. (1991). Photosensitive and photostable pigments in the retinae of Old World monkeys. *Journal of Experimental Biology, 156*, 1–19.

Bowmaker, J. K., Jacobs, G. H., Spiegelhalter, D. J., & Mollon, J. D. (1985). Two types of trichromatic squirrel monkey share a pigment in the red-green spectral region. *Vision Research, 25*, 1937–46.

Brainard, D. H., Roorda, A., Yamauchi, Y., Calderone, J. B., Metha, A., Neitz, M., Neitz, J., Williams, D. R., & Jacobs, G. H. (2000). Functional consequences of the relative numbers of L and M cones. *Journal of The Optical Society of America A, 17*, 607–14.

Carroll, J., McMahon, C., Neitz, M., & Neitz, J. (2000). Flicker-photometric electroretinogram estimates of L : M cone photoreceptor ratio in men with photopigment spectra derived from genetics. *Journal of The Optical Society of America A, 17*, 499–509.

Cicerone, C. M. (1990). Color appearance and cone mosaic in trichromacy and dichromacy. In: *Color Vision Deficiencies. Proceedings of the Symposium of the International Research Group on Color Vision Deficiencies* (pp. 1–12). Amsterdam: Kugler & Ghedini.

Cicerone, C. M. & Nerger, J. L. (1989). The relative numbers of long-wavelength-sensitive to middle-wavelength-sensitive cones in the human fovea centralis. *Vision Research, 29*, 115–28.

Dacey, D. M., Diller, L. C., Verweij, J., & Williams, D. R. (2000). Physiology of L- and M-cone inputs to H1 horizontal cells in the primate retina. *Journal of The Optical Society of America A, 17*, 589–96.

Dartnall, H. J. A., Bowmaker, J. K., & Mollon, J. D. (1983a). Human visual pigments: microspectrophotometric results from the eyes of seven persons. *Proceedings of the Royal Society of London B, 220*, 115–30.

Dartnall, H. J. A., Bowmaker, J. K., & Mollon, J. D. (1983b). Microspectrophotometry of human receptors. In: J. D. Mollon & L. T. Sharpe (Eds) *Colour Vision: Physiology and Psychophysics*, (pp. 69–80). London: Academic Press.

Deeb, S. S., Diller, L. C., Williams, D. R., & Dacey, D. M. (2000). Interindividual and topographical variation of L : M cone ratios in monkey retinas. *Journal of The Optical Society of America A, 17*, 538–44.

De Vries, H. (1947). The heredity of the relative numbers of red and green receptors in the human eye. *Genetica, 24*, 199–212.

Dobkins, K. R., Thiele, A., & Albright, T. D. (2000). Comparison of red-green equiluminance points in humans and macaques: evidence for different L : M cone ratios between species. *Journal of The Optical Society of America A, 17,* 545–56.

Dulai, K. S., Bowmaker, J. K., Mollon, J. D., & Hunt, D. M. (1994). Sequence divergence, polymorphism and evolution of the middle-wave and long-wave visual pigment genes of Great Apes and Old World monkeys. *Vision Research, 34,* 2483–91.

Dulai, K. S., von Dornum, M., Mollon, J. D., & Hunt, D. M. (1999). The evolution of trichromatic color vision by opsin gene duplication in New World and Old World primates. *Genome Research, 9,* 629–38.

Hagstrom, S. A., Neitz, J., & Neitz, M. (1998). Variations in cone populations for red-green color vision examined by analysis of mRNA. *Neuroreport, 9,* 1963–67.

Hagstrom, S. A., Neitz, M., & Neitz, J. (2000). Cone pigment gene expression in individual photoreceptors and the chromatic topography of the retina. *Journal of The Optical Society of America A, 17,* 527–37.

Jacobs, G. H. & Deegan, J. F. (1997). Spectral sensitivity of macaque monkeys measured with ERG flicker photometry. *Visual Neuroscience, 14,* 921–8.

Jacobs, G. H., Deegan, K. F., & Moran, J. L. (1996). ERG measurements of the spectral sensitivity of common chimpanzee (*Pan troglodytes*). *Vision Research, 36,* 2587–94.

Knowles, A. & Dartnall, H. J. A. (1977). The Photobiology of Vision. In: H. Davson, *The Eye, 2B,* (pp. 1–689). New York: Academic Press.

Lennie, P., Haake, P. W., & Williams, D. R. (1991). The design of chromatically opponent receptive fields. In: *Computational Models of Visual Processing* (pp. 71–82). Cambridge MA: MIT Press.

Liebman, P. A. & Entine, G. (1964). Sensitive low-light-level microspectrophotometer: detection of photosensitive pigments of retinal cones. *Journal of the Optical Society of America, 54,* 1451–9.

Miyahara, E., Pokorny, J., Smith, V. C., Baron, R., & Baron, E. (1998). Color vision in two observers with highly biased LWS/MWS cone ratios. *Vision Research, 38,* 601–12.

Mollon, J. D. & Bowmaker, J. K. (1992). The spatial arrangement of cones in the primate fovea. *Nature, 360,* 677–9.

Mollon, J. D., Bowmaker, J. K., & Jacobs, G. H. (1984). Variations of colour vision in a New World primate can be explained by polymorphism of retinal photopigments. *Proceedings of the Royal Society of London B, 222,* 373–99.

Mollon, J. D. & Jordan, G. (1988). Eine evolutionäre Interpretation des menschlichen Farbensehens. *Die Farbe, 35/36,* 139–70.

Mollon, J. D. & Jordan, G. (1997). On the nature of unique hues. In: C.M. Dickinson, I.T. Murray, & D. Carden (Eds), *John Dalton's Colour Vision Legacy* (pp. 381–92). London: Taylor and Francis.

Nathans, J., Thomas, D., & Hogness, D. S. (1986). Molecular genetics of human color vision: the genes encoding blue, green, and red pigments. *Science, 232,* 193–202.

Neitz, M., Hagstrom, S. A., Kainz, P. M., & Neitz, J. (1996). L-cone and M-cone opsin gene expression in the human retina: relationship with gene order and retinal eccentricity. *Investigative Ophthalmology & Visual Science, 37,* 2045.

Onishi, A., Koike, S., Ida, M., Imai, H., Shichida, Y., Takenaka, O., Hanazawa, A., Konatsu, H., Mikami, A., Goto, S., Suryobroto, B., Kitahara, K., & Yamamori, T. (1999). Vision—Dichromatism in macaque monkeys. *Nature, 402*, 139–40.

Parry, J. W. L. & Bowmaker, J. K. (2000). Visual pigment reconstitution in intact goldfish retina using synthetic retinaldehyde isomers. *Vision Research, 40*, 2241–7.

Pokorny, J., Smith, V. C., & Wesner, M. F. (1991). Variability of cone populations and implications. In: A. Valberg & B. B. Lee (Eds) *From Pigments to Perception*, (pp. 23–34). New York: Plenum.

Reid, R. C. & Shapley, R. M. (1992). Spatial structure of cone inputs to receptive fields in primate lateral geniculate nucleus. *Nature, 356*, 716–18.

Roorda, A., Metha, A. B., Lennie, P., & Williams, D. R. (2001). Packing arrangement of the three cone classes in primate retina. *Vision Research, 41*, 1291–306.

Roorda, A. & Williams, D. R. (1999). The arrangement of the three cone classes in the living human eye. *Nature, 397*, 520–2.

Rushton, W. A. H., & Baker, H. D. (1964). Red/green sensitivity in normal vision. *Vision Research, 4*, 75–85.

Vos, J. J. & Walraven, P. L. (1971). On the derivation of the foveal receptor primaries. *Vision Research, 11*, 799–818.

Wang, Y., Macke, J. P., Merbs, S. L., Zack, D. J., Klaunberg, B., Bennett, J., Gearhart, J., & Nathans, J. (1992). A locus control region adjacent to the human red and green visual pigment genes. *Neuron, 9*, 429–40.

Wang, Y., Smallwood, P. M., Cowan, M., Blesh, D., Lawler, A., & Nathans, J. (1999). Mutually exclusive expression of human red and green visual pigment-reporter transgenes occurs at high frequency in murine cone photoreceptors. *Proceedings of the National Academy of Sciences, 96*, 5251–6.

Winderickx, J., Battisti, L., Motulsky, A. G., & Deeb, S. S. (1992). Selective expression of human X chromosome-linked green opsin genes. *Proceedings of the National Academy of Sciences, 89*, 9710–14.

Yamaguchi, T., Motulsky, A. G., & Deeb, S. S. (1997). Visual pigment gene structure and expression in human retinae. *Human Molecular Genetics, 6*, 981–90.

CHAPTER 6

COMPARISON OF HUMAN AND MONKEY PIGMENT GENE PROMOTERS TO EVALUATE DNA SEQUENCES PROPOSED TO GOVERN L:M CONE RATIO

C. McMAHON, J. NEITZ, AND M. NEITZ

Introduction

Genes encoding the long (L)- and middle (M)-wavelength sensitive cone photopigments are tandemly arrayed on the X-chromosome. Each L or M cone exclusively expresses one gene from the array (Hagstrom *et al.* 2000). A simple and attractive theory is that a stochastic process determines the choice to express one gene from the array, and this alone determines the identity of each cone as M or L (Wang *et al.* 1999).

It has been hypothesized that a necessary enhancer element, termed the locus control region (LCR), located upstream of the first gene of the array (Nathans *et al.* 1989; Wang *et al.* 1992) acts as the stochastic selector by forming an irreversible complex with the promoter of one gene in the array, thereby activating expression from only one X-chromosome visual pigment gene per L/M cone cell.

The L:M cone ratio averages about 2:1 in humans (Carroll *et al.* 2000; Hagstrom *et al.* 1998; Schnapf *et al.* 1987), and the human L pigment gene is normally first in the array (Sjoberg *et al.* 1998; Vollrath *et al.* 1988). Thus, although the choice is considered random, it has been proposed that the probability that a gene within the array will be chosen for expression decreases with increasing distance from the LCR, thereby explaining the biased L:M cone ratio observed in humans (Hayashi *et al.* 1999; Winderickx *et al.* 1992).

The LCR appears to be essential for normal levels of L and M pigment gene expression *in vivo* (Nathans *et al.* 1989; Wang *et al.* 1992). However, conclusive evidence that the LCR is the stochastic selector is lacking, as is evidence that the relative proximity of a gene to the LCR influences the probability of its being expressed. The latter idea is weakened by evidence from Old World primates. In other primates the L gene is first but it is not expressed in the most cones. We analyzed the structures of the L/M photopigment gene arrays in four species of Old World monkey (*M. fascicularis, M. nemestrina, P.c. anubis and C. aethiops*; to be published elsewhere). As for humans, arrays from all species had

Table 6.1 Previously published measurements of percentage of L cones ($L/(L+M) \times 100$) using microspectrophotometric, biochemical and direct imaging techniques

Reference	Species	$L/(L+M) \times 100$
Marc and Sperling (1977), *Science*	*Papio cynocephalus*	38
Bowmaker *et al.* (1983), *Colour Vision*	*Macaca mulatta*	42
	Macaca fascicularis	39
	Papio papio	43
Baylor *et al.* (1987), *J. Phys.*	*Macaca fascicularis*	44
Harosi (1987), *J. Gen. Phys.*	*Macaca fascicularis*	48
	Macaca mulatta	50
Mollon and Bowmaker (1992), *Nature*	*Cercopithecus talapoin*	47
Roorda *et al.* (2001), *Vision Research*	*Macaca fascicularis*	58
	Average	**45**

an L gene first, and a single LCR with the conserved 37-bp LCR core element. The approximate spacing between the LCR core element and the array was also conserved. However, while humans rarely have an L : M cone ratio below 1 : 1, the ratio in Old World monkeys is usually near or below 1 : 1 (see Table 6.1) (Baylor *et al.* 1987; Bowmaker *et al.* 1991; Bowmaker *et al.* 1978, 1980; Deeb *et al.* 2000; Harosi 1987; Marc and Sperling 1977; Mollon and Bowmaker 1992; Roorda *et al.* 2001; Bowmaker *et al.* 1983).

We are interested in understanding the genetic mechanisms responsible for the difference in cone ratio between monkeys and man. If a random choice for pigment gene expression determines whether a cone will be L or M, then it is logical that sequences physically associated with the genes might be responsible for biasing that choice. Since gene order and L gene proximity to the LCR are not different between monkey and man, we have to look to other sequence differences associated with the L and M genes as candidate factors that govern L : M ratio.

Earlier, results from *in vitro* experiments using the WERI human retinoblastoma cell line led to the proposal that differences in the promoters of the M and L pigment genes play a role in controlling cone ratios (Shaaban and Deeb 1998). Shaaban *et al.* (1998) found that the M promoter was more active than the L promoter and changing the nucleotide at position -3 from T (normally found in L) to C (normally found in M) increases the activity of the L promoter *in vitro*. This led them to propose that the C at -3 of the M gene promoter enhances the proportion of M cones *in vivo*.

There are normally 15 nucleotide differences between the human L and M gene promoter regions in the 236-bp immediately upstream of the start codons (we identified one that was not previously reported) (Nathans *et al.* 1986). In contrast, in the present study, the monkey L and M gene promoters only differed by 5–7 nucleotides. Eleven nucleotide positions, including the -3 position, that differ between human M and L also differ between bonobo M and L gene promoter regions, but not between monkey

M and L gene promoters. The monkeys were identical to the human L at all 11 of these positions in both M and L promoters. The differences in promoter sequences between monkeys and man reported here are candidates for playing a role in the difference in cone ratio between the two. However, if T at the −3 position reduced the proportion of M cones, as proposed from *in vitro* studies, one might expect the monkeys to have a higher proportion of L cones than humans instead of a lower proportion, as has been observed.

Methods

Tissue and nucleic acid extraction. Retinas from 2 *Macaca fascicularis*, 2 *Macaca nemestrina*, and 1 *Papio cynocephalus anubis* were obtained from the Regional Primate Research Center at the University of Washington-Seattle. COS-1 cells (*Cercopithecus aethiops*) were obtained from the American Type Culture Center (ATCC CRL-1650). Muscle from 1 *Pan paniscus* was obtained from a zoo. Nucleic acids were extracted as previously described (Hagstrom *et al.* 1997).

Polymerase chain reaction (PCR), and sequencing

A reverse primer (5′TGGGTGCTGTCCTCATAGCTG) corresponding to sequences within exon 1 that are shared by human M and L genes was paired with different forward primers to specifically amplify M and L pigment gene promoter regions. A 531-bp fragment containing the L pigment gene promoter region was amplified using a forward primer (5′CCTGGGCTTTCAAGAGAACCACATG) to sequences that lay 459-bp upstream of the start codon of the L gene. A 463-bp DNA segment containing the M gene promoter was amplified with a forward primer (5′AGGCGTGTGCCACTGTGCC) corresponding to sequences that lie about 390-bp upstream of the start codon of M genes. Hot start PCR was done using AmpliWax gems and the XL PCR kit (ABI). Each reaction contained 200 µM each of dATP, dCTP, dGTP, and dTTP, and 1.5 mM magnesium acetate. Primer concentrations were 300 nM each for the L promoter amplification, and 100 nM each for the M promoter amplification. Reactions were incubated at 94 °C for 5 min, followed by 40 cycles of 94 °C for 1 min, 63 °C for 1 min, 72 °C for 1 min, and a final incubation at 72 °C for 10 min. PCR products were directly sequenced using the ABI BigDye terminator cycle sequencing version 2.0 kit. M pigment gene promoter segments were also sequenced after cloning. Sequencing reactions were analyzed on an ABI Prism 310 Genetic Analyzer.

In order to compare our results to those reported by Dulai, von Dornum, Mollon and Hunt (1999) for the promoter region of the M genes for two other Cercopithecid species (*Cercopithecus Diana, Erythrocebus patas*), we amplified and directly sequenced a 748-bp fragment from upstream of the M genes using primers MW+ and MW− described by those authors. MW+ and MW− correspond to human sequences, and amplify a PCR product that overlaps the 463-bp M gene promoter fragment described above.

Results

The aligned sequences for the region extending from −195 to +41 of the L and M pigment gene promoters for human, bonobo (*P. paniscus*), macaque (*M. fascicularis* and *M. nemestrina*), baboon (*P.c. anubis*), and African green monkey (*C. aethiops*) are shown in Table 6.2(a). Over the region shown, 15 nucleotide positions differed between L and M for both human and bonobo, but only 5–7 positions differed between L and M in the monkeys (Table 6.2b). The Cercopithecid species (*M. fascicularis*, *M. nemestrina*, *P.c. anubis*, *C. aethiops*) we examined maintained only 4 of the 15 differences (nucleotide positions −78, −163, −165, and −191) found in humans, plus they differed at one additional position (−156). There were 11 nucleotide positions (−166, −144, −141, −134, −88, −86, −36, −31, −21, −3, and +1) that differed between human L and M promoters, but all of the Old World monkey L and M promoters we sequenced were identical to human L at these positions. Also, species-specific sequence variations were observed among the monkeys. For example, polymorphisms occurred in *M. fascicularis* at position −124, *M. nemestrina* at position +19 and *C. aethiops* at positions −40 and −48.

The sequences in Table 6.2(a) from the M promoter regions for the Cercopithecid species we examined differed from those reported by Dulai *et al.* (1999) for two other Cercopithecid species at positions −166, −144, −141, −134, −88, −86, −36, −31, −21, and −3, and +1. Dulai *et al.* (1999) reported that Diana and patas monkeys matched human M at these positions, whereas, the Cercopithecid animals we examined did not. Two of these positions (−88 and −86) lie within the primer, MW−, that was used by Dulai *et al.* (1999) to amplify this region, and that was designed to match human sequence. The M and L gene promoters for Diana and patas monkeys differed at four positions (−191, −165, −163, and −78) that also distinguish M and L promoters of the Cercopithecid species reported here.

To confirm the authenticity of our Cercopithecid M gene promoter sequences, we used primers MW+ and MW− described by Dulai *et al.* (1999) to amplify and sequence a 748-bp fragment upstream of the M genes for 6 Cercopithecid monkeys, a bonobo and a human. This PCR product overlaps the 463-bp M gene promoter fragments for which sequences are shown in Table 6.2(a). The overlap includes positions −96 through −348. The sequences from −96 to −195 for the 748-bp and the 463-bp PCR products were identical. The segment from −348 to −195 was also present on both the 748-bp and the 463-bp PCR products, and we sequenced this region for the Cercopithecid monkeys, a bonobo, and a human. The sequences, shown in Table 6.3(a), were identical for both PCR products from each animal (Table 6.3a), and were very similar to Diana monkey sequence reported by Dulai *et al.* (1999). It is important to note that on the 463-bp PCR product from the M gene promoters of our 6 Cercopithecid monkeys the segment from +41 to −195 that does not match Diana monkey sequence is physically contiguous with the segment from −194 to −348 that does match the Diana monkey sequence. This result confirms the authenticity of our M gene promoter sequences.

Table 6.2 Nucleotide sequences of the L(gray) and M (black) pigment gene proximal promoters. (a) L and M pigment gene proximal promoter sequences from 2 *Macaca fascicularis*, 2 *Macaca nemestrina*, 1 *P.c. anubis*, 1 *Cercopithecus aethiops*, 1 *Pan paniscus* (bonobo) and 1 human. *C. diana* sequences are from Dulai *et al.* (1999). The TATA box, -3 position, and the ATG start codon are outlined. The transcriptional start site is numbered +1. The Y at position +19 of *M. nemestrina* indicates a C/T polymorphism. (b) Comparison of the number of nucleotide differences between the L and M pigment gene proximal promoters in human and Old World monkey species.

(a)

```
               -195   -191                           -166,-165 -163      -156              -144 -141
                ↓      ↓                                ↓↓   ↓              ↓                  ↓    ↓
H.sapiens  M   GGTTTCCAGCAAATCCCTCTGAGCCGCCCCCGGGGGCTCGCCTCAGGAGCAAGGAA
H.sapiens  L   ....C........................TT.C..............G..G.
P.paniscus M   ...................................................
P.paniscus L   ....C........................TT.C..............G..G.
M.fascicularis M ...........................T..........A.........G..G.
M.fascicularis L ...C.........................TT.C..............G..G.
M.nemestrina M ...........................T..........A.........G..G.
M.nemestrina L ....C........................TT.C..............G..G.
P.c. anubis  M ...........................T..........A.........G..G.
P.c. anubis  L ....C........................TT.C..............G..G.
C.aethiops   M ...........................T..........A.........G..G.
C.aethiops   L ...C.........................TT.C..............G..G.
C. diana     M ......................................A.............
C. diana     L ....C........................TT.C..............G..G.
```

```
    -134           -124                              -88 -86      -78
     ↓              ↓                                 ↓↓  ↓        ↓
GCAAGGGGTGGGAGGAGGAGGTCTAAGTCCCAGGCCCAATTAAGAGATCAGATGGTGTAGGATTTGGGAGCTTTTAA
.....A...................................G.A......G..............
.....A...................................G.A......G..............
.....A...............T...................G.A....................
.....A...................................G.A......G..............
.....A...................................G.A....................
.....A...................................G.A......G..............
.....A...................................G.A....................
.....A...................................G.A......G..............
.....A...................................G.A....................
...................C.....................................
A....A...................................G.A......G......A......
```

```
    -48       -40  -36    -31          -21                    -3  +1        +9
     ↓         ↓    ↓      ↓             ↓                      ↓   ↓         ↓
GGTGAAGAGGCCCGGGCTGATCCCACTGGCCGG TATAAA GCACCGTGACCCTCAGGTGA C GCACCAGGGCCGGCTGC
.......................A....A........G...........| T |..T.......
...........................................G...........| T |.G.......
...........................A....A........G...........| T |.G.......T.....
...........................A....A........G...........| T |.G.......T.....
...........................A....A........G...........| T |.G.......T.....
...........................A....A........G...........| T |.G.......T.....
...........................A....A........G...........| T |.G.......T.....
...........................A....A........G...........| T |.G.......T.....
.................A.......T...A....A........G...........| T |.G.......T.....
...........................A....A........G...........| T |.G.......T.....
...................................G...........| T |...........
.A.......T.....T...........A....A........G...........|[T]|.....A.T.A.AA.
```

```
  +19                   +41
   ↓                     ↓ Start codon
CGTCGGGGACAGGGCTTTCCATAGCCATG
.............................
.............................
.............................
.............................
...Y.........................
...Y.........................
.............................
.............................
.............................
.............................
.......................A.....
.............................
```

(b)

	# differences between L and M promotors -195 to +41	# animals sequenced
Human	15	1
P. paniscus	15	1
M. fascicularis	6	2
M. nemestrina	5	2
P.c. anubis	5	1
C. aethiops	7	1
C. diana	28	?

Table 6.3 Nucleotide sequences upstream of Old World monkey L and M pigment gene proximal promoters. (a) Sequence upstream of the M pigment gene proximal promoter from 1 human, 1 *Pan paniscus*, 2 *Macaca fascicularis*, 2 *Macaca nemestrina*, 1 *P.c. anubis*, and 1 *Cercopithecus aethiops*, all shown in black. *Cercopithecus diana* sequence (gray) is from Dulai *et al.* (1999). The S at position -234 indicates a A/G polymorphism in *M. nemestrina*. (b) Sequence upstream of the L pigment gene proximal promoter sequences from 1 human, 1 *Pan paniscus*, 2 *Macaca fascicularis*, 2 *Macaca nemestrina*, 1 *P.c. anubis*, and 1 *Cercopithecus aethiops*. The sequence upstream of the C. *diana* L promoter is unknown. The same numbering convention used in Table 6.2 is used here. The shaded sequence overlaps the sequences given in Table 6.2A.

```
                -321                -304  -298        -288 -283              -268
(a) H.sapiens M  ----AGACAGAGTCTTGGTCTGTTGCCCAGGCTAGAGTTCAGTGGCGCCATCTCAGC
    P. paniscus M ----..........CC.........................................
    M.fascicularis M TTTC...TG........T.....C.........G....G..............TG..
    M.nemestrina M ................C.....A.........G....G..............TG..
    P.c. anubis M ........G.......C.....C.........G....G..............TG..
    C. aethiops M ........G.......T.....C.........G....G.......T.......TG..
    C. diana M*   ............C.T.....C.........G....G......T....C..TG..
```

```
    -246 -243 -241  -235              -219,-218                      -195
    TCACTGCAACCTCCGCCTCCCAGATTCAAGCGATTCTCCTGCCTCGACCTCCCAGTAGCTGGGATTACAGGTTT
    .....A......................................................................
    ............T....T..G.G.....C................AG............................
    ............T..G.G.....CS...................AG............................
    ............T..G.G.....C....A...............AG............................
    ............T..G.G.....C...................AG............A...............
    ............T..G.G.....C...A...............AG............................
```

```
         -348        -338       -329 -326 -322              -304 -302 -299
(b) H.sapiens L  AGTCTGCAAATCCTGACCCGTGGGTCCACCTGCCCCAAAGGCGGACGCAGGACAGTA
    P. paniscus L ..........................................................
    M. fascicularis L ..........A.......T..A...................G.A..A.......
    M.nemestrina L ..........A.......T..A...T...............G.A..A.......
    P.c. anubis L ..........A.......T..A...................G.A..A.......
    C. aethiops L ..........A.......T..A...T...............G.A..A.......
```

```
    -278                       -251               -234      -227
    GAAGGGAACAGAGAACACATAAACACAGAGAGGGCCACAGCGGCTCCCACAGTCACCGCCACCTTCCTGGCGGGGAT
    ....................................................................................
    ...........G...........................A..........T......G.............
    ...........G...........................A..........T......G.............
    ...........G...........................A..........T......G.............
    ...........G....................C......A..........T......G.............
```

```
    -195
    GGGTGGGGCGTCTGAGTTTGGTTC
    ........................
    ........................
    ........................
    ........................
    ........................
```

For the L gene promoter region shown in Table 6.2(a) Dulai *et al.* (1999) reported 14 differences between human and Diana/patas monkey (positions $-139, -70, -61, -53, -47, -21, -2 + 1, +7, +11, +13, +14,$ and $+39$); however only one of these (-61) differed between human and the Cercopithecid species we examined. To confirm the authenticity of our Cercopithecid L gene promoter sequences, we also sequenced the adjacent ~150-bp extending from -348 to -194 for all of our animals, and the data are shown in Table 6.3(b). There were 11 polymorphic positions ($-338, -329, -326, -322, -309, -302, -299, -278, -251, -234,$ and -227) that distinguished humans and apes from Cercopithecids. Two positions -322 and -258 were polymorphic among the Cercopithecid species examined.

Two pieces of evidence further confirm the authenticity of our Cercopithecid L and M gene promoter sequences. First, the data was consistent for 6 individual Cercopithecid monkeys whose DNA was isolated and sequenced at different times. Second, the M gene promoter sequences from -321 to $+41$ were more homologous among Cercopithecid species (100–97 per cent) than between Cercopithecids and humans or bonobo (91–93 per cent). This was also true for L promoters, which from -348 to $+41$ shared 99.5–100 per cent homology among Cercopithecids, but only 97 per cent homology between Cercopithecids and humans or bonobo. Human and bonobo M gene promoters were nearly identical over the region sequenced, as were their L gene promoters.

The breakdown in homology between the M promoter sequences for the Cercopithecid species we examined and the Diana monkey occurs at a location that corresponds to the position of one of the PCR primers used by Dulai *et al.* (1999) (Op $+$ 1, which extends from -216 to -205) to obtain the sequence reported for positions -195 to $+41$ region.

Discussion

It has been hypothesized that DNA sequence differences between the L and M promoters affect the L : M cone ratio. Here we used a comparative approach to identify candidate positions in the promoters of the L and M genes that may be involved in determining the cone ratio. We sequenced $\sim$500-bp upstream of the coding sequence for the L gene, and $\sim$360-bp upstream of the M gene for six monkeys representing four Cercopithecid species, a bonobo, and a human.

Shaaban *et al.* (1998) observed that in a reporter gene assay in WERI cell cultures the M gene promoter was more active than the L gene promoter. Mutating the nucleotide at position -3 from T (normally found in human L) to C (normally found in human M) increased the activity of the L promoter, making it similar in activity to the wild-type M promoter. It was proposed that the cell culture results are relevant to what happens in the human eye. The -3 nucleotide difference was proposed to have evolved to enhance M gene expression in order to offset the disadvantage in competing for binding to the LCR experienced by the M gene due to its greater distance from the LCR. If this were correct, it would predict that the -3 difference between L and M promoters would be maintained in the monkeys and perhaps additional differences that further enhance M gene expression might be present to account for the higher relative number of M cones in the monkey compared to human. Instead however, the monkey promoters did not differ at the -3 position and, over the region sequenced the monkey L and M pigment gene promoters are 97–98 per cent identical to each other and 96–97 per cent identical to human L, whereas the human L and M promoters are only 94 per cent identical.

In the WERI cell line, transfection assays showed differences in the activities of human L and M pigment gene promoter constructs. However, the WERI cell assays cannot provide information about the mechanisms that govern the ratio of L : M cones in the normal primate eye because the assays do not measure the ratio of cells that choose to express L versus M.

It is quite possible that sequences of the L and M gene promoter regions influence the L versus M cone decision-making process during development. We speculate that the similarity between the L and M promoters in Old World monkeys may be related to the nearly equal numbers of L and M cones in these animals and that some of the additional differences between the human L and M promoters may play a role in producing the difference in L and M cone numbers in human retinas. It is also possible that other differences between L and M genes, for example differences within the introns, may play a role in determining the L : M ratio.

Acknowledgements

M. N. is the recipient of the RPB Lew Wasserman Merit Award. This work was supported by Research to Prevent Blindness, NIH grants EY09620, EY09303, EY01931, and RR10066. We thank Dr Dennis Dacey and Dr Anita Hendrickson, both from the University of Washington, Seattle for providing monkey retinal tissue.

References

Baylor, D. A., Nunn, B. J., & Schnapf, J. L. (1987). Spectral sensitivity of cones of the monkey *Macaca fascicularis. Journal of Physiology 390*, 145–60.

Bowmaker, J. K. & Mollon, J. D. (1983). Microspectrophotometric results for Old and New World primates. In J. D. Mollon & L. T. Sharpe (Eds.), *Colour Vision Physiology and Psychophysics* London, Academic Press.

Bowmaker, J. K., Astell, S., Hunt, D. M., & Mollon, J. D. (1991). Photosensitive and photostable pigments in the retinae of Old World monkeys. *Journal of Experimental Biology 156*, 1–19.

Bowmaker, J. K., Dartnall, H. J. A., Lythgoe, J. N., & Mollon, J. D. (1978). The visual pigments of rods and cones in the rhesus monkey, *Macaca mulatta. Journal of Physiology 274*, 329–48.

Bowmaker, J. K., Dartnall, H. J. A., & Mollon, J. D. (1980). Microspectrophotometric demonstration of four classes of photoreceptor in an Old World primate, *Macaca fascicularis. Journal of Physiology 298*, 131–43.

Carroll, J., McMahon, C., Neitz, M., & Neitz, J. (2000). Flicker-photometric electroretinogram estimates of L : M cone photoreceptor ratio in men with photopigment spectra derived from genetics. *Journal of the Optical Society of America A 17*, 499–509.

Deeb, S. S., Diller, L. C., Williams, D. R., & Dacey, D. M. (2000). Interindividual and topographical variation of L :M cone ratios in monkey retinas. *Journal of the Optical Society of America A 17*, 538–44.

Dulai, K. S., von Dornum, M., Mollon, J. D., & Hunt, D. M. (1999). The evolution of trichromatic color vision by opsin gene duplication in new world and old world primates. *Genome Research 9*, 629–38.

Hagstrom, S. A., Neitz, J., & Neitz, M. (1997). Ratio of M/L pigment gene expression decreases with retinal eccentricity. In Colour Vision Deficiencies XIII, Cavonius, C. R., (Ed.) Dordrecht: Kluwer Academic Publishers, pp. 59–66.

Hagstrom, S. A., Neitz, J., & Neitz, M. (1998). Variations in cone populations for red–green color vision examined by analysis of mRNA. *NeuroReport 9*, 1963–7.

Hagstrom, S. A., Neitz, M., & Neitz, J. (2000). Cone pigment gene expression in individual photoreceptors and the chromatic topography of the retina. *Journal of the Optical Society of America A 17*, 527–37.

Harosi, F. I. (1987). Cynomolgus and rhesus monkey visual pigments. The *Journal of General Physiology 89*, 717–43.

Hayashi, T., Motulsky, A. G., & Deeb, S. S. (1999). Position of a 'green–red' hybrid gene in the visual pigment array determines colour-vision phenotype. *Nature Genetics 22*, 90–3.

Marc, R. E. & Sperling, H. G. (1977). Chromatic organization of primate cones. *Science 196*, 454–6.

Mollon, J. D. & Bowmaker, J. K. (1992). The spatial arrangement of cones in the primate fovea. *Nature 360*, 677–9.

Nathans, J., Davenport, C. M., Maumenee, I. H., Lewis, R. A., Hejtmancik, J. F., Litt, M., Lovrien, E., Weleber, R., Bachynski, B., Zwas, F., Klingaman, R., & Fishman, G. (1989). Molecular genetics of blue cone monochromacy. *Science 245*, 831–8.

Nathans, J., Thomas, D., & Hogness, D. S. (1986). Molecular genetics of human color vision: the genes encoding blue, green, and red pigments. *Science 232*, 193–202.

Roorda, A., Metha, A., Lennie, P., & Williams, D. R. (2001). Packing arrangement of the three cone classes in primate retina. *Vision Research 41*, 1291–306.

Schnapf, J. L., Kraft, T. W., & Baylor, D. A. (1987). Spectral sensitivity of human cone photoreceptors. *Nature 325*, 439–41.

Shaaban, S. A. & Deeb, S. S. (1998). Functional analysis of the promoters of the human red and green visual pigment genes. *Investigative Ophthalmology* & *Visual Science 39*, 885–96.

Sjoberg, S. A., Neitz, M., Balding, S. D., & Neitz, J. (1998). L-cone pigment genes expressed in normal colour vision. *Vision Research 38*, 3213–19.

Vollrath, D., Nathans, J., & Davis, R. W. (1988). Tandem array of human visual pigment genes at Xq28. *Science 240*, 1669–72.

Wang, Y., Macke, J. P., Merbs, S. L., Zack, D. J., Klaunberg, B., Bennett, J., Gearhart, J., & Nathans, J. (1992). A locus control region adjacent to the human red and green visual pigment genes. *Neuron 9*, 429–40.

Wang, Y., Smallwood, P. M., Cowan, M., Blesh, D., Lawler, A., & Nathans, J. (1999). Mutually exclusive expression of human red and green visual pigment-reporter transgenes occurs at high frequency in murine cone photoreceptors. *Proceedings of the National Academy of Sciences, USA 96*, 5251–6.

Winderickx, J., Battisti, L., Motulsky, A. G., & Deeb, S. S. (1992). Selective expression of human X chromosome-linked green opsin genes. *Proceedings of the National Academy of Sciences USA 89*, 9710–14.

RETINAL PROCESSES

CHAPTER 7

STRUCTURE OF RECEPTIVE FIELD CENTERS OF MIDGET RETINAL GANGLION CELLS

BARRY B. LEE

Introduction

The midget ganglion cells of the parvocellular (PC) pathway have been shown to receive antagonistic input from the middle- (M-) and long- (L-) wavelength sensitive cones (Derrington *et al.* 1984; Lee *et al.* 1987). Although it has been proposed that an alternative pathway may exist for red-green color vision (Calkins and Sterling 1999), PC-cells display properties, such as detection contours in an M, L-cone space (Lee *et al.* 1993), which strongly resemble those of the chromatic channel responsible for psychophysical detection along this dimension (Cole *et al.* 1993).

Classical anatomical studies (Boycott and Dowling 1969; Polyak 1941) suggest that, up to 10° of eccentricity, single cones contact single midget bipolar cells, which contact single midget ganglion cells. Beyond 10°, two or more midget bipolars contact a single ganglion cell's dendritic tree. By 20–30°, eccentricity the "midget" dendritic tree may encompass the axonal arbors of 20–30 midget bipolars (Dacey 1993; Goodchild *et al.* 1996). In central retina, one-to-one connectivity would provide a single cone input to the receptive field center, necessarily generating cone specificity. The source of the opponent cone input to the surround is contentious; it is theoretically feasible that full cone opponency could arise solely through a cone-specific input to the receptive field center with mixed cone input to the surround (Lennie *et al.* 1991), but physiological evidence suggests that some degree of cone-specificity is present (Lee *et al.* 1998; Reid and Shapley 1992), although no anatomical evidence for cone-specific input to the surround has been found (Calkins and Sterling 1996).

Recent evidence has indicated that even the hypothesis of a single-cone input to the receptive field center of a midget ganglion cell may be an over-simplification. This brief review discusses factors influencing measurement of midget ganglion cell receptive field centers and relevant recent physiological evidence.

Measurements of center size and optical blur

The primary evidence for single-cone connectivity to the centers of midget ganglion cells is the unique anatomy of the midget system. Much larger center sizes are indicated by physiological data; a summary of the literature is shown in Fig. 7.1(a). In some of these papers (Croner and Kaplan 1995; Derrington and Lennie 1984), receptive field center Gaussian radii were derived from spatial frequency tuning curves to which a difference-of-Gaussians receptive field model was fitted. In such fits, the center radius parameter is largely determined by the high spatial frequency cut-off, of which the period is approximately equivalent to center radius (Peichl and Wassle 1979). This approximation was used for other papers in which cut-off alone is given (Blakemore and Vital-Durand 1986; Crook et al. 1988). Still other papers used other techniques to estimate radius (de Monasterio and Gouras 1975; Lee et al. 1998). The physiological data show considerable overlap but yield center radii much larger than that expected of a center deriving from a single cone. This latter curve was derived from anatomical measurements of cone diameter as a function of eccentricity (Packer et al. 1989). The Gaussian radius of cone sampling aperture relative to cone diameter has been determined in the fovea using interference fringes (MacLeod et al. 1992) and it is assumed this result holds at other eccentricities. The curve is terminated at 10° eccentricity since beyond this point ganglion cells may receive input from more than one midget bipolar.

A major factor in enlargement of centers beyond cone dimensions is optical blur. Figure 7.1(c) shows the optical transmission of the eye as a function of spatial frequency taken from Navarro et al. (1993). The spatial frequency response expected of a single foveal cone is plotted in Fig. 7.1(d) and extends to several hundred cycles per degree. When the eye's optics are bypassed by use of interference fringes, aliased images are observed due to the regularity of the foveal cone mosaic (Williams 1985), and these can seen up to frequencies well above one hundred cycles/degree.

The combination of the optical transfer function with that of a single cone results in a tuning curve largely determined by the former. The resolution limit expected of single cone centers after optical blur is also drawn in Fig. 7.1(a). It forms a lower bound to the experimental estimates.

The shape of a tuning curve modulated by optical blur differs from that expected of a Gaussian profile; the tuning curve of a Gaussian profile with similar cut-off is shown for comparison. After low-frequency roll-off due to the surround is included (not shown), the most obvious difference in shape to be expected is in the slope of the descending limb of the curve, which is shallower when determined by optical blur. Data in the literature have not commented on this feature of PC-cell tuning curves. However, in a recent series of measurements (Passaglia et al. 2000) we found no evidence of systematic deviations from the slope expected of a Gaussian center at high spatial frequencies. Such negative evidence is not necessarily conclusive, but does lead to a consideration of physiological factors that might enlarge center size.

Physiological factors influencing center size and shape

Although the results from different studies overlap in Fig. 7.1(a), there is considerable variability from study to study in PC-cell center size estimates. This is unlikely to be

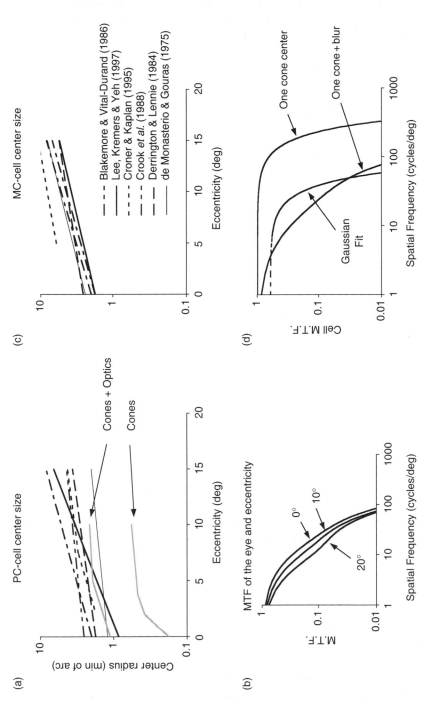

Figure 7.1 (a) Receptive field Gaussian radii of PC-cells as estimated from reports in the literature. Also shown is the estimated Gaussian radius expected of a receptive field constructed from a single cone, and the expected radius of a single cone center after blurring by the optics of the eye. (b) Receptive field Gaussian radii of MC-cells. (c) Optical transfer function of the eye taken from Navarro *et al.* (1993). (d) Expected spatial frequency tuning curve of a single cone center with and without optical blur. The shape expected of the curve with blur has a shallower slope than expected of a Gaussian profile (superimposed for comparison). Low-frequency roll-off expected from the receptive field surround has been neglected for this demonstration.

entirely due to differences in method, since a comparison of data sets for MC-cells from the same authors shows more consistency, except for the data of Croner and Kaplan (1995), which was based on a small cell sample. It is noteworthy that the center sizes of estimates for PC- and MC-cells (Fig. 7.1b) show considerable overlap. The frequent statement that MC-cells have much larger center sizes than PC-cells is extrapolated from anatomical evidence and is generally not borne out by the physiological data; the $1:3$ ratio of PC- to MC-cells center sizes cited by Derrington *et al.* (1984), for example, was based on the ratio of the smallest PC-cell centers to the average MC-cell data, and this is unlikely to be a reliable population estimate.

Three recent sets of physiological data suggest that physiological factors may also contribute to the enlargement of PC-cell center size beyond that of a single cone. McMahon *et al.* (2000) measured spatial frequency tuning curves of foveal PC-cells using interference fringes so as to avoid blur due to the eye's optics. Almost all cells showed tuning curves with multiple peaks at high spatial frequencies, and curve shape was strongly dependent on grating orientation. The authors attributed these irregular shapes to input from multiple cones, which causes aliasing among these multiple inputs at high spatial frequencies which would give rise to irregular tuning curves and irregular phase behavior. Calculations show that these irregularities cease to be significant with receptive field centers 4–5 cones across. This is approximately the dimension of a MC-cell receptive field center and so these cells' tuning curves are not expected to suffer from these irregularities.

The anatomical wiring responsible for these multiple cone inputs to PC-cell centers remains to be determined. One possibility would be inter-cone coupling in the outer retina. McMahon *et al.* (2000) considered this possibility and rejected it, favoring an inner retinal rather than an outer retinal origin. In one electron microscopical study (Kolb and Dekorver 1991), direct input to midget ganglion cells from neighboring midget bipolars comprised very few synaptic boutons whereas another study (Calkins *et al.* 1994) could not find any such input. These results are consistent with the light microscopy and thus midget bipolar convergence onto ganglion cells would seem unlikely to be responsible for the large aliased responses observed. It is uncertain whether the multiple cone inputs derive from just one cone type (that of the main center input) or from both M- and L-cones, although the latter alternative would cause a loss of cone specificity. The strong orientation specificity of curve shapes in McMahon *et al.* (2000) might suggest a spatial anisotropy which might derive from cone specificity. If so, a cone-specific amacrine cell circuit would be an obvious substrate, although this has not been detected anatomically (Calkins and Sterling 1996).

Recent data from peripheral retina suggest that there are cone-specific mechanisms which support the PC-cell receptive field center. In peripheral retina characteristic midget morphology is lost and the dendritic trees of this ganglion cell type encompass many (20–30) cones (Dacey 1993; Goodchild *et al.* 1996). If this cone sample were drawn from a random cone mosaic, then little cone specificity would be expected. It has been suggested that the loss of psychophysical sensitivity to red–green chromatic modulation in peripheral compared to central vision is due to a loss of chromatic opponency in midget ganglion cells because of the cone convergence onto the dendritic tree (Mullen and Kingdom 1996). However, recent direct electrophysiological measurement has shown that peripheral midget ganglion cells are as responsive to red–green chromatic modulation as are central cells (Martin *et al.* 2001). It was possible to show that this was incompatible with random connectivity to the M,L-cone array and that some mechanism promoting cone-specific connectivity must exist. It was speculated that the often anisotropic (i.e. elliptical) shape of peripheral midget dendritic fields was a result of some developmental mechanism providing cone specific connectivity to the center, either through a Hebbian learning process or through some chemical marker. It is not known if such a mechanism is restricted to peripheral retina. However, since the high chromatic responsivity of peripheral midget cells is not psychophysically utilized, restriction of such a mechanism to peripheral retina is unlikely.

The anisotropic dendritic trees of peripheral midget cells would be expected to lead to elliptical receptive field centers. Although this was not systematically studied by Martin *et al.* (2001) receptive field plots with hand-held stimuli often revealed an elliptical shape. If some mechanism provides multiple cone inputs to the centers of even central PC-cells, then anisotropic receptive field centers may also be present in central retina. In a recent series of experiments (Passaglia *et al.* 2002), we measured responses of PC- and MC-cells in the parafovea to achromatic sine-wave gratings drifted across the receptive field at different spatial frequencies and orientations. We reasoned that in the parafovea, where cone size and separation is larger than in central retina but optical quality is largely preserved, some degree of anisotropy due to multiple cone connectivity might survive optical blur.

At each orientation, the spatial frequency tuning curve was fitted with a difference-of-Gaussians model and the Gaussian radius for that orientation estimated. Figure 7.2(a) shows shapes of centers of typical PC- and MC-cells derived in this way. Each set of data was fitted with an ellipse. The center of the MC-cell is almost circular in shape but that of the PC-cell is elliptical. Figure 7.2(b) compares the major-to-minor axis ratios of the fitted ellipses for PC- and MC-cells. The distribution of major-to-minor ellipse ratio shows a systematic difference between the cell types. The distribution for MC-cells is similar to that reported for cat ganglion cells (Levick and Thibos 1982), but PC-cells have more elliptical receptive fields; this difference was significant at the 5 per cent level. Some cells also showed evidence for irregularities in tuning curves at high spatial frequencies as reported by McMahon *et al.*, although they were much smaller in amplitude than in these authors' data, presumably due to optical attenuation. These results are thus consistent with that earlier study. In summary, the data of McMahon *et al.* and of Passaglia *et al.* suggest the presence of physiological factors expanding size and shape of PC-cell centers beyond the size of a single cone. The mechanism of this unexpected degree of complexity remains unknown.

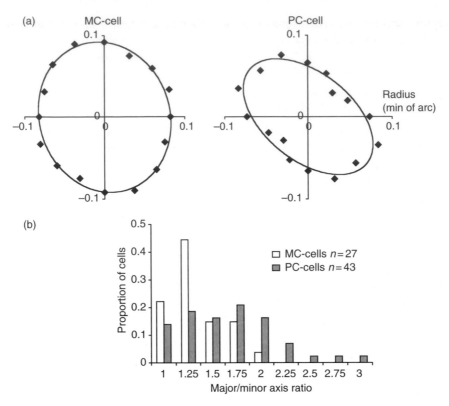

Figure 7.2 (a) Receptive field center radii estimated with drifting gratings of different orientations for a MC- and a PC-cell. Data points were fitted with ellipses. (b) Distribution of major-to-minor ellipse ratio of PC- and MC-cells. The two groups differ significantly at the 5% level.

Conclusions

Receptive field center size of midget ganglion cells is much larger than the aperture of a single cone. This is partly due to the effects of optical blur. The cone-specific midget anatomy may not have evolved to achieve a small center size, since this would be lost by optical blurring anyway, but to help provide cone specificity. On the other hand, recent physiological data suggest that the center structure of midget ganglion cells may derive from more than one cone even in central retina, and that cone-specific mechanisms exist which contribute to center structure. In any event, it appears that the center structure of these cells is more complex than anticipated from the anatomy.

Acknowledgements

I would like to thank numerous co-workers for permission to use data obtained in collaborative experiments. In particular, I would like to thank Chris Passaglia and John

Troy for permission to cite unpublished data on receptive field anisotropy in central retina. This work was partially supported by NEI 13112.

References

Blakemore, C. & Vital-Durand, F. (1986). Organization and post-natal development of the monkey's lateral geniculate nucleus. *Journal of Physiology, 380*, 453–92.

Boycott, B. B. & Dowling, J. E. (1969). Organization of the primate retina: light microscopy. *Philosophical Transactions of the Royal Society of London B, 255*, 109–84.

Calkins, D. J., Schein, S. J., Tsukamoto, Y., & Sterling, P. (1994). M and L cones in macaque fovea connect to midget ganglion cells by different numbers of excitatory synapses. *Nature, 37*, 70–2.

Calkins, D. J. & Sterling, P. (1996). Absence of spectrally specific lateral inputs to midget ganglion cells in primate retina. *Nature, 381*, 613–15.

Calkins, D. J. & Sterling, P. (1999). Evidence that circuits for spatial and color vision segregate at the first retinal synapse. *Neuron, 24*, 313–21.

Cole, G. R., Hine, T., & McIlhagga, W. (1993). Detection mechanisms in L-, M- and S-cone contrast space. *Journal of the Optical Society of America A, 10*, 38–51.

Croner, L. J. & Kaplan, E. (1995). Receptive fields of P and M ganglion cells across the primate retina. *Vision Research, 35*, 7–24.

Crook, J. M., Lange-Malecki, B., Lee, B. B., & Valberg, A. (1988). Visual resolution of macaque retinal ganglion cells. *Journal of Physiology, 396*, 205–24.

Dacey, D. M. (1993). The mosaic of midget ganglion cells in the human retina. *Journal of Neuroscience, 13*, 5334–55.

de Monasterio, F. M., & Gouras, P. (1975). Functional properties of ganglion cells of the rhesus monkey retina. *Journal of Physiology, 251*, 167–95.

Derrington, A. M., Krauskopf, J., & Lennie, P. (1984). Chromatic mechanisms in lateral geniculate nucleus of macaque. *Journal of Physiology, 357*, 241–65.

Derrington, A. M. & Lennie, P. (1984). Spatial and temporal contrast sensitivities of neurones in lateral geniculate nucleus of macaque. *Journal of Physiology, 357*, 219–40.

Goodchild, A. K., Ghosh, K. K., & Martin, P. R. (1996). A comparison of photoreceptor spatial density and ganglion cell morphology in the retina of human, macaque monkey, cat and the marmoset. *Journal of Comparative Neurology, 366*, 55–75.

Kolb, H. & Dekorver, L. (1991). Midget ganglion cells of the parafovea of the human retina: a study by electron microscopy and serial section reconstructions. *Journal of Comparative Neurology, 303*, 617–36.

Lee, B. B., Kremers, J., & Yeh, T. (1998). Receptive fields of primate ganglion cells studied with a novel technique. *Visual Neuroscience, 15*, 161–75.

Lee, B. B., Martin, P. R., Valberg, A., & Kremers, J. (1993). Physiological mechanisms underlying psychophysical sensitivity to combined luminance and chromatic modulation. *Journal of the Optical Society of America A, 10*, 1403–12.

Lee, B. B., Valberg, A., Tigwell, D. A., & Tryti, J. (1987). An account of responses of spectrally opponent neurons in macaque lateral geniculate nucleus to successive contrast. *Proceedings of the Royal Society B, 230,* 293–314.

Lennie, P., Haake, P. W., & Williams, D. R. (1991). The design of chromatically opponent receptive fields. In: M.S. Landy & J.A. Movshon (Eds) *Computational Models of Visual Processing* (pp. 71–82). Cambridge, MA, USA: MIT Press.

Levick, W. R. & Thibos, L. N. (1982). Analysis of orientation bias in cat retina. *Journal of Physiology, 329,* 243–61.

MacLeod, D. I. A., Williams, D. R., & Makous, W. (1992). A visual non-linearity fed by single cones. *Vision Research, 32,* 347–63.

Martin, P. R., Lee, B. B., White, A. J., Solomon, S. G., & Rüttiger, L. (2001). Chromatic sensitivity of ganglion cells in peripheral primate retina. *Nature, 410,* 933–6.

McMahon, M. J., Lankheet, M. J., Lennie, P., & Williams, D. R. (2000). Fine structure of parvocellular receptive fields in the primate fovea revealed by laser interferometry. *Journal of Neuroscience, 20,* 2043–53.

Mullen, K. T. & Kingdom, F. A. (1996). Losses in peripheral colour sensitivity predicted from "hit or miss" post-receptoral cone connections. *Vision Research, 36,* 1995–2000.

Navarro, R., Artal, P., & Williams, D. R. (1993). Modulation transfer of the human eye as a function of retinal eccentricity. *Journal of the Optical Society of America A, 10,* 201–12.

Packer, O., Hendrickson, A. E., & Curcio, C. A. (1989). Photoreceptor topography of the retina in the adult pigtail macaque (Macaca nemestrina). *Journal of Comparative Neurology, 288,* 165–83.

Passaglia, C. L., Troy, J. B., Rüttiger, L., & Lee, B. B. (2002). Orientation sensitivity of ganglion cells in primate retina. *Vision Research, 42,* 683–94.

Peichl, L. & Wassle, H. (1979). Size, scatter and coverage of ganglion cell receptive field centres in the cat retina. *Journal of Physiology, 291,* 117–41.

Polyak, S. L. (1941). The Retina. Chicago: University of Chicago Press.

Reid, R. C. & Shapley, R. M. (1992). Spatial structure of cone inputs to receptive fields in primate lateral geniculate nucleus. *Nature, 356,* 716–18.

Williams, D. R. (1985). Aliasing in human foveal vision. *Vision Research, 25,* 195–205.

CHAPTER 8

THE NEURAL CIRCUIT PROVIDING INPUT TO MIDGET GANGLION CELLS

DAVID W. MARSHAK

Midget ganglion cells are the most common type of ganglion cell in the primate retina, and they are also known as P cells because they project to the parvocellular layers of the lateral geniculate nucleus. In the central retina, they receive an excitatory input from a single midget bipolar cell which, in turn, receives input from a single long (L) or middle (M) wavelength sensitive cone. The midget ganglion cells become larger with increasing eccentricity, receiving input from two or more midget bipolar cells in the peripheral retina, but they retain their characteristic morphology (Rodieck 1998). Midget ganglion cells with dendrites in the proximal half of the inner plexiform layer (IPL) have ON responses, being excited by increments in light intensity in their receptive field centers and inhibited by that stimulus in the surrounding area; midget ganglion cells branching in the distal half of the IPL have the opposite, or OFF, responses (Dacey and Lee 1994).

In electrophysiological studies, most midget ganglion cells within the central 50° have responses of opposite polarity to stimulation of the L or the M wavelength cones. Figure 8.1 shows an example of such a response, an intracellular recording from a neuron that was subsequently injected with Neurobiotin and identified morphologically as a midget ganglion cell (Dacey and Lee 1994). In the central 10°, the input from a single midget bipolar cell accounts for the specificity of the excitatory input (Kolb and DeKorver 1991; Calkins *et al.* 1994). However, there is evidence that midget ganglion cells receive excitatory input from more than one cone, even in the central retina (McMahon *et al.* 2000; Kolb and Marshak 2002). In those instances and in the mid-peripheral retina, there are two possible explanations for the cone-selectivity of the response. First, the midget ganglion cells might selectively contact a single subtype of midget bipolar cell, and the elliptical shape of the dendritic arbors of midget ganglion cells provides some support for this hypothesis (Dacey 1993; Martin *et al.* 2001). A second possibility is that there is no selectivity in the synaptic contacts, but due to chance, all the midget bipolar cells presynaptic to the midget ganglion cell receive input from the same type of cone (Calkins and Sterling 1999). This is possible because L and M cones are randomly arranged, and cones of the same type are clustered (Mollon and Bowmaker 1992; Roorda *et al.* 2001). However, there is no obvious anatomical explanation for the selective inhibitory input

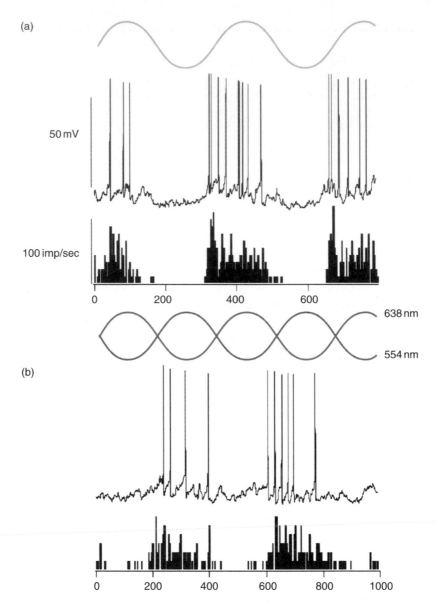

(a)

50 mV

100 imp/sec

0   200   400   600

638 nm

554 nm

(b)

0   200   400   600   800   1000

Figure 8.1(a),(b) Responses recorded intracellularly from a peripheral midget ganglion cell in the macaque retina by Dacey and Lee (1994). The stimulus is represented above each set of responses and the histograms below are the averages of 20 stimulus presentations for (a) ON responses to sinusoidal luminance modulation at 3.3 Hz and (b) sinusoidal, heterochromatic flicker at 3.3 Hz. The cell increases its firing rate in response to increments in light intensity and has branches in the inner half of the IPL. The cell is excited by increments in the green (554 nm) and inhibited by increments in the red light (638 nm).

in any part of the retina. Horizontal cells are unselective in their contacts with L and M cones, and their light responses indicate that the input from both cones is of the same polarity (Dacey *et al.* 1996). Amacrine cells are also unselective in their contacts with bipolar cells (Calkins and Sterling 1996). This negative evidence from anatomical studies led to the hypothesis that midget ganglion cells with responses like those in Fig. 8.1 occurred only by chance and that red–green color opponent responses were mediated by another type of ganglion cell that has not yet been identified morphologically (Calkins and Sterling 1999). I propose, instead, that interactions between amacrine cells in the pathway providing input to the midget ganglion cells produce responses that are more selective than would be predicted from the distribution of L and M cones.

Midget ganglion cells receive half of their input from amacrine cells in the central retina (Kolb and DeKorver 1991; Calkins and Sterling 1994), and in the peripheral retina, a larger proportion of their input comes from amacrine cells (Kolb *et al.* 2000). Kolb and DeKorver (1991) distinguished two types of amacrine cells in the pathway based on their ultrastructure and synaptic connections. Calkins and Sterling (1996) reconstructed four of the amacrine cells presynaptic to midget ganglion cells, two narrow field and two wide field, and they also described frequent contacts between the presynaptic amacrine cells. The main features of the input pathway I am proposing are illustrated in Fig. 8.2. The narrow field amacrine cells are unselective in their contacts with bipolar cells, but because their dendritic arbors are so small, their responses tend to be biased toward L or M cones, the same type that provides input to most of the nearby midget bipolar cells. The narrow field amacrine cells make inhibitory synapses onto wide field amacrine cells.

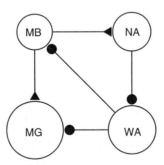

Figure 8.2 A simplified, schematic diagram of the neural circuit providing input to a central midget ganglion cell. The midget bipolar cell (MB) receives input from a single cone, and it makes an excitatory synapse (triangle) onto a midget ganglion cell (MG). The narrow-field amacrine cell also receives an excitatory input from the midget bipolar cell and from neighboring bipolar cells, and it is often biased toward one cone type, either L or M. The wide-field amacrine cell (WA) receives input from equal numbers of L and M cones; it makes inhibitory synapses (circles) on both the midget ganglion cell and the midget bipolar cell, providing the classical surround. The key to the model is that the narrow-field amacrine cell strongly inhibits the wide field amacrine cell. The difference between the spectral sensitivities of the two types provides a color opponent surround when both types are active, despite the fact that neither amacrine cell is selective in its contacts with bipolar cells.

The wide field amacrine cells inhibit the midget ganglion cells and midget bipolar cells, and they provide the classical, spatially antagonistic surround, as originally proposed by Dowling and Boycott (1966). Because the wide field amacrine cells have much larger dendritic trees, their input reflects the ratio of L to M cones in the entire region of the retina. A key assumption is that the output of the wide field amacrine cell can be inhibited locally without producing a major change in the spectral sensitivity of its light responses. Presynaptic inhibition of the terminal processes of the wide field amacrine cell is a possible mechanism. Because of the differences in the spectral sensitivities of the two types of amacrine cells, this circuit essentially computes the difference between the activity of the local cones and those in a much larger area. This signal is potentially more cone-specific than the response of any single type of cell. If the small amacrine cell is biased toward one cone type, the strength of surround inhibition will depend on the wavelength of the stimulus, despite the fact that the amacrine cells that produce the surround are unselective in their contacts with bipolar cells. However, if the stimulus is not effective in driving the narrow-field amacrine cells, the light responses of the midget ganglion cell will reflect the distribution of cones in the receptive field.

To illustrate how inhibition from narrow field amacrine cells onto wide field amacrine cells might produce L or M cone selective surrounds, consider a midget ganglion cell with M-ON responses in an area where the majority of midget bipolar cells receive inputs from M cones. A middle wavelength stimulus produces an ON response in the midget ganglion cell and narrow-field amacrine cells. Surround antagonism is relatively weak because the narrow-field amacrine cells inhibit the wide-field amacrine cells. The surround appears to be driven selectively by L cones because, with long wavelength stimuli, the narrow field amacrine cells are not as active and surround antagonism is stronger. This mechanism could not produce cone selectivity in an area with equal numbers of L and M cones in the receptive field, and this may account for the 20 per cent of mid-peripheral midget ganglion cells that are not spectrally opponent (Martin et al. 2001). This circuit would not promote spectral opponency the far periphery, where the receptive field centers receive input from a large number of L and M cones, and this is also consistent with the physiological results (Dacey 1999).

Another model has been proposed in which some spectral opponency arose from irregularities in the cone mosaic, but the surround had only one component, and the interaction with the center was linear (Lennie et al. 1991). An H1 horizontal cell or a single type of amacrine cell could produce such a surround. However, a recent physiological study indicates that there are nonlinear components in the interaction between the L and M cone responses in midget ganglion cells (Benardete and Kaplan 1999). One possible source of this nonlinearity is a positive feedback loop that would develop when (1) narrow field amacrine cells are excited via the cone type that predominates locally, (2) the narrow field amacrine cells inhibit wide field amacrine cells, (3) midget bipolar cells receive less inhibition, and (4) narrow field amacrine cells are excited further. Another possible source of nonlinearity is the convergence of several midget bipolar cells onto one narrow field amacrine cell (Fig. 8.3). The amacrine cells presynaptic to midget ganglion cells are

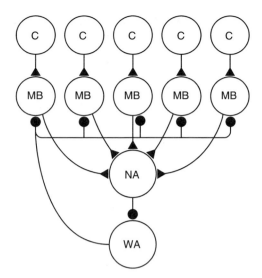

Figure 8.3 Convergence of midget bipolar cells onto narrow-field amacrine cells. Each midget bipolar cell (MB) receives excitatory input (triangle) from a single cone (C). Five midget bipolar cells make excitatory synapses onto a narrow-field amacrine cell (NA). The narrow-field amacrine cell makes an inhibitory synapse (circle) on the wide-field amacrine cell (WA). The wide field amacrine cell makes inhibitory synapses onto all of the midget bipolar cells. If the synapses made by the wide-field amacrine cell were tonically active, this circuit would account for the observation that the receptive field centers of midget bipolar cells are larger than their dendritic fields. Stimuli to cones outside the dendritic field would excite narrow-field amacrine cell, inhibit the wide-field amacrine cell and enhance the response of the midget bipolar cell via disinhibition.

known to receive input from 4 to 6 midget bipolar cells (Calkins and Sterling 1996). If the wide field amacrine cells also tonically inhibit the midget bipolar cells, this circuit might also explain why the receptive field centers of midget bipolar cells are 2–3 times larger than their dendritic fields (Dacey *et al.* 2000). Stimulation of neighboring midget bipolar cells would activate the narrow field amacrine cell because of the convergence, and the result would be to stimulate the midget bipolar cell through disinhibition. A third source of nonlinearity might be divergence of one midget bipolar cell onto several narrow field amacrine cells, which has the potential to greatly enhance the effect of a single midget bipolar cell (Fig. 8.4). Stimuli selective for L or M cones would tend to promote these nonlinear interactions. Because of the existence of clusters of one cone type, neighboring narrow field amacrine cells would also tend to have similar spectral sensitivities. These nonlinear interactions would amplify the effect of the predominant cone type, and they may also contribute to the cone selectivity in the centers of the midget ganglion cell receptive fields in the mid-periphery.

This circuit could also explain the discrepancy between the results of early studies of the color opponent responses of midget ganglion cells with simple stimuli and the more recent studies with complex stimuli. The early studies used chromatic adaptation

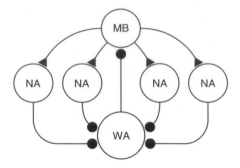

Figure 8.4 Divergence of a midget bipolar onto narrow-field amacrine cells. A midget bipolar cell (MB) makes excitatory synapses (triangles) onto several narrow-field amacrine cells (NA). The narrow-field amacrine cell makes an inhibitory synapse (circle) onto a wide-field amacrine cell (WA). This circuit can amplify the effect of a stimulus to a single bipolar cell and promote cooperative interactions between narrow-field amacrine cells.

and small spots to characterize the receptive field centers or annuli to characterize the surrounds (Zrenner 1983). Stimuli like these might not drive the narrow field amacrine cells in the pathway providing input to midget ganglion cells, and this may account for the variability in opponency observed in these studies. The more recent studies used stimuli that were more complex and changed continuously, and these stimuli might be more effective for amacrine cells. These stimuli include: full-field, heterochromatic flicker (Smith *et al.* 1992; Dacey and Lee 1994; Martin *et al.* 2001); a checkerboard with flickering, cone-isolating stimuli (Reid and Shapley 1992); a bipartite field with the two sides modulated in counterphase (Lee *et al.* 1998), and two sine wave gratings presented simultaneously (Benardete and Kaplan 1999). In a study of the macaque lateral geniculate nucleus, there is evidence for a loss of color selectivity in the responses of individual neurons when the stimulus changed from a full field to a moving spot (Kruger 1977), and the same may be true of midget ganglion cells. It should also be possible to test this hypothesis more directly. Because the narrow-field amacrine cells are critical for generating opponent responses and the smaller amacrine cells in primate retinas use glycine as their neurotransmitter (Koontz *et al.* 1993), the glycine antagonist strychnine should reduce the strength of opponent interactions between L and M cones in response to these complex stimuli to the level predicted from the cone mosaic.

Acknowledgements

Figure 8.1 was provided by Dr. Dennis Dacey, University of Washington. Supported by grant EY06472 from the National Eye Institute.

References

Benardete, E. A. & Kaplan, E. (1999) Dynamics of primate P retinal ganglion cells: responses to chromatic and achromatic stimuli. *Journal of Physiology* 519: 775–90.

Calkins, D. J., Schein, S. J., Tsukamoto, Y., & Sterling, P. (1994) M and L cones in macaque fovea connect to midget ganglion cells by different numbers of excitatory synapses. *Nature* 371: 70–2.

Calkins, D. J. & Sterling, P. (1996) Absence of spectrally specific lateral inputs to midget ganglion cells in primate retina. *Nature* 381: 613–15.

Calkins, D. J. & Sterling, P. (1999) Evidence that circuits for spatial and color vision segregate at the first retinal synapse. *Neuron* 24: 313–21.

Dacey, D. M. (1993) The mosaic of midget ganglion cells in the human retina. *Journal of Neuroscience* 13: 5334–35.

Dacey, D. M. (1999) Primate retina: cell types, circuits and color opponency. *Progress in Retinal and Eye Research* 18: 737–63.

Dacey, D. M. & Lee, B. B. (1994) The "blue-on" opponent pathway in primate retina originates from a distinct Bistratified ganglion cell type. *Nature* 367: 731–5.

Dacey, D. M., Lee, B. B., Stafford, D. K., Pokorny, J., & Smith, V. (1996) Horizontal cells of the primate retina: cone specificity without spectral opponency. *Science* 271: 656–9.

Dacey, D. M., Packer, O. S., Diller, L., Brainard, D., Peterson, B., & Lee, B. B. (2000) Center surround receptive field structure of cone bipolar cells in primate retina. *Vision Research* 40: 1801–11.

Dowling, J. E. & Boycott, B. B. (1996) Organization of the primate retina: electron microscopy. *Proceedings of the Royal Society Series B* 166: 80–11.

Koontz, M. A., Hendrickson, L. E., Brace, S. T., & Hendrickson, A. E. (1993) Immunocytochemical localization of GABA and glycine in amacrine and displaced amacrine cells of macaque monkey retina. *Vision Research* 33: 2617–28.

Kolb, H. & DeKorver, L. (1991) Midget ganglion cells of the parafovea of the human retina: a study by electron microscopy and serial section reconstructions. *Journal of Comparative Neurology* 303: 617–36.

Kolb, H., DeKorver, L., Yamada, E., & Marshak, D. (2000) EM reconstruction of an ON midget ganglion cell in central monkey retina. *Investigative Ophthalmology and Visual Science* 41: S936.

Kolb, H. E., & Marshak, D. W. (2002) The midget pathways of the primate retina. *Documenta Ophthalmologica* in press.

Kruger, J. (1977) Stimulus dependent colour specificity of monkey lateral geniculate neurons. *Experimental Brain Research* 30: 297–311.

Lee, B. B., Kremers, J., & Yeh, T. (1998) Receptive fields of primate retinal ganglion cells studied with a novel technique. *Visual Neuroscience* 15: 161–75.

Lennie, P., Haake W., & Williams, D. R. (1991) The design of chromatically opponent receptive fields. In M.S. Landy and J.A. Movshon, eds. *Computational Models of Visual Processing*. MIT Press, Cambridge, MA.

Martin, P. R., Lee, B. B., White, A. J. R., Solomon, S. G., & Ruttiger, L. (2001) Chromatic sensitivity of ganglion cells in the peripheral primate retina. *Nature* 410: 923–36.

McMahon, M. J., Lankheet, M. J., Lennie, P., & Williams, D. R. (2000) Fine structure of parvocellular receptive fields in the primate fovea revealed by laser interferometry. *Journal of Neuroscience* 20: 2043–53.

Mollon, J. D. & Bowmaker, J. K. (1992) The spatial arrangement of cones in the primate fovea. *Nature* 360: 677–9.

Reid, R. C. & Shapley, R. M. (1992) Spatial structure of cone inputs to receptive fields in primate lateral geniculate nucleus. *Nature* 356: 716–18.

Rodieck, R. W. (1998) *The First Steps in Seeing.* Sinauer Associates, Sunderland, MA.

Roorda, A., Metha, A. B., Lennie, P. & Williams, D. R. (2001) Packing arrangement of the three cone classes in primate retina. *Vision Research* 41: 1291–1306.

Smith, V., Lee, B. B., Pokorny, J., Martin, P. R. & Valberg, A. (1992) Responses of macaque ganglion cells to the relative phase of heterochromatically modulated lights. *Journal of Physiology* 458: 191–221.

Zrenner, E. (1983) *Neurophysiological Aspects of Color Vision in Primates.* Springer-Verlag, Berlin.

CHAPTER 9

CODING OF POSITION OF ACHROMATIC AND CHROMATIC EDGES BY RETINAL GANGLION CELLS

HAO SUN, BARRY B. LEE, AND LUKAS RÜTTIGER

Introduction

In studies concerning vernier performance, achromatic stimuli have been used much more often than chromatic targets (e.g. Levi and Klein 1982; Levi 1996; McKee 1991; Morgan *et al.* 1983; Morgan and Aiba 1985*a,b*; Westheimer and Hauske 1975; Westheimer and McKee 1975, 1977*a,b*; Westheimer 1979, 1981). However, Morgan and Aiba (1985*a,b*) measured vernier thresholds for two bars with varying chromaticity and luminance. They found a deterioration of vernier threshold with bars set in an equiluminant surround, and showed vernier thresholds displayed properties consistent with photometric additivity when lights of different chromaticity were combined, as might be expected if a luminance channel mediated performance. For another hyperacuity task, Rüttiger and Lee (2000) showed that for displacement thresholds of edges with incremental chromatic and luminance contrasts, performance was strictly determined by luminance contrast, consistent with magnocellular (MC-) pathway cells playing a more important role than parvocellular (PC-) cells in this task. On the other hand, Krauskopf and Farell (1991) measured vernier thresholds for either luminance or equiluminant chromatic Gaussian and Gabor patterns. They found that, except for narrow Gaussian patterns, vernier thresholds were approximately equal when the modulation contrasts were equal multiples of detection threshold. Their results imply that chromatic and luminance channels can be equally effective in providing a vernier signal.

It has been shown that the spatial precision of MC-cells' responses to achromatic targets, analyzed with a template matching procedure, is independent of target velocity over a wide range (Rüttiger and Lee 1998). We ask here how accurately ganglion cells carry positional information about chromatic and achromatic moving edges, and compare results with psychophysical thresholds to similar stimuli. We do not suggest that mechanisms for vernier performance are located at the retinal level; we are only concerned here with the accuracy of the spatial signal a single ganglion cell can deliver.

We used edges of different luminance and chromatic contrasts. The physiological data showed that spatial precision of MC-cells' responses was determined solely by luminance contrast, but that of PC-cells was dependent on chromatic contrast. Psychophysical vernier thresholds for edges of the same luminance, but different chromatic contrasts were similar when plotted as a function of luminance contrast, but were different when plotted in detection threshold units. Taken together, the physiological and psychophysical data suggest that positional information delivered by MC-cells is important for vernier performance.

Methods

Physiology

Stimuli

Visual stimuli were generated with a Cambridge Research VSG 3 System controlled by a Macintosh 950 computer, and presented on a Barco CRT video display (frame rate: 195 Hz, luminance resolution of RGB gun: 15 bit) 2.6 m away from the monkey. The stimulus was a horizontal edge moving downwards at a speed of 2°/s. The luminance of the background was fixed at 40 cd/m², and the luminance of the test, which was added to the background, was varied to change either the luminance contrast alone (when chromaticities of the test and background are the same) or both the luminance and chromatic contrasts (when chromaticities of the test and background are different) of the edge. For the pure-luminance condition (edges with luminance contrast alone), the chromaticity of both test and background was (0.45, 0.47) in CIE (x, y) coordinates, which appeared yellowish to observers with normal color vision. For the luminance–chromatic conditions (edges with both luminance and chromatic contrasts), the chromaticity of the test or background was one of the following (0.625, 0.34), (0.28, 0.595) or (0.153, 0.07), which appeared reddish, greenish or bluish to observers with normal color vision. The following test/background combinations were chosen in order to favor different cone opponent cells; red-on-green (a reddish test on a greenish background for +L−M cells), green-on-red (a greenish test on a reddish background for +M−L cells), and blue-on-red (a bluish test on a reddish background for +M−L and +S−ML cells). For all conditions, the luminance contrast was varied from about 1–33 per cent (Weber contrast). For luminance–chromatic edges, at the maximal luminance contrast the L- and M-cone contrasts were about (39, 18 per cent) and (28, 52 per cent) for red-on-green and green-on-red edges, respectively, and the L-, M-, and S-cone contrasts were (20, 50, 95 per cent) for the blue-on-red edge.

Procedure

Ganglion cell responses to edge stimuli were recorded from the retinae of three anesthetized macaques (Lee *et al.* 1989). Receptive field eccentricities were between 4° and 8°. Times of spike occurrence were recorded to an accuracy of 100 μs. Binwidth in histograms was 6 ms, with 20 or 40 sweeps for each histogram.

The spatial precision of a cell's impulse trains was estimated using a template matching procedure (Rüttiger and Lee 1998). For each edge condition, the response histogram at

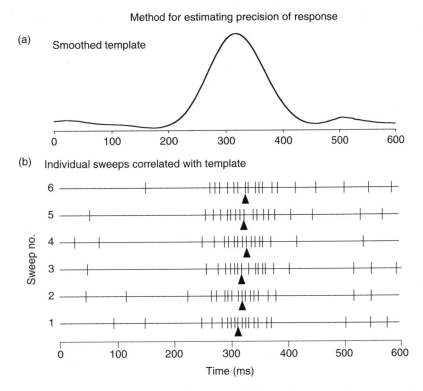

Figure 9.1 (a) The template matching procedure. A matching template was obtained by smoothing the cell's response histogram at maximal contrast; the same template was used at different contrast levels of the same edge condition. (b) The impulse train was shifted over the template until the matching positions (arrows) that gave maximal correlation between impulse train and template were found. This procedure was repeated for each individual impulse train. The standard deviation of the matching positions was a measure of the reliability of spatial localization by the cell.

maximal contrast was smoothed, and used as a template for that edge condition at all contrast levels. Each impulse train was shifted over the template to find the matching location that gave maximal correlation between the impulse train and the template. This procedure was repeated for each individual impulse train, and the standard deviation of the matching locations was taken as a measure of the reliability of spatial localization by the cell. The method is illustrated in Fig. 9.1.

Psychophysics

Stimuli

The same display system was used as in the physiological experiments. The viewing distance was extended to 11.4 m by means of two surface-silvered mirrors. The vernier stimulus consisted of two vertical edges (separated by 4 arcmin), moving rightward or leftward for 188 ms. The luminance, chromaticity, and speed of the edge were the same as in physiological experiments.

To achieve a sub-pixel resolution (theoretically 0.1 arcsec at a physical CRT pixel size of 10.7 arcsec), the intensities of a row of pixels at the border of the edge were adjusted so as to shift the contour of the edge by the required amount (Morgan and Aiba 1985*b*). To ensure that relative positional information could not be derived from stimulus onset or offset locations, a 50 ms masking edge was presented at both onset and offset of the stimulus in some sets of experiments. For our experimental conditions, presence or absence of the masks had no effect on thresholds.

Procedure

The vernier threshold was measured with staircase method. The observer viewed the visual target monocularly. A fixation point was presented before each trial; at the onset of each trial, the fixation point disappeared and the stimulus appeared, and the observer's task was to indicate if the top edge was to the left or right of the bottom one. An auditory feedback was given after each trial. Each run included two randomly interleaved staircases. The direction of movement was leftward in one staircase and rightward in the other. Threshold of each staircase was the average of six reversals. Thresholds plotted were the averages of six staircases.

We also measured detection thresholds for each edge condition using a four-alternative forced-choice procedure. A moving edge was presented in one of the four quadrants. The observer's task was to indicate in which quadrant the stimulus was presented. Thresholds were estimated with the same staircase method as in the vernier experiment.

Observer

Two observers participated in the experiments, both with normal color vision as assessed with Neitz Anomaloscope, Ishihara pseudoisochromatic plates and Farnsworth-Munsell 100-Hue Test. Both observers are myopic and wore contact lens during experiments.

Results

Physiology

Responses of macaque ganglion cells were measured for 6 MC-cells, 14 L/M cone opponent PC-cells, and 2 +S−ML cells. For each cell, we recorded responses to four types of edges at five luminance contrasts. Figure 9.2 shows response histograms at ~33 per cent luminance contrast. The MC-cells gave similar transient responses to all drifting edges. +L−M PC-cells gave strong sustained responses only to red-on-green edges, and were suppressed by green-on-red edges. +M−L cells gave strong sustained responses to green-on-red and blue-on-red edges, and were suppressed by red-on-green edges. +S−ML cells responded only to blue-on-red edges.

Figure 9.3a shows the standard deviations of the maximal correlation loci (the measure of spatial reliability) as a function of luminance contrast. Four plots represent data

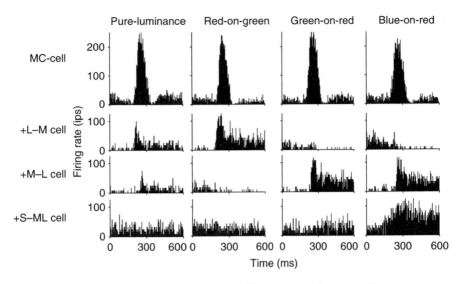

Figure 9.2 Histograms of ganglion cells' responses to different types of edges at ~33 per cent luminance contrast. Four rows show responses of MC−, +L−M, +M−L, and +S−ML cells. Four columns represent responses to pure-luminance, red-on-green, green-on-red, and blue-on-red edges, respectively. The binwidth was 6 ms, with 20 or 40 sweeps each histogram.

for MC-, +L−M, +M−L, and +S−ML cells. Data are shown for pure-luminance (squares), red-on-green (erect triangles), green-on-red (inverted triangles) and blue-on-red (circles) edges. Lines represent linear fits. Arrows indicate the standard deviation of the maximal correlation positions in the absence of stimulation, that is, at 0 per cent contrast, and data points near this level indicate chance performance by the neurometric algorithm.

For PC-cells, only excitatory responses yielded positional information. Inhibitory responses did not provide any spatial cue. This was also the case for MC-cells, for example, off-center cells gave little spatial information as to the location of the incremental edges used here (data not shown). The spatial precision of MC-cell spike trains was similar for all four types of edges. This is expected for stimuli of the same luminance contrasts. The spatial precision increased with contrast; the slopes of linear fits were between −0.83 to −1.0. L/M opponent PC-cells and +S−ML cells gave spatial information only with edges with the appropriate chromatic components.

Psychophysics

There is evidence that MC- and PC-pathways form the physiological basis for psychophysical luminance and chromatic channels (Crook *et al.* 1987; Kaiser *et al.* 1990; Lee *et al.* 1988). If so, we expect psychophysical vernier thresholds for edges of the same luminance but different chromatic contrast to be similar if the luminance mechanism underlies vernier performance, but vernier thresholds may differ if chromatic pathways

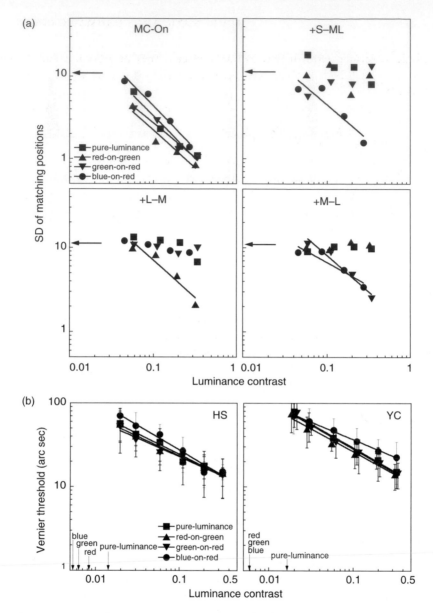

Figure 9.3 Comparison of spatial precision of the cells' responses and human vernier thresholds.
(a) SD of the matching positions of ganglion cells at different luminance contrasts. Four plots represent
data for MC-, +L−M, +M−L, and +S−ML cells. Data are shown for pure-luminance (squares),
red-on-green (erect triangles), green-on-red (inverted triangles) and blue-on-red (circles) edges. Lines
represent linear fits where appropriate. Arrows indicate the standard deviation of the maximal
correlation positions at 0 per cent contrast. At the maximal luminance contrast, the L- and M-cone
contrasts were about (39, 18 per cent) and (28, 52 per cent) for red-on-green and green-on-red edges,
respectively, and the L-, M-, and S-cone contrasts were (20, 50, 95 per cent) for the blue-on-red edge.
(b) Vernier thresholds from two observers. Data are shown for pure-luminance (squares),
red-on-green (erect triangles), green-on-red (inverted triangles) and blue-on-red (circles) edges. Lines
represent linear fits. Arrows indicate the detection thresholds for each edge condition.

contribute to vernier performance. In the latter case, they may become similar when contrast is normalized to detection threshold, following the suggestion of Krauskopf and Farell (1991).

The vernier thresholds from human observers are shown in Fig. 9.3b. Data are shown for pure-luminance (squares), red-on-green (erect triangles), green-on-red (inverted triangles) and blue-on-red (circles) edges. Lines represent linear fits. Arrows indicate the detection thresholds for each edge condition. Detection thresholds were highest for the pure-luminance edge and lower in the luminance–chromatic edge conditions.

For all edges, the vernier thresholds decreased steadily as the luminance contrast increased, with a slope of about −0.5. Vernier threshold curves overlapped when plotted against luminance contrast, but did not overlap when plotted in detection threshold units. This is consistent with a luminance mechanism determining performance.

Discussion

To identify the roles of achromatic and chromatic mechanisms, we chose to use incremental edges with both luminance and chromatic contrast as chromatic stimuli rather than equiluminance edges for two reasons (Morgan and Ingle 1994). One was to avoid the non-linear MC-cell chromatic response which can occur with equiluminance edges (Kaiser *et al*. 1990; Valberg *et al*. 1992). The other was to avoid luminance artifacts arising from chromatic aberration with equiluminance edges. These factors are not expected to play a role with the stimuli used here.

Our result is consistent with earlier psychophysical experiments (Morgan and Aiba 1985*a*, *b*) which suggested involvement of a luminance mechanism in vernier performance, but inconsistent with Krauskopft and Farell (1991) who showed that, with a Gaussian or Garbor patterns, the luminance and chromatic channels can make equivalent contributions to vernier thresholds. Our data are also consistent with previous results (Lee *et al*. 1995) employing achromatic stimuli which also suggested a dominant role for the MC-pathway in a vernier task.

Detection of targets of different wavelengths on a white background has been attributed to different chromatic and achromatic mechanisms (King-Smith 1975; Sperling and Harwerth 1971), and different cell types of the PC- and MC-pathways are thought to underlie these mechanisms (Crook *et al*. 1987). In these experiments we used different backgrounds to enhance chromatic contrast. We suggest that the differences in detection thresholds between pure-luminance and luminance–chromatic edges result from detection by a luminance mechanism for the pure-luminance edge and by chromatic mechanisms for the luminance–chromatic edges.

The physiological data showed that with pure-luminance moving edges, the spatial information delivered by the MC-cells was more precise than that of PC-cells. PC-cells can only yield accurate spatial information with chromatic contrasts that cause an increase in firing rate. Chromatic contrasts that cause a cessation of maintained activity do not appear to generate a useful spatial signal. It has been proposed that a combination of +M−L and +L−M cell responses could yield a mechanism with a spectral sensitivity similar to the luminosity function (Ingling and Martinez-Uriegas 1983; Lennie and D'Zmura 1988). However, the responses shown in Fig. 9.2 do not combine to produce such a mechanism due to the rectification associated with zero firing rate for some of the chromatic combinations.

Acknowledgements

This work was partially supported by DFG Le 524-14/2 and NEI 13112. We would like to thank Linda Glennie for providing part of the programs. We also thank William Swanson, Qasim Zaidi, and Harry Wyatt for their helpful suggestions and observer YC for her time.

References

Crook, J. M., B. B. Lee, D. A. Tigwell & A. Valberg (1987). Thresholds to chromatic spots of cells in the macaque geniculate nucleus as compared to detection sensitivity in man. *Journal of Physiology*, *392*, 193–211.

Ingling, C. R. & E. Martinez-Uriegas (1983). The relationship between spectral sensitivity and spatial sensitivity for the primate r-g X channel. *Vision Research*, *23*, 1495–500.

Kaiser, P. K., B. B. Lee, P. R. Martin & A. Valberg (1990). The physiological basis of the minimally distinct border demonstrated in the ganglion cells of the macaque retina. *Journal of Physiology*, *422*, 153–83.

King-Smith, P. E. (1975). Visual detection analysed in terms of luminance and chromatic signals. *Nature*, *255*, 69–70.

Krauskopf, J. & B. Farell (1991). Vernier acuity: effects of chromatic content, blur and contrast. *Vision Research*, *31*, 735–49.

Lee, B. B., P. R. Martin & A. Valberg (1988). The physiological basis of heterochromatic flicker photometry demonstrated in the ganglion cells of the macaque retina. *Journal of Physiology*, *404*, 323–47.

Lee, B. B., P. R. Martin & A. Valberg (1989). Sensitivity of macaque retinal ganglion cells to chromatic and luminance flicker. *Journal of Physiology*, *414*, 223–43.

Lee, B. B., C. Wehrhahn, G. Westheimer & J. Kremers (1995). The spatial precision of macaque ganglion cell responses in relation to Vernier acuity of human observers. *Vision Research*, *35*, 2743–58.

Lennie, P. & M. D. D'Zmura (1988). Mechanisms of color vision. *CRC Critical Reviews in Neurobiology*, *3*, 333–400.

Levi, D. M. (1996). Pattern perception at high velocities. *Current Biology*, *6*, 1020–4.

Levi, D. M. & S. Klein (1982). Hyperacuity and amblyopia. *Nature*, *298*, 268–70.

McKee, S. P. (1991). The physical constraints on visual hyperacuity. In: J. J. Kulikowski, V. Walsh & I. J. Murray (Eds) *Limits of Vision* (pp. 221–33). Macmillan Press.

Morgan, M. J. & T. S. Aiba (1985*a*). Positional acuity with chromatic stimuli. *Vision Research, 25,* 689–95.

Morgan, M. J. & T. S. Aiba (1985*b*). Vernier acuity predicted from changes in the light distribution of the retinal image. *Spatial Vision, 1,* 151–61.

Morgan, M. J. & G. Ingle (1994). What direction of motion do we see if luminance but not colour contrast is reversed during displacement? Psychophysical evidence for a signed-colour input to motion detection. *Vision Research, 34,* 2527–35.

Morgan, M. J., R. J. Watt & S. P. McKee (1983). Exposure duration affects the sensitivity of vernier acuity to target motion. *Vision Research, 23,* 541–6.

Rüttiger, L. & B. B. Lee (2000). Chromatic and luminance contributions to a hyperacuity task. *Vision Research, 40,* 817–32.

Rüttiger, L. R. & B. B. Lee (1998). Vernier signals derived from primate ganglion cells: effects of motion speed and contrast. *Investigative Ophthalmology and Visual Science Supplement, 39,* S564.

Sperling, H. G. & R. S. Harwerth (1971). Red-green cone interaction in the increment-threshold spectral sensitivity of primates. *Science, 172,* 180–4.

Valberg, A., B. B. Lee, P. K. Kaiser & J. Kremers (1992). Responses of macaque ganglion cells to movement of chromatic borders. *Journal of Physiology, 458,* 579–602.

Westheimer, G. (1979). The spatial sense of the eye. *Investigative Ophthalmology and Visual Science, 18,* 893–912.

Westheimer, G. (1981). Visual Hyperacuity. In: D. Ottoson (Ed.) *Progress in Sensory Physiology* (pp. 1–30). Berlin: Springer.

Westheimer, G. & G. Hauske (1975). Temporal and spatial interference with Vernier acuity. *Vision Research, 15,* 1137–41.

Westheimer, G. & S. P. McKee (1975). Visual acuity in the presence of retinal-image motion. *Journal of the Optical Society of America, 65,* 847–50.

Westheimer, G. & S. P. McKee (1977*a*). Perception of temporal order in adjacent visual stimuli. *Vision Research, 17,* 887–92.

Westheimer, G. & S. P. McKee (1977*b*). Spatial configurations for visual hyperacuity. *Vision Research, 17,* 941–7.

SPATIAL AND TEMPORAL ASPECTS OF COLOUR PERCEPTION

PSYCHOPHYSICAL CORRELATES OF PARVO- AND MAGNOCELLULAR FUNCTION

VIVIANNE C. SMITH AND JOEL POKORNY

Introduction

Modern studies of anatomy and physiology have distinguished three major pathways that transmit information about visual stimuli from the retina to the lateral geniculate nucleus and thence to primary visual cortex (Dacey 2000). These pathways, the Parvocellular (PC-), Magnocellular (MC-) and Koniocellular (KC-) were named according to their structure in the lateral geniculate nucleus. The anatomical basis for the pathways is evident however at the level of the bipolar cells, the second cell in the transmission of information from photoreceptor to visual cortex. The PC-pathway has its origin in the midget bipolar cells that transmit information to the midget ganglion cells. The MC-pathway has its origin in the diffuse bipolar cells that transmit information to the parasol ganglion cells. Both these pathways have on- and off-units that are distinguished anatomically by the level at which the ganglion cell dendrites ramify in the outer nuclear level. The input to the bipolar cells is from the long wavelength sensitive (LWS) and middle wavelength sensitive (MWS) cones. Short wavelength sensitive (SWS) cones are associated with the KC-pathway, which is not discussed further in this review.

Physiological studies have delineated differences in the characteristic cell responses in the PC- and MC-pathway. The PC-pathway shows center-surround behavior in which one cone type mediates the center and the other mediates the surround of both on-center and off-center cells (Derrington *et al.* 1984; Lee *et al.* 1990; Reid and Shapley 1992). Thus there are four subtypes of PC-cell designated by the type and sign of the center cone: $+L-M$, $-L+M$, $+M-L$, $-M+L$. PC-cells have low-pass characteristics to both temporal and spatial sinusoids for equiluminant stimuli modulated in chromaticity and band-pass characteristics for stimuli modulated in luminance. The contrast response function for equiluminant chromatic stimuli shows high sensitivity and can be characterized by a saturating response function. For achromatic stimuli, the PC-cells are insensitive, giving an almost linear response with increasing contrast. The MC-pathway shows center–surround behavior in which both the LWS and MWS cones have inputs to both the on- and off-diffuse bipolar cells. MC-cells respond primarily to luminance stimuli, showing a band-pass characteristic to both temporal and spatial sinusoids

(Derrington and Lennie 1984; Lee *et al.* 1990; Purpura *et al.* 1990). MC cells are highly sensitive to small contrast variation and to luminance transients and show a rapidly saturating contrast response function (Kaplan and Shapley 1986).

There has been a sustained interest in relating these early retinal pathways to psycho-physical data. One way to isolate the PC-pathway is by use of equiluminant chromatic stimuli. This has proved a useful way to study chromatic vision. However the method ignores the possible role of the PC-pathway in achromatic vision. A second way is by use of temporal waveforms to take advantage of the differences in temporal processing. Near threshold, slowly ramped or long pulses favor PC-pathway processing; brief pulses are an efficient way to isolate the MC-pathway with its preference for luminance transients. These techniques have been used to study both spectral (King-Smith and Carden 1976) and spatial sensitivity (Legge 1978).

In our laboratory, we introduced a contrast discrimination technique (Pokorny and Smith 1997) that reveals PC- and MC-pathway function by taking advantage of their differences in achromatic contrast response. Our paradigms allow us to evaluate spatio-temporal processing for these pathways using achromatic stimuli. It is important to note that we do not claim that the psychophysical functions we describe are mediated at the retina. The signals leaving the retina are subject to considerable further processing by higher visual processes. By biasing the early retinal processing to one or other pathway, we can access different properties of higher order processes. The goal of this paper is to review these studies, indicating the possible clinical applications of the approach.

Rationale for this approach

The contrast response function has been measured either with achromatic drifting sine wave gratings (Kaplan and Shapley 1986) to compare PC- and MC-cell behavior or with temporal sinusoidal full-field stimuli (Lee *et al.* 1990) to compare achromatic and chromatic properties of PC- and MC-cells. For chromatic stimuli, two chromatic lights are modulated out of phase and contrast is expressed relative to unity. In both types of study the individual cell data could be fit with saturation functions showing the response in impulses per second (ips) as a function of stimulus contrast.

$$R = R_0 + R_{\max} C/(C + C_{\text{sat}}) \tag{1}$$

where R is the response rate to the sinusoidal stimulus, R_0 is the resting response at the average retinal illuminance, and C is the Michelson contrast of the sinusoidal stimulus. The function is characterized by two free parameters: $R_{\max}$ is the maximal response rate and C_{sat} is the contrast at which response reaches half $R_{\max}$. Figure 10.1(a) shows typical contrast saturation functions obtained for PC-cells responding to chromatic and luminance stimuli at a low temporal frequency (1 Hz) and for MC-cells responding to luminance stimuli near 10 Hz. As noted above, PC-cells show a vigorous response to chromatic contrast and a lesser response to luminance contrast while MC-cells show a vigorous response to luminance stimuli. In electrophysiological studies, these functions

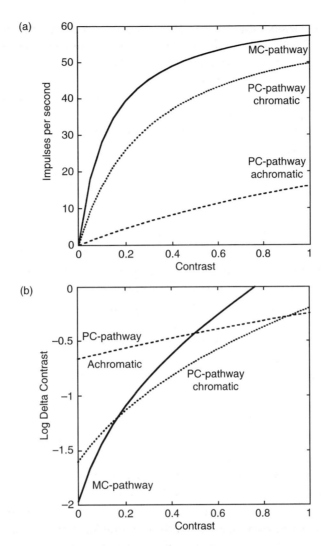

Figure 10.1 (a) Examples of the contrast saturation response for MC- and PC-pathway cells plotted as a function of Michelson contrast for achromatic stimuli and relative contrast for chromatic stimuli. Equation (1) in the text was used for this calculation. (b) Predicted contrast detection and discrimination for the MC-pathway and PC-pathway cells plotted as a function of contrast. Equation (2) in the text was used for this calculation.

are often characterized by their initial slope (R_{max}/C_{sat}), or contrast gain. Figure 10.1(b) shows that contrast gain is much higher for the MC-pathway than for the PC-pathway.

For sinusoidal modulation, on- and off-cells are differentiated by their response phase not by their amplitude response. However contrast responses can also be measured to pulses incremented or decremented from the average retinal illuminance, and a maximal response rate can be calculated in the few milliseconds following pulse onset (Lee *et al.* 1994). In a pulse paradigm, on- and off-amplitude responses are differentiated since the cell types increment their firing rate to their preferred contrast. On-cells respond to luminance increments and off-cells respond to luminance decrements. Contrast saturation functions can be fit for on-cells to contrast increments, and for off-cells to contrast decrements.

Contrast discrimination can be calculated from contrast saturation functions for a criterion increase in firing rate, δ:

$$\Delta C = \delta/R_{max}(C + C_{sat})^2/[C_{sat} - (\delta/R_{max})(C + C_{sat})] \tag{2}$$

where the terms are as described for eqn (1). Figure 10.1 (also) shows the results of eqn (2) using the parameters of eqn (1) and a criterion δ of 5 ips. The absolute contrast threshold is lowest where contrast gain is highest but contrast discrimination deteriorates rapidly as a cell saturates. Thus the MC-cell shows the lowest absolute contrast threshold, but a steeply deteriorating contrast discrimination function. The PC-cell shows a poor absolute contrast threshold to an achromatic stimulus with a very shallow contrast discrimination function. Achromatic contrast discrimination in the PC-cell remains good for a wide range of contrasts. The PC-cell chromatic response is intermediate between the MC- and PC-cell achromatic responses.

In a single cell, the three parameters δ, R_{max}, and C_{sat}, uniquely determine contrast discrimination. In psychophysics however, the psychophysical threshold involves higher order processes that combine inputs from arrays of retinal cells. Therefore, to compare contrast discrimination in humans to single cell data, we considered only the shapes of the contrast discrimination functions not the absolute levels. Further, to make clear the need to differentiate on- and off-response behavior, we considered pulse data and plotted the off-cell responses to decrements and on-cell responses to increments from the background. Figure 10.2 shows predictions that can be compared with psychophysical data.

Figure 10.2 is plotted in a threshold versus illuminance (TVI) format with logarithmic axes. The TVI format is a variant of that proposed by Stiles (1978) for chromatic adaptation. Data plotted in this format obey the Stiles Displacement laws, provided contrast threshold is invariant with luminance level. The position of the data on the abscissa reflects the adapting properties of the background. The position of the data on the ordinate reflects the sensitivity of the observer to the chromaticity and spatio-temporal properties of the test pulse. Figure 10.2 shows predictions taken from Fig. 10.1 with an arbitrary normalization for both axes. The abscissa shows contrast multiplied by retinal illuminance normalized to the background. The ordinate is normalized to an absolute contrast threshold of 1 td. Figure 10.2 shows a two-fold variation of increment and decrement pulses relative to the background. It is clear that PC- and MC-pathway behavior can be differentiated by the characteristic slopes of their contrast discrimination function. Our approach therefore was to measure contrast discrimination on fixed surrounds or backgrounds.

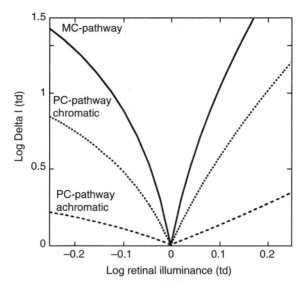

Figure 10.2 Predicted contrast detection and discrimination for MC-pathway to achromatic and PC-pathway cells to achromatic and chromatic pulsed increments or decrements expressed in retinal illuminance rather than contrast. A V-shape function occurs. The abscissa is normalized to the background and the thresholds are normalized to 1 td to allow comparison of the initial slopes in a double logarithmic format.

Methods

The experiment displays

The experimental display was generated on a color monitor system (Miyahara *et al.* 1993; Smith and Pokorny 1996; Pokorny and Smith 1997). Here, we summarize data from several studies conducted over a 6-year period. During this time we employed a diversity of display systems, all calibrated in a uniform manner. Data have proved replicable between display systems. We report our data in a cone troland system (Boynton and Kambe 1980) referable to the Judd (1951) colorimetric system. In this system an L cone troland is the l-chromaticity of a given stimulus multiplied by the luminance in trolands. The surround chromaticity was metameric to the equal energy spectrum. The luminance of the surround was kept at $12 \, \text{cd/m}^2$ throughout the experiments. This luminance corresponded to 115 effective trolands (Le Grand 1968). We used different temporal waveforms. In one experiment the temporal waveform slowly increased and decreased with a period of 1.5 s. In other experiments we used pulsed stimuli that were multiples of the screen refresh rate. The monitor screen was viewed binocularly at 1 m. The observer adapted to the uniform screen at $12 \, \text{cd/m}^2$ for 2 min before the protocols began.

The stimulus array was a ca. 2° square and appeared in a larger surround. The stimulus array consisted of four 1° squares with small separations. One square was designated as the test square; its position changed randomly from trial to trial.

The Paradigms: three paradigms were established

Paradigm 1, the Pulsed-Pedestal condition. The four squares appeared only during the trial period as a pulsed pedestal, with the test square at a higher or a lower retinal illuminance than the other three (Fig. 10.3, upper panel). The observer maintained adaptation to a uniform 115 td screen between trials.

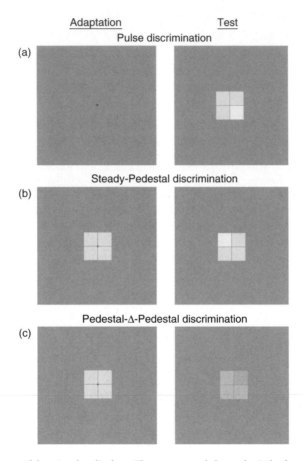

Figure 10.3 Diagram of the stimulus displays. The upper panel shows the Pulsed paradigm in which the observer viewed a homogeneous adaptation field. The stimulus array, three identical squares and a fourth that was either an increment or a decrement from the other three, was pulsed on during a trial. The center panel shows the Steady-Pedestal paradigm. A stimulus array consisting of four identical squares was viewed during the adaptation period. Conditions were run in which the four squares were dimmer than, equal to, and brighter than the surround. On a trial, one of the four squares changed either as an increment or a decrement. The lower panel shows the Pedestal-Δ-Pedestal paradigm. Adaptation is the same as for the Steady-Pedestal paradigm, but on a trial all four squares changed, three in an identical fashion and the fourth as either an increment or a decrement (Δ-Pedestal) from the other three.

Paradigm 2, the Steady-Pedestal condition.   The four squares were present as a steady pedestal within the surround during the entire protocol and the observer adapted for one minute to the surround plus steady pedestal before a measurement began. In this paradigm only the retinal illuminance of the test square changed during the trial period (Fig. 10.3, center panel).

Paradigm 3, the Pedestal-Δ -Pedestal condition.   The protocol was identical to the Steady-Pedestal condition in all respects except that during the trial, the retinal illuminance of the all four squares was incremented or decremented, (a Pedestal-Δ-Pedestal), with the test square incremented or decremented by a different amount (Fig. 10.3, lower panel).

Procedures

All the data were collected combining adaptive staircase procedures with a spatial four-alternative forced choice. These have been described fully (Pokorny and Smith 1997; Smith *et al.* 2000). Two staircases were alternated, allowing thresholds to be assessed in both increment and decrement directions. For the Pulsed- and Steady-Pedestal Paradigms, the pedestal retinal illuminance was fixed for each pair of staircases. For the Pedestal-Δ-Pedestal Paradigm, the pedestal-Δ-pedestal retinal illuminance was fixed for each pair of staircases. The threshold was defined as the average of 10 reversals per staircase. A 45-min protocol allowed measurement of increment and decrement thresholds at four or five pedestal retinal illuminances. The Protocols were repeated and the plotted thresholds represent averages of 4–6 increment/decrement staircases.

Observers

The observers included the authors, graduate students, and naïve observers. All observers had normal visual acuity, with correction and had normal color vision. Rayleigh matches were normal and observers showed superior discrimination ability (FM 100 Hue error scores less than 40). Data were collected from at least three observers for every paradigm. In this summary, data for author VCS are shown in Fig. 10.4; data for naïve observer AC (male, aged 30) are shown in Figs 10.5–10.7. Data for naïve observer IY (female, aged 25) are shown in Figs 10.6 and 10.7; and data for graduate student EK (female, aged 24) are shown in Fig. 10.8.

Results

Chromatic and achromatic data with a 1.5-s raised cosine

In this work, we used a 2.05° square array of four 1° squares with 3.25′ separations. The surround was 9.2° by 8.7° and filled the separations between the squares. The temporal presentation was one cycle of a 1.5-s raised cosine (Pokorny and Smith 1997; Smith *et al.* 2000). These stimulus presentations involved gradual changes in time; there were no abrupt temporal transients. The Pulsed- and Steady-Pedestal Pedestal

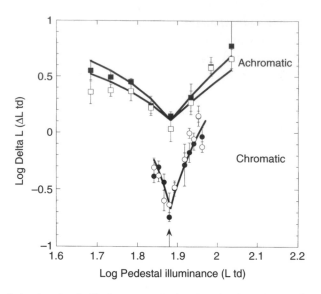

Figure 10.4 Discrimination thresholds for a 1.5-s raised cosine stimulus using equiluminant chromatic or luminance stimuli. Data are expressed in L trolands to facilitate comparison of chromatic and achromatic data. The circles show the data for equiluminant chromatic stimuli, squares show data for achromatic luminance stimuli. Solid symbols show data for the Pulsed-Pedestal Paradigm. Open symbols show data for the Steady-Pedestal Paradigm. The lines represent V-shapes generated by a saturation equation (see text for further explanation). An arrow shows the retinal illuminance of the surround.

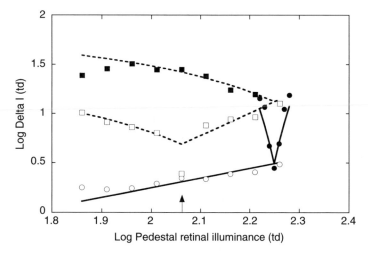

Figure 10.5 Comparison of the discrimination thresholds for the three Paradigms using a 33.33 ms pulse. Open squares show data for the Pulsed-Pedestal Paradigm; open circles show data for the Steady Pedestal Paradigm. Solid symbols show data for the Pedestal-Δ-Pedestal Paradigm. The lines represent fits described in the text. An arrow shows the retinal illuminance of the surround.

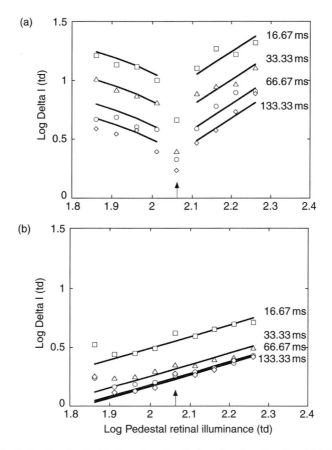

Figure 10.6 Discrimination thresholds for pulse stimuli of varying duration. Panel (a) shows data for the Pulsed-Pedestal Paradigm. Panel (b) shows data for the Steady-Pedestal Paradigm. The solid lines represent fits described in the text.

paradigms were used. In one set of protocols, the pedestal varied in chromaticity at a constant retinal illuminance, equivalent to the 115 td surround. These pedestals appeared greenish (70 L td) to reddish (90 L td) in the achromatic surround. There were 76.5 L td at the surround luminance. In a second set of protocols the pedestal was achromatic and varied in retinal illuminance from 72.5 to 182 td giving a series of luminance contrasts, including decrements and increments from the surround. The graph is plotted in L td and ΔL td to enable comparison of the chromatic and achromatic protocols.

Figure 10.4 shows data for the Pulsed- and Steady-Pedestal Paradigms for chromaticity and luminance variation. Chromatic discrimination data are shown by circles and achromatic discrimination data are shown by squares. Closed symbols are used for the Pulsed-Paradigm and open symbols are used for the Steady-Pedestal Paradigm. All four data sets showed a V-shape with minimum threshold at the 115 td, achromatic

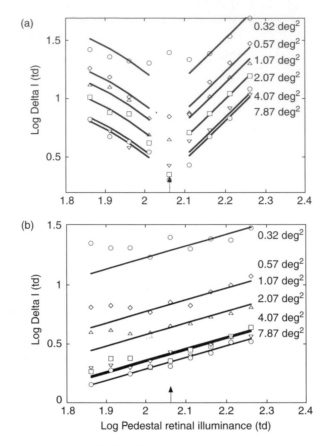

Figure 10.7 Discrimination thresholds for pulse stimuli of varying stimulus array area. Panel (a) shows data for the Pulsed-Pedestal Paradigm. Panel (b) shows data for the Steady-Pedestal Paradigm. The solid lines represent fits described in the text.

surround. The V-shape was steeper for the chromatic than the achromatic data. The thresholds were about one log unit more sensitive for chromatic than for achromatic thresholds. The Pulsed- and Steady-Pedestal paradigms gave very similar data. There was no difference for the chromatic data and a small widening of the V-shape for the achromatic data. Four other observers also showed only small differences between the Pulsed- and Steady-Pedestal Paradigms for both the chromatic (Smith *et al.* 2000) and the achromatic conditions.

The solid lines fit to the data represent two different models. The lines fit to the chromatic data are from a model of chromatic discrimination (Smith *et al.* 2000) that was based specifically on PC-physiology. Since the rest of the paper shows achromatic data, this model will not be further discussed. The lines fit to the achromatic data are based on eqn (2), and will be discussed further below. The use of equiluminant chromatic contrast

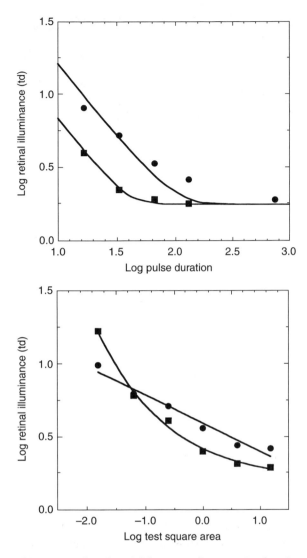

Figure 10.8 Temporal (upper panel) and spatial (lower panel) summation functions for the Pulsed- and Steady-Pedestal Paradigms. For each graph data were averaged from three observers. The upper panel shows predicted thresholds for a 115-td pulse based on the fits of Fig. 10.6, plotted as a function of pulse duration. The solid lines are predicted pulse detection functions derived from temporal sensitivity data (Swanson *et al.* 1987). The lower panel shows predicted thresholds for a 115 td pulse based on the fits of Fig. 10.7 plotted as a function of the area of one square of the four square array. The solid lines have no theoretical basis.

was designed to isolate PC-pathway function. The differences between the chromatic and achromatic contrast discrimination functions are consistent with differences in PC-pathway single cell data for chromatic and achromatic stimuli. We interpret the achromatic data to reveal PC-pathway achromatic contrast behavior. Of note is that the PC-pathway responds to spatio-temporal contrast of the stimulus array in both the Pulsed- and the Steady-Pedestal Paradigms (Smith *et al.* 2000).

Achromatic data with a brief pulse

The use of a 1.5-s raised cosine waveform gave data consistent with PC-pathway mediation for both chromatic and achromatic contrast. This temporal waveform was chosen originally to favor PC-pathway sensitivity, by eliminating temporal transients. We next used a brief, 33.33 ms stimulus better suited to MC-pathway sensitivity (2 refreshes at a 60 Hz frame rate). Data were collected for all three paradigms and are plotted in a TVI format with I in trolands in Fig. 10.5. Different symbols indicate different paradigms. The arrow shows the steady background at 115 td.

Open squares show data for the Pulsed-Pedestal Paradigm. For the Pulsed-Pedestal Paradigm a V-shape was obtained with minimum at the adapting chromaticity. The slope of the arms of the V was shallow similar to the achromatic data of Fig. 10.4. The dashed lines fit to these data points are based on eqn (2), but allowing a free vertical scaling parameter K.

$$\log \Delta I = \log (KI) + \log[(C + C_{sat})^2] - \log\{[C_{sat} - (k)(C + C_{sat})]\} \qquad (3)$$

where I is the surround retinal illuminance (115 td), and k incorporates (δ/R_{max}). The term, k is expected to be small. It is needed primarily for data that start to show saturation. Our data did not show saturation and the term was either set at 0.01 or left at zero for most observers. The fits allowed 2 free parameters, K and C_{sat}. The value of C_{sat} was similar to that of Fig. 10.4 for an achromatic raised cosine, in the range for individual PC-pathway cells. There was a discontinuity at the surround retinal illuminance of 115 td. The data point at 115 td was more sensitive than predicted by the V-shape.

Open circles show the Steady-Pedestal Paradigm. For the Steady-Pedestal Paradigm, the thresholds increased monotonically with the Pedestal retinal illuminance. The solid line fitting these data had a slope of unity with a single vertical scaling constant. These data were quite different from the Steady-Pedestal data of Fig. 10.4 and we interpreted the result to indicate that a different mechanism was mediating the thresholds. The data indicated that this mechanism was yielding thresholds adapted to the Steady-Pedestal luminance; and was not affected by the spatio-temporal contrast signals at the edges of the stimulus array. We postulated that the MC-pathway mediated the Steady-Pedestal data for the brief pulse.

Why did the MC-pathway not respond to the Pulsed-Paradigm when we had chosen a temporal waveform to render it more sensitive than the PC-pathway? Our interpretation is that the pulse step briefly saturated the MC-pathway response. We therefore chose to look at smaller Pedestal contrasts, using the Pedestal-Δ-Pedestal Paradigm. We used a fixed Pedestal of 178 td. Closed circles show data for six small pedestals near 178 td, plotted as a function of total pedestal illuminance. The data (solid circles) showed a steep V-shape. The solid line fit to these data was from eqn (3) and the value of C_{sat} was in the range for individual MC-pathway cells. Closed squares show data for 7 larger Δ Pedestals, pedestal steps expected to saturate the MC-pathway response. The data for these pedestals were fit (dashed line) with eqn (3) and the value of C_{sat} used for the Pulsed-Pedestal data. The data and fits indicated a change in pathway as the Δ Pedestal increased. Pulsed-Pedestal contrasts of 0.02 log unit were sufficient to saturate the MC-pathway for a brief period following pulse onset.

Temporal and spatial summation

Temporal and spatial summation can be assessed for the Pulsed- and Steady-Pedestal paradigms by varying spatio-temporal parameters of the test. According to the vertical displacement laws, these manipulations should displace the psychophysical functions vertically on the threshold axis without changing their shape. To evaluate temporal summation, we varied the pulse duration from 16.6 to 128 ms (Pokorny and Smith 1997). To evaluate spatial summation, we varied the stimulus array size from 0.32° to 7.87° using a fixed 8° surround (Smith *et al.* 2001). Figures 10.6 and 10.7 show the data for temporal and spatial variation respectively with the Pulsed-Pedestal Paradigm in the upper panels and the Steady-Pedestal Paradigm in the lower panels. As expected, the data showed parallel displacements. For both temporal and spatial variation, sensitivity increased as duration or pulse area increased. The Pulsed-Pedestal Paradigm data could be fit using eqn (2) merely by varying the sensitivity scaling factor K in eqn (3). The Steady-Pedestal Paradigm data could similarly be fit by lines of unit slope changing only the sensitivity scaling factor. The data deviated from the Weber line for Pedestal decrements. This effect was more pronounced for smaller test arrays and attributed to preretinal spread light (Smith *et al.* 2001).

The forms of the summation functions could be derived by plotting the predicted thresholds at the background retinal illuminance, as shown in Fig. 10.8. This calculation was based on the average of three observers, and revealed differing temporal (upper panel) and spatial (lower panel) summation properties for the presumed PC- and MC-pathways. Temporal summation extends over 200 ms for the presumed PC-pathway data but is complete within 80 ms for the presumed MC-pathway data. Spatial summation extends continuously for the presumed PC-pathway data but shows a steep decrease with test square area with minimal summation above 1° square for the presumed MC-pathway data. Smith *et al.* (2001) noted that the temporal and spatial summation properties for the presumed MC-pathway are consistent with the classical threshold data in the literature.

Detection and identification

When equiluminant chromatic stimuli are used, the observers can identify the color direction of the pulse at detection threshold (Gille 1984; Mullen and Kulikowski 1990). On a white background, a pulse having a higher l-chromaticity appears "reddish" and a pulse having a lower l-chromaticity appears "greenish". We have noted no difference in detection and identification for chromatic contrast discrimination. If an observer makes the discrimination, he or she also correctly identifies the polarity of the test relative to the Pedestal. Conversely, for achromatic contrast detection the polarity of the contrast ("brighter" or "darker") cannot be identified at detection threshold (Tolhurst and Dealy 1975); a slightly greater luminance (about 0.10 log unit) is needed for polarity identification. A natural question is thus what is the nature of polarity identification for achromatic stimuli using the Pulsed- and Steady-Pedestal Paradigms.

To study this question, we used four interleaved staircases, interleaving a detection criterion and a polarity criterion for both the increment and decrement staircases. On each trial the observer identified the test square and responded whether the test square was brighter or darker than the three Pedestal squares. Figure 10.9 shows the data for a 26.67 ms pulse (two refreshes at a 75-Hz frame rate). For the Pulsed-Pedestal condition, the pulse polarity was correctly identified at the detection threshold. For the Steady-Pedestal Paradigm, the pulse polarity was rarely identified at detection. Polarity identification required approximately 0.15 log unit more contrast than detection of the correct square.

These data suggested that when the PC-pathway is involved in a detection or discrimination, it signals also the polarity both for chromaticity and luminance. This result in turn suggests the existence of cortical centers that can combine information from the four

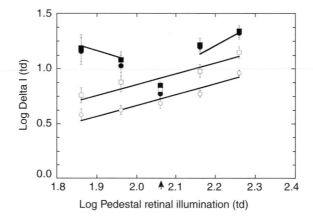

Figure 10.9 Detection/Identification for the Pulsed- and Steady-Pedestal Paradigms. Solid symbols show data for the Pulsed-Pedestal Paradigm. Open symbols show data for the Steady-Pedestal Paradigm. Circles show detection; squares show identification. The solid lines represent fits described in the text.

separate PC-pathway sub-units so that their luminance and chromaticity signals are separated. This concept is sometimes referred to as "demultiplexing". Studies of early visual cortex have not revealed the physiological basis for demultiplexing (Lennie *et al.* 1990). The data for the Steady-Pedestal Paradigm concur with Tolhurst and Dealy (1975). In the Steady-Pedestal Paradigm, both on- and off-channels are at their adaptation point. The stimulus may be detected in either channel. Perhaps a delta Pedestal is required to separate the channels. Alternatively, the MC-pathway may have more noise that could limit the ability to perform identification.

Discussion

In this summary of a 5-year psychophysical study, it is clear that the Pulsed- and Steady-Pedestal Paradigms designed to study contrast discrimination consistently reveal activity in two independent visual processing pathways. We have associated these Paradigms with the PC- and MC-pathway processing streams primarily because of our ability to link psychophysical contrast discrimination ability to the characteristic contrast processing signatures of these retinal pathways.

These studies have revealed achromatic processing abilities of the PC-pathway. The PC-pathway shows excellent contrast discrimination over a wide range of achromatic contrasts. Our studies of equiluminant chromatic discrimination showed that discrimination is controlled by the contrast edge that by virtue of ongoing eye movements generates a continuous retinal contrast signal (Smith *et al.* 2000). Higher order processing is able to make use of these contrast signals. The pathway shows temporal summation over a long time period and spatial summation over a large area. As shown in another paper in this volume (Leonova *et al.*, chapter 11, this volume), the PC-pathway is capable of processing high spatial frequencies. The spatial summation is not matched to the spatial frequency ability and strengthens our conclusion that spatial summation occurs over edge contrasts not field area.

Temporal summation for the Steady-Pedestal paradigm matched temporal resolution for achromatic sinusoidal modulation and temporal summation for the Pulsed-Pedestal paradigm matched temporal resolution for chromatic sinusoidal modulation (Pokorny and Smith 1997). Lee *et al.* (1990) showed that retinal ganglion cells show better temporal resolution than human psychophysics. For the MC-pathway comparison, the difference in both temporal resolution and predicted critical duration was small. These differences might be explained by additional temporal processing of the optic tracts and cells in the primary visual cortex (Lee *et al.* 1990). The difference for the PC-pathway is large. One possibility is that the cortical summation of signal information over extended edges comes at the expense of temporal resolution.

The Pulsed- and Steady-Pedestal Paradigms can be adapted for use in clinical studies. The paradigms were applied to the study of early changes in Retinitis Pigmentosa (Alexander *et al.* 2001). The data revealed deficits in the Steady-Pedestal Paradigm while thresholds in the Pulsed-Pedestal Paradigm were normal. The protocols proved easy to adapt for the clinical use and patients completed the tasks without difficulty. We conclude that these techniques can find use in study of eye disease.

Acknowledgements

We thank our students Hao Sun, Vincent C. W. Sun and Emily Kachinsky who made these studies possible, our other observers for their patience, and Linda Glennie for help in programming and calibrating the monitor systems. This research was supported by USPH Research grants NEI EY07390 and EY00901.

References

Alexander, K. R., Pokorny, J., Smith, V. C., Fishman, G. A., & Barnes, C. S. (2001). Contrast discrimination deficits in retinitis pigmentosa are greater for stimuli that favor the magnocellular pathway. *Vision Research, 41*, 671–83.

Boynton, R. M. & Kambe, N. (1980). Chromatic difference steps of moderate size measured along theoretically critical axes. *Color Research and Application, 5*, 13–23.

Dacey, D. M. (2000). Parallel pathways for spectral coding in primate retina. *Annual Review of Neuroscience, 23*, 743–75.

Derrington, A. M., Krauskopf, J., & Lennie, P. (1984). Chromatic mechanisms in lateral geniculate nucleus of macaque. *Journal of Physiology (London), 357*, 241–65.

Derrington, A. M. & Lennie, P. (1984). Spatial and temporal contrast sensitivities of neurones in lateral geniculate nucleus of macaque. *Journal of Physiology (London), 357*, 219–40.

Gille, J. L. (1984). Evaluation of a general model of color vision using detection and identification of narrowband increments to a neutral background. *Dissertation, University of California, Los Angeles.*

Judd, D. B. (1951). Colorimetry and artificial daylight, in Technical Committee No. 7 Report of Secretariat United States Commission, International Commission on Illumination, Twelfth Session, Stockholm, pp. 1–60.

Kaplan, E. & Shapley, R. M. (1986). The primate retina contains two types of ganglion cells, with high and low contrast sensitivity. *Proceedings of the National Academy of Sciences, USA, 83*, 2755–57.

King-Smith, P. E. & Garden, D. (1976). Luminance and opponent-color contributions to visual detection and adaptation and to temporal and spatial integration. *Journal of the Optical Society of America, 66*, 709–17.

Le Grand, Y. (1968). *Light, Colour, and Vision.* Second Edition (pp. 1–564). London: Chapman and Hall.

Lee, B. B., Pokorny, J., Smith, V. C., & Kremers, J. (1994). Responses to pulses and sinusoids in macaque ganglion cells. *Vision Research, 34*, 3081–96.

Lee, B. B., Pokorny, J., Smith, V. C., Martin, P. R., & Valberg, A. (1990). Luminance and chromatic modulation sensitivity of macaque ganglion cells and human observers. *Journal of the Optical Society of America A, 7*, 2223–36.

Legge, G. (1978). Sustained and transient mechanisms in human vision: temporal and spatial properties. *Vision Research, 18,* 69–81.

Lennie, P., Krauskopf, J., & Sclar, G. (1990). Chromatic mechanisms in striate cortex of macaque. *Journal of Neuroscience, 10*(2), 649–69.

Leonova, A., Pokorny, J., & Smith, V. C. (this volume). Spatial Contrast Sensitivity for Pulsed and Steady-Pedestal Stimuli, Chapter 11.

Miyahara, E., Smith, V. C., & Pokorny, J. (1993). How surrounds affect chromaticity discrimination. *Journal of the Optical Society of America A, 10,* 545–53.

Mullen, K. T. & Kulikowski, J. J. (1990). Wavelength discrimination at detection threshold. *Journal of the Optical Society of America A, 7,* 733–42.

Pokorny, J. & Smith, V. C. (1997). Psychophysical signatures associated with magnocellular and parvocellular pathway contrast gain. *Journal of the Optical Society of America A, 14,* 2477–86.

Purpura, K., Tranchina, D., Kaplan, E., & Shapley, R. M. (1990). Light adaptation in the primate retina: analysis of changes in gain and dynamics of monkey retinal ganglion cells. *Visual Neuroscience, 4,* 75–93.

Reid, R. C. & Shapley, R. M. (1992). Spatial structure of cone inputs to receptive fields in primate lateral geniculate nucleus. *Nature, 356,* 716–18.

Smith, V. C., & Pokorny, J. (1996). Color contrast under controlled chromatic adaptation reveals opponent rectification. *Vision Research, 36,* 3087–105.

Smith, V. C., Pokorny, J., & Sun, H. (2000). Chromatic contrast discrimination: Data and prediction for stimuli varying in L and M cone excitation. *Color Research and Application, 25,* 105–15.

Smith, V. C., Sun, V. C., & Pokorny, J. (2001). Pulse and steady-pedestal contrast discrimination: effect of spatial parameters. *Vision Research, 41,* 2079–88.

Stiles, W. S. (1978). *Mechanisms of Colour Vision.* London: Academic Press.

Swanson, W. H., Ueno, T., Smith, V. C., & Pokorny, J. (1987). Temporal modulation sensitivity and pulse detection thresholds for chromatic and luminance perturbations. *Journal of the Optical Society of America A, 4,* 1992–2005.

Tolhurst, D. J. & Dealy, R. S. (1975). The detection and identification of lines and edges. *Vision Research, 15,* 1367–72.

CHAPTER 11

SPATIAL CONTRAST SENSITIVITY FOR PULSED- AND STEADY-PEDESTAL STIMULI

ANNA LEONOVA, JOEL POKORNY, AND
VIVIANNE C. SMITH

Introduction

Modern studies suggest that spatial vision is mediated by higher order mechanisms tuned to both spatial frequency and orientation (DeValois and DeValois 1988; Graham 1989). The role of the Magnocellular (MC) and Parvocellular (PC) processing streams in providing input to these higher order mechanisms has not been delineated. The spatial modulation contrast sensitivity function shows evidence of both transient and sustained properties (Legge 1978), suggesting involvement of both pathways. Lennie (1993) suggested that processing of luminance information is mediated at low spatial frequencies by the MC-pathway, and at high spatial frequencies by the PC-pathway. This point of view implies that the PC-pathway participates not only in the processing of chromatic information but also of luminance patterns, while the MC-pathway mediates luminance information only. An alternative view is that the MC-pathway alone may mediate processing of low contrast luminance patterns (Shapley and Perry 1986; Lee et al. 1993) while the PC-pathway is engaged principally in chromatic spatial tasks (Lee 1993).

  Evidence differentiating these two hypotheses is controversial. Anatomical evidence indicates that PC-cells maintain the spatial resolution afforded by single cones in the central retina (McMahon et al. 2000). The receptive field centers of PC-cells allow individual cell resolution up to 40 cycles/deg (Lee 1993). The network of the PC-cells has high sampling density and is capable of transmitting high spatial frequency information beyond the retina. The limitation of the PC-cells is their low achromatic contrast sensitivity. Summation at higher levels in the visual system would be needed to match individual cell performance to the psychophysical contrast sensitivity function. The MC-ganglion cells exhibit response properties consistent with human behavior on heterochromatic flicker and minimally distinct border photometric tasks (Lee et al. 1988; Kaiser et al. 1990), suggesting that the MC-system is the physiological substrate for the luminance channel. The MC-cells have high contrast sensitivity and single cells in the fovea show spatial resolution in a similar range to that observed for the PC-cells.

The goal of this study was to evaluate spatial modulation sensitivity under conditions inferred to favor the MC- and PC-pathways.

Methods

Pulsed- and Steady-Pedestal Paradigms

Pokorny and Smith (1997) developed Pulsed- and Steady-Pedestal Paradigms that were interpreted to reflect contrast discrimination mediated by the PC- and MC-pathways. The strategy was to separate the pathways on the basis of their different contrast gain properties. In order to study spatial contrast sensitivity, we modified the paradigms used in the previous work (Pokorny and Smith 1997; Smith *et al.* 2001). We used a large uniform pedestal and superimposed narrow-band spatially localized test patterns of various spatial frequencies. In the Pulsed-Pedestal Paradigm, the pedestal and the test pattern appeared only during the test period. In this case, the pedestal introduces an overall luminance increment or decrement, which is intended to saturate the MC-pathway (see Smith and Pokorny, Chapter 10, this volume). The spatio-temporal step in luminance produced by the pedestal is designed to decrease sensitivity of the entire population of the MC-cells (Crook *et al.* 1987). Thus, detection in the Pulsed-Pedestal Paradigm was inferred to be mediated by the PC-pathway. In the Steady-Pedestal Paradigm the pedestal was displayed for the entire experimental protocol. The use of a uniform pedestal allows adaptation to the pedestal for both pathways. Thus we used temporal presentation to bias activity in the two pathways for the Steady-Pedestal Paradigm. A brief pulse favors mediation by the MC-pathway. A long stimulus without temporal transients favors mediation by the PC-pathway (Pokorny and Smith 1997; Smith and Pokorny, Chapter 10 this volume). The test array was identical in both paradigms; the paradigms differed only in the inter-stimulus adaptation.

Stimuli

The stimuli were generated by a Macintosh PowerPC Computer with a 10-bit Radius video card and were displayed on a 17 NEC MultiSync FE750 color monitor. The display resolution was set at 832×624 and the refresh rate was 75 Hz. The monitor screen was viewed binocularly at 1 m. Observers used a chin rest for head stabilization.

We used a spatially localized, narrow-band pattern and measured contrast detection thresholds as a function of the peak spatial frequency of the pattern. The luminance profile of the pattern was defined by the sixth spatial derivative of a Gaussian (Swanson and Wilson 1985) in the horizontal dimension, with a Gaussian envelope in the vertical dimension.

$$D6 = C/15\{15 - 90(x/\sigma)^2 + 60(x/\sigma)^4 - 8(x/\sigma)^6\}e^{(-x^2/\sigma_x^2)}e^{(-y^2/\sigma_y^2)} \tag{1a}$$

where σ_x and σ_y define spatial frequency components. The effective contrast, C is given by:

$$C = (L_{max} - L_{pedestal})/L_{pedestal} \tag{1b}$$

And the peak spatial frequency is given by:

$$SF_{D6} = 1.73/\pi\sigma_x \qquad (1c)$$

The D6 patterns have a narrow spatial frequency bandwidth: 1.0 octave at half height. The D6 test pattern was presented on a 4° by 4° uniform pedestal. We tested seven peak D6 spatial frequencies: 0.25, 0.5, 1, 2, 4, 8, and 16 cycles deg. The vertical dimension was fixed at 2.5°. The temporal presentation of the test pattern was either a brief pulse of 26.6 ms duration (2 refreshes at the 75 Hz screen rate) or 1 s temporal raised cosine.

The observer first adapted for 2 min to a uniform 12 cd/m² (approximately 115 td, Le Grand 1968) display (in the Pulsed-Pedestal Paradigm) or to the 162 td uniform pedestal presented on the 115 td display (in the Steady-Pedestal Paradigm). Detection thresholds for the D6 pattern were then measured on the 162 td pedestal. A two-interval temporal forced-choice procedure was used in which the pedestal appeared in one interval and the pedestal plus the D6 appeared in another with a 700-ms pause between the two. Double random alternating 3-yes-1-no staircases were used to determine contrast thresholds. Staircases terminated after 10 reversals. Data for the Pulsed- and Steady-Pedestal Paradigms at the two temporal presentation profiles were investigated in separate runs for each temporal presentation and included three replications. The threshold was calculated as the average reversal, averaged over the three replications.

Observers

Three observers with normal color vision and normal visual acuity served as observers. Color vision was assessed with the Ishihara pseudoisochromatic plates and the Neitz OT anomaloscope. Data are shown for one observer, EK (female, aged 25). Results from the other two observers were closely similar.

Results and discussion

In the first experiment, we used Pulsed- and Steady-Pedestal Paradigms with a brief (26.6 ms) stimulus presentation time. In Fig. 11.1, contrast sensitivity is plotted versus the peak spatial frequency of the test pattern. Filled circles show results for the Steady-Pedestal Paradigm and open circles show results for the Pulsed-Pedestal Paradigm. Error bars represent +/− one SE for the three replications. The lines are descriptive fits to the data using sums of exponentials. In the Steady-Pedestal Paradigm, the curve had a predominantly low-pass shape and the sensitivity fell off abruptly beyond the frequency of 8 cycles/deg. In the Pulsed-Pedestal Paradigm, the curve showed a bandpass shape with peak sensitivity near 2 cycles/deg.

The greatest difference between the two curves occurred at low spatial frequencies, while the two curves merged at the higher spatial frequencies. This difference suggested that there are two separable early pathways that mediate processing of spatial frequency up to about 2 cycles/deg. At 8 and 16 cycles/deg, observers showed overlapping sensitivity for the two paradigms, though all three observers showed slightly

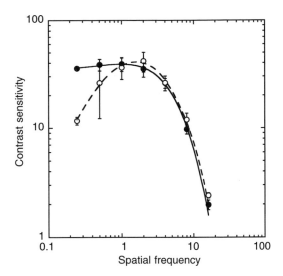

Figure 11.1 Contrast sensitivity for the D6 pattern using the Pulsed- and Steady-Pedestal Paradigms and a 26.6-ms pulse. Data for the Pulsed-Pedestal Paradigm are shown by open circles and dashed line; filled circles and solid line show data for the Steady-Pedestal Paradigm. Error bars represent ±1 SE.

greater sensitivity for the Pulsed-Pedestal Paradigm. We interpreted these results to indicate that the MC-pathway mediated spatial contrast sensitivity at low spatial frequencies while the PC-pathway was more sensitive than the MC-pathway at high spatial frequencies.

Another way to isolate the PC- and MC-pathways is by use of temporal waveforms which take advantage of the differences in the temporal processing between the pathways. Slowly ramped or long stimuli are efficient in isolating the PC-pathway, since MC-pathway units show bandpass temporal contrast sensitivity functions (Lee *et al.* 1990). We examined the sensitivity of the PC-pathway at high spatial frequencies in the second experiment using a 1-s temporal raised cosine to bias sensitivity to the PC-pathway. In Fig. 11.2, filled squares show the results for the Steady-Pedestal Paradigm and open squares show the results for the Pulsed-Pedestal Paradigm. Both functions showed bandpass characteristics with peak spatial frequency near 4 cpd and reflect activity in the inferred PC-pathway. Results depicted by circles are replotted from Fig. 11.1 for comparison.

The bandpass shape of the contrast sensitivity functions in the raised cosine condition resembled closely the curve obtained with the Pulsed-Pedestal Paradigm at short durations. The overall improvement in sensitivity for the Pulsed-Pedestal Paradigm with increased pulse duration is due to temporal summation (Pokorny and Smith 1997). The similarity of the shapes between the curves in the temporal raised cosine condition and the curve obtained with the Pulsed-Pedestal Paradigm (at short durations) supports the hypothesis that high spatial frequency processing is mediated by the PC-pathway.

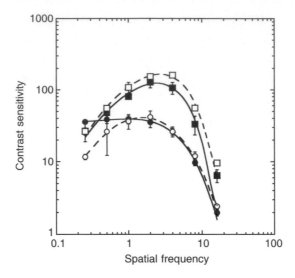

Figure 11.2 Contrast sensitivity for the D6 pattern using a 1 s temporal raised cosine. Data for the Pulsed-Pedestal Paradigm are shown by open squares and dashed line; filled squares and solid line show data for the Steady-Pedestal Paradigm. Results from Fig. 11.1 are replotted for comparison.

For both paradigms the spatial contrast sensitivity functions do not resemble single cell data. For the MC-pathway, single cell data have bandpass characteristics (Derrington and Lennie 1984). The contrast sensitivity functions we showed are the envelope of the sensitivities of the underlying spatial frequency channels. The slight improvement in peak spatial frequency with increased duration might indicate the recruitment of high spatial frequency channels in the raised cosine condition.

In conclusion, the Pulsed- and Steady-Pedestal Paradigms revealed characteristic difference in spatial frequency processing. Our results suggest that Pulsed-Pedestal D6 spatial contrast sensitivity functions are mediated by the PC-pathway. Steady-Pedestal contrast sensitivity functions are mediated by the MC-pathway at low spatial frequencies and by the PC-pathway above ~4 cycles/deg. These data support the hypothesis of a major role for the PC-pathway in achromatic spatial vision.

Acknowledgments

NEI Research Grant EY00901 supported this research.

References

Crook, J. M., Lee, B. B., Tigwell, D. A., & Valberg, A. (1987). Thresholds to chromatic spots of cells in the macaque geniculate nucleus as compared to detection sensitivity in man. *Journal of Physiology: London, 392,* 193–211.

Derrington A. M. & Lennie, P. (1984). Spatial and temporal contrast sensitivities of neurones in lateral geniculate nucleus of macaque. *Journal of Physiology (London)*, *357*, 219–40.

DeValois, R. L. & DeValois, K. K. (1988). *Spatial Vision*. New York: Oxford University Press.

Graham, N. V. S. (1989). *Visual Pattern Analyzers*. New York: Oxford University Press.

Kaiser, P. K., Lee, B. B., Martin, P. R., & Valberg, A. (1990). The physiological basis of the minimally distinct border demonstrated in the ganglion cells of the macaque retina. *Journal of Physiology (London)*, *422*, 153–83.

Le Grand, Y. (1968). *Light, Colour and Vision*. Second Edition, (pp. 1–564). London: Chapman and Hall.

Lee, B. B. (1993). Macaque ganglion cells and spatial vision. *Progress in Brain Research*, *95*, 33–43.

Lee, B. B., Martin, P. R., & Valberg, A. (1988). The physiological basis of heterochromatic flicker photometry demonstrated in the ganglion cells of the macaque retina. *Journal of Physiology (London)*, *404*, 323–47.

Lee, B. B., Martin, P. R., Valberg, A., & Kremers, J. (1993). Physiological mechanisms underlying psychophysical sensitivity to combined luminance and chromatic modulation. *Journal of the Optical Society of America A*, *10*, 1403–12.

Lee, B. B., Pokorny, J., Smith, V. C., Martin, P. R., & Valberg, A. (1990). Luminance and chromatic modulation sensitivity of macaque ganglion cells and human observers. *Journal of the Optical Society of America A*, *7*, 2223–36.

Legge, G. (1978). Sustained and transient mechanisms in human vision: temporal and spatial properties. *Vision Research*, *18*, 69–81.

Lennie, P. (1993). Roles of M and P Pathways. In R. Shapley & D. M. K. Lam (Eds), *Contrast Sensitivity*, (pp. 201–13). Cambridge, MA: MIT Press.

McMahon, M. J., Lankheet, M. J., Lennie, P., & Williams, D. R. (2000). Fine structure of parvocellular receptive fields in the primate fovea revealed by laser interferometry. *Journal of Neuroscience*, *20*(5), 2043–53.

Pokorny, J. & Smith, V. C. (1997). Psychophysical signatures associated with magnocellular and parvocellular pathway contrast gain. *Journal of the Optical Society of America A*, *14*, 2477–86.

Shapley R. & Perry, V. H. (1986). Cat and monkey retinal ganglion cells and their visual functional roles. *Trends in Neurosciences*, *9*, 229–35.

Smith, V. C., Sun, V. C., & Pokorny, J. (2001). Pulse and steady-pedestal contrast discrimination: effect of spatial parameters. *Vision Research*, *41*, 2079–88.

Swanson, W. H. & Wilson, H. R. (1985). Eccentricity dependence of contrast matching and oblique masking. *Vision Research*, *25*, 1285–95.

CHAPTER 12

CHROMATIC ASSIMILATION: EVIDENCE FOR A NEURAL MECHANISM

STEVEN K. SHEVELL AND DINGCAI CAO

Introduction

A single wavelength presented on a dark background has a characteristic color but the same wavelength can appear a very different hue when seen within a context of other nearby light. Context affects the neural representation of the visual stimulus, and thus its appearance.

Chromatic induction is the shift in color appearance caused by nearby light. Most research on chromatic induction has focused on *color contrast*, which is a shift in appearance away from the color of the nearby light (e.g. Jameson and Hurvich 1964; Ware and Cowan 1982; Shevell 1987; Zaidi *et al.* 1992). For example, a patch that appears achromatic in the dark is perceived as greenish when viewed within a large long-wavelength, red-appearing surround. With more complex context composed of repetitive patterns, however, appearance can shift in the opposite direction, toward the color of nearby light (Wyszecki 1986); this is *chromatic assimilation*. Assimilation has been studied surprisingly little, despite the clear shifts in appearance that it causes (Fig. 12.1).

Two general classes of explanation have been proposed for assimilation: non-neural and neural. Non-neural explanations include eye movements, chromatic aberration, and spread light. These factors cause a fraction of the contextual light to fall in the retinal area of the stimulus judged in color. Smith *et al.* (2001) found that assimilation from isoluminant square-wave gratings at higher spatial frequencies can be accounted for by spread light. Most studies of assimilation, however, conclude that neural processes contribute to it (Helson 1963; Fach and Sharpe 1986; Moulden *et al.* 1993; De Weert and Spillmann 1995). The nature of the neural mechanism, however, is often vague or untested.

The present study has two aims. First, a new stimulus is introduced to minimize the influence of prereceptoral factors. Most previous studies of assimilation used contextual light covering half or more of the whole stimulus area (e.g. inducing and test fields that were alternating bars of a square-wave grating). In comparison, the inducing light in various conditions here covers only 9–37 per cent of the whole area. The measurements

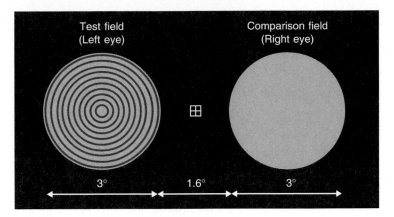

Figure 12.1 See also colour plate section. Schematic of haploscopically presented test and comparison fields. Observers set the uniform comparison field to match the appearance of the test background.

show that chromatic assimilation from this contextual light cannot be explained by prereceptoral factors. Second, the proportion of the whole area covered by inducing light was varied systematically to test for neural summation over the stimulus area. The measurements are generally consistent with neural summation.

Method

Apparatus

Stimuli were presented on a colorimetrically calibrated Radius PressView 17-inch video display, which was controlled by a Macintosh G4 computer. The resolution was 832×624 pixels and the refresh rate was 75 Hz non-interlaced. Stimuli on the display were viewed through a haploscope (viewing distance 115 cm). An adjustable chin and forehead rest was used to maintain a stable head position. For details of calibration, see Shevell and Wei (1998).

Stimuli

Separate comparison and test fields were perceived to appear side by side, separated by 1.6° (Fig. 12.1). The comparison field was a uniform circular disk with diameter 3°. The test field was a circle of the same diameter but with inserted inducing light composed of thin concentric rings. The test field had luminance 4 cd/m² and l, s chromaticity 0.62, 0.14 (MacLeod and Boynton 1979; units of s here are normalized to 1.0 for equal energy white). Without the inducing-rings, the circular test appeared green. Test luminance and chromaticity were held fixed throughout the experiments.

Inducing-rings inserted into the circular test were varied in width, spacing, chromaticity, and luminance. Ring width was 2 or 4 min, and spacing between rings was 4, 6, 8, 12, or 16 min. For the 2-min-wide rings, the proportion of the stimulus covered by inducing light ranged from 9 per cent (16-min separation) to 32 per cent (4-min separation); for 4-min-wide rings, the analogous values were 13–37 per cent (the smallest separation was 6 min with 4-min-wide inducing-rings). The inducing-rings appeared either blue (l, s chromaticity 0.53, 9.5) or red (l, s chromaticity 0.83, 0.09). The luminance of the rings was 3, 5, or 8 cd/m^2.

Procedure

The appearance of the test field with inserted inducing-rings was measured by haplo-scopic matching. In each session, the rings' width and separation were fixed, with chro-maticity and luminance varied randomly from trial to trial. Observers dark adapted for 3 min at the beginning of each run. Each chromaticity and luminance combination then was repeated four times within the session. At the beginning of each trial, the comparison field was assigned a random starting chromaticity and luminance. Observers matched the perceived color of the test by adjusting the hue, saturation and brightness of the uni-form, haploscopically presented comparison field, by pressing buttons on a pad sensed by the computer. Each condition was repeated in four separate sessions, on different days. The order of sessions was randomized. Results from the four days' measurements were averaged for each inducing-ring width, separation, chromaticity, and luminance. Standard errors were calculated using the mean value from each of the four sessions.

Observers

Two observers participated in the study. Both D. C., an author, and P. M., who was naïve about the purpose of the experiments, were experienced psychophysical observers. The observers were age 30 and 32, and had normal color vision as determined using an anomaloscope.

Results and discussion

Inducing-field luminance

Prereceptoral processes cause some fraction of the inducing light to fall in the retinal area of the test region judged in color. This implies that scaling the luminance of inducing light has a lawful effect on light in the test region, so if this light mediates chromatic assimilation then matches set by the observer will lawfully follow the inducing-light luminance. Measurements for two observers, however, show that the inducing luminance fails to show this lawful relation (Fig. 12.2).

Consider the magnitude of assimilation with "blue" 2-min-wide inducing-rings (4-min spacing between rings) at luminance 3 cd/m^2 (smallest open square). Calculation shows that increasing inducing luminance 2.67 times from 3 to 8 cd/m^2, should increase the matching s coordinate by at least two-fold, if prereceptoral processes mediate assim-ilation (see Appendix). For both observers, the measured increase is far less (31 per cent for observer P. M., 36 per cent for D. C.; large open squares in Fig. 12.2). For the "red"

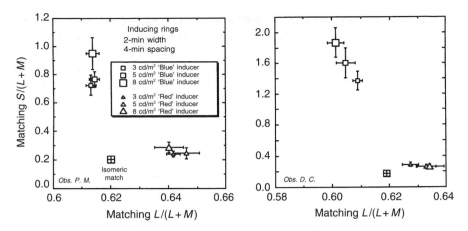

Figure 12.2 Haploscopic matches to the test background, presented with no inducing rings (isomeric match, square-with-plus), "blue" inducing rings (squares) or "red" inducing rings (triangles). Inducing rings were 2-min wide and spaced 4 min apart, at luminance 3, 5, or 8 cd/m² (see legend). Each panel shows results for a different observer.

inducing rings, the color matches do not differ significantly as a function of inducing luminance (triangles); for observer P. M., assimilation did not increase monotonically with inducing luminance. A similar conclusion follows from results with 4-min-wide "blue" inducing rings (data not shown): rather than the lawful increase of at least two-fold, the increase with 6-min spacing was −0.08 per cent (nonmonotonic) for P. M. and 41 per cent for D. C.; with 8-min spacing, analogous values were 7 per cent for P. M. and 40 per cent for D. C. None of these measurements is consistent with a prereceptoral explanation for assimilation.

Inducing-field relative area

Several authors have suggested assimilation is mediated by some kind of neural summation (Helson 1963; Hurvich and Jameson 1974; Moulden *et al.* 1993). This can be tested directly by varying the fraction of the test-eye stimulus covered by inducing light, using a fixed inducing chromaticity and luminance ("blue" inducing-rings at 5 cd/m² are used here). While simple spatial averaging of light cannot account for assimilation, because physical averaging implies a lawful effect of inducing luminance that was not found in Fig. 12.2, averaging of neural signals that do *not* linearly increase with luminance is a viable model. For example, inducing luminance would not affect the appearance of the test if neural averaging occurs in luminance-independent chromatic pathways $s = S/(L + M)$ and $l = L/(L + M)$. More generally, measurements of color appearance with fixed inducing-light chromaticity, width, and luminance (but with varying ring spacing) can be used to test for neural spatial averaging, regardless of the relation between neural response and luminance.

Suppose the neural signal mediating the appearance of the test is the spatial average of neural response $f(I)$ for inducing light I of fixed size, chromaticity, and luminance; and response $g(T)$ for light T in the test region. The neural responses $f(I)$ and $g(T)$ can be arbitrary nonlinear functions. If the inducing light covers proportion P of the whole area, then the average neural response over the whole area is $f(I) \times P + g(T) \times (1 - P)$. Rearranging terms, the neural average is $g(T) + P[f(I) - g(T)]$, a linear function of the proportion of area, P, covered by the inducing light. With no inducing light ($P = 0$), the neural "average" is simply $g(T)$. Thus, the change in the neural average caused by introducing inducing light covering area P is $\{g(T) + P[f(I) - g(T)]\} - \{g(T)\} = P[f(I) - g(T)]$.

A parameter free test of the neural summation model follows from normalizing each change in neural average by the change in the neural average when P is largest (P_{max}). For example, with the 4-min-wide inducing-ring, P_{max} is 0.37. Normalizing in this way gives the relative change in average neural response for inducing light that covers area P:

$$\{P[f(I) - g(T)]\}/\{P_{max}[f(I) - g(T)]\} = P/P_{max}. \tag{1}$$

Thus, if chromatic assimilation depends on the average of the neural responses from inducing light and test light, weighted by their relative areas, then the shift in appearance should be directly proportional to P/P_{max}.

This can be tested directly with the color assimilation measurements, which were found to be in the direction of the inducing chromaticity. The magnitude of assimilation, therefore, can be quantified by the distance between the appearance match with a particular inducing light and the match with no inducing light (isomeric match). The neural summation model implies greatest assimilation when the inducing light covers the largest proportion of the test area (i.e. at P_{max}). This was indeed the case empirically. Color shifts for other areas of inducing light were normalized to this value, giving relative measurements of assimilation scaled between 0 (no inducing light, isomeric match) and 1.0 (P_{max}). The relative magnitude of assimilation is plotted in Fig. 12.3 as a function of P/P_{max}, for 2-min-wide and 4-min-wide inducing-rings (open and solid circles, respectively). The values fall close to the 45° line, as required by the neural summation model.

In sum, chromatic assimilation scales closely with inducing-light relative area but not with luminance. While assimilation tends to increase with inducing luminance, the magnitude of increase is far less than predicted by prereceptoral factors. Assimilation, therefore, depends on a neural process. Failure of the lawful relation between color appearance and inducing luminance, however, does not imply that no inducing light falls in the test area. The combined effects of (i) neural summation within luminance-independent chromatic pathways and (ii) non-neural factors that cause a fraction of inducing light to fall in the test area may account for the proportional relation between assimilation and relative inducing area, and the weak relation between assimilation and luminance.

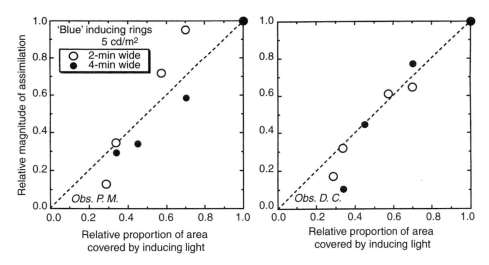

Figure 12.3 Relative magnitude of assimilation (defined in text) as a function of the relative proportion of the test-field area covered by inducing light. Results are shown for 5 cd/m^2 "blue" inducing rings, 2-min wide (open circles) or 4-min wide (solid circles). Each panel shows results for a different observer.

Acknowledgment

This research was supported by NIH grant EY-04802. Publication supported in part by an unrestricted grant to the Department of Ophthalmology & Visual Science from Research to Prevent Blindness.

Appendix

Let the L-, M-, and S-cone stimulations from the test (inducing) light be L_T, M_T, and S_T (L_I, M_I, and S_I). Prereceptoral processes cause some of the inducing light to fall in the retinal area of the test. If the fraction of inducing light, α, that falls in the test region is independent of wavelength (an assumption relaxed below), then the total cone stimulations in the test region are $L_{TOTAL} = L_T + \alpha L_I$, $M_{TOTAL} = M_T + \alpha M_I$ and $S_{TOTAL} = S_T + \alpha S_I$. As $s = S/(L + M)$ by definition, and $L + M$ is luminance (LUM), $S = s$ LUM. Therefore,

$$s_{TOTAL} = (S_T + \alpha S_I)/(L_T + \alpha L_I + M_T + \alpha M_I)$$

$$= (s_T \text{LUM}_T + \alpha s_I \text{LUM}_I)/(\text{LUM}_T + \alpha \text{LUM}_I) \tag{1}$$

The lawful prediction concerns the level of s that should be set with inducing level 8 cd/m^2 ($s_{TOTAL,8}$), given the setting of s with inducing level 3 cd/m^2 ($s_{TOTAL,3}$). With the measurement of $s_{TOTAL,3}$ and known quantities s_T, s_I, LUM_T, and LUM_I set by the experimenter, the value of α can be determined from eqn (1).

The ratio of the s settings, $s_{\text{TOTAL},8}/s_{\text{TOTAL},3}$, predicted by prereceptoral processes is specified from eqn (1), given the value of α determined from the measurement $s_{\text{TOTAL},3}$. Substituting the luminance of the test (4 cd/m^2), the ratio is

$$s_{\text{TOTAL},8}/s_{\text{TOTAL},3} = [(4s_T + 8\alpha s_I)/(4 + 8\alpha)]/[(4s_T + 3\alpha s_I)/(4 + 3\alpha)]. \quad (2)$$

The range of α determined for all of the 'blue' inducing-ring conditions at luminance 3 cd/m^2 over both observers is 0.050–0.235, which from eqn (2) gives a smallest predicted ratio $s_{\text{TOTAL},8}/s_{\text{TOTAL},3}$ of 2.03 (more than a two-fold increase).

As a generalization, suppose that prereceptoral processes result in a larger proportion of inducing light absorbed by S cones than M or L cones in the test area. Then, $L_{\text{TOTAL}} = L_T + \alpha L_I$ and $M_{\text{TOTAL}} = M_T + \alpha M_I$ are unchanged, but S_{TOTAL} can be larger: $S_{\text{TOTAL}} = S_T + (\alpha + \delta)S_I$, where $0 \leq \delta$. Now the ratio is

$$s_{\text{TOTAL},8}/s_{\text{TOTAL},3} = [(4s_T + 8(\alpha+\delta)s_I)/(4+8\alpha)]/[(4s_T + 3(\alpha+\delta)s_I)/(4+3\alpha)]. \quad (3)$$

For all values of δ greater than 0, the value of the ratio $s_{\text{TOTAL},8}/s_{\text{TOTAL},3}$ increases with δ (i.e. $d(s_{\text{TOTAL},8}/s_{\text{TOTAL},3})/d\delta > 0$). Therefore, if a larger proportion of inducing light is absorbed by S than by M or L cones in the test area, the ratio $s_{\text{TOTAL},8}/s_{\text{TOTAL},3}$ will be even larger than the ratio found by assuming α is identical for all three cone-types.

References

De Weert, C. M. M. & Spillmann, L. (1995) Assimilation: Asymmetry between brightness and darkness? *Vision Research*, **35**, 1413–19.

Fach, C. & Sharpe, L. T. (1986) Assimilative hue shifts in color gratings depend on bar width. *Perception & Psychophysics*, **40**, 412–18.

Helson, H. (1963) Studies of anomalous contrast and assimilation. *Journal of the Optical Society of America*, **53**, 179–84.

Hurvich, L. M. & Jameson, D. (1974) Opponent processes as a model of neural organization. *American Psychologist*, **29**, 88–102.

Jameson, D. & Hurvich, L. M. (1964) Theory of brightness and color contrast in human vision. *Vision Research*, **4**, 135–54.

MacLeod, D. I. A. & Boynton, R. M. (1979) Chromaticity diagram showing cone excitation by stimuli of equal luminance. *Journal of the Optical Society of America*, **69**, 1183–5.

Moulden, B., Kingdom, F., & Wink, B. (1993) Colour pools, brightness pools, assimilation and the spatial resolving power of the human colour-vision system. *Perception*, **22**, 343–51.

Shevell, S. K. (1987) Processes mediating color contrast. *Die Farbe*, **34**, 261–8.

Shevell, S. K. & Wei, J. (1998) Chromatic induction: Border contrast or adaptation to surrounding light? *Vision Research*, **38**, 1561–6.

Smith, V. C., Jin, P., & Pokorny, J. (2001) The role of spatial frequency in color induction. *Vision Research*, **41**, 1007–21.

Ware, C. & Cowan, W. (1982) Changes in perceived color due to chromatic interactions. *Vision Research*, **22**, 1353–62.

Wyszecki, G. (1986) Color Appearance. In K. R. Boff, L. Kaufman, and J.P. Thomas (Eds) *Handbook of Perception and Human Performance, Vol I: Sensory Processes and Perception*, pp. 9-1–9-57. New York: Wiley.

Zaidi, Q., Yoshimi, B., Flanigan, N., & Canova, A. (1992) Lateral interactions within color mechanisms in simultaneous induced contrast. *Vision Research*, 32, 1695–707.

CHAPTER 13

REACTION TIMES TO STIMULI IN ISOLUMINANT COLOUR SPACE

D. J. MCKEEFRY, N. R. A. PARRY, AND I. J. MURRAY

Introduction

Simple Reaction Times (RTs) are a useful measure of supra-threshold information processing. In this paper we investigate the relationship between RTs and stimulus chromaticity. Central to this is the efficiency with which the stimulus isolates the sustained activity of the chromatic system and minimizes contributions from the luminance system. For example, in studies where chromatic stimuli were confounded with luminance increments or flickered at fast rates ($\approx$15 Hz), RT was shown to be independent of wavelength (Holmes 1926; Lit *et al.* 1971; Ueno *et al.* 1985). Better isolation of the chromatic visual system can be achieved by manipulation of stimulus parameters (see: Piéron 1932; Mollon and Krauskopf 1973; Nissen and Pokorny 1977; Schwartz and Loop 1983; Ueno *et al.* 1985; Parry 2001). When this is achieved under neutral adaptation, RTs exhibit a strong dependence on wavelength, with the longest RTs occurring at approximately 570 nm and decreasing at longer and shorter wavelengths (Nissen and Pokorny 1977; Ueno *et al.* 1985). However, recent experiments cast doubt on the view that there is a strong dependency of RT on stimulus chromaticity even when achromatic or luminance intrusions are strictly controlled (Smithson and Mollon 2001*a*).

   In this study we re-examine the issue of RT variation with stimulus chromaticity and explore how it relates to the properties of the physiological pathways that process chromatic information. When utilizing chromatic stimuli that modulate along different axes in colour space it is important, particularly when looking at the effects of supra-threshold stimuli, to consider how to scale stimulus intensity. Previous experiments have generally assessed the effects of wavelength on RT using saturated (often spectral) stimuli. Therefore, a specific aim of this study was to examine how the metric used to scale coloured stimuli influences the variation in RT with chromaticity. There are several approaches to equating chromatic stimuli and in this series of experiments we examined the effects of chromaticity on RT when stimuli were scaled in one of three ways. First, we employed a metric that has been adopted in numerous physiological experiments where the stimuli were scaled in terms of the maximum excursion permitted by the colour gamut of the monitor (e.g. Derrington *et al.* 1984; Rabin *et al.* 1994). In the second experiment the stimuli were equated in terms of the modulation of cone excitation produced. In a third experiment, chromatic stimuli were scaled in terms of equal multiples above detection threshold.

Methods

Simple reaction times (RTs) were recorded to the onset of a coloured patch on an isoluminant neutral background (CIE 1931 chromaticity co-ordinates $x = 0.310, y = 0.316$, mean luminance 12.5 cd/m^2). Stimuli were presented foveally on a high-resolution colour graphics monitor (Sony GDM500) by means of a Cambridge Research Systems VSG 2/5 card which has an on board timer allowing RTs to be measured with a resolution of <1 ms.

Stimuli

The chromatic stimuli lay on an isoluminant plane that is analogous to the MBDKL colour space (MacLeod and Boynton 1979; Derrington *et al.* 1984). In this space, the angle ϕ defines a specific chromatic axis (see Fig. 13.1(a)). Eight axes in total were investigated ($\phi = 0°, 53°, 90°, 130°, 180°, 233°, 270°$, and $310°$), four of which are of particular importance. $0°$ and $180°$ produce stimuli that minimally activate S-cones and produce only L- and M-cone excitation. Conversely, $90°$ and $270°$ isolate S-cone activity whilst minimally activating L- and M-cones. Four other axes were also used where the relative activation of the L-, M-, and S-cones varied (see Fig. 13.1(b)).

Stimulus contrasts were specified using the equation:

$$\text{RMS cone contrast} = \sqrt{((L_c^2 + M_c^2 + S_c^2)/3)} \tag{1}$$

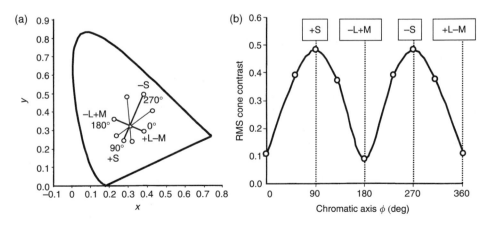

Figure 13.1 (a) 1931 CIE chromaticity diagram showing the location in colour space of the eight chromatic axes that were tested. Open circles represent the gamut limit in each direction. The location of the background (illuminant C, $x = 0.310$, $y = 0.316$) is also indicated. (b) RMS cone contrast of the eight stimuli expressed as a function of chromatic axis, ϕ (see text for details).

where L_c, M_c, and S_c are the Weber cone contrasts produced by each stimulus on the neutral background. Cone excitations were calculated using the Judd-modified 1931 CIE values in conjunction with the Smith and Pokorny (1975) fundamentals. Stimuli were calibrated with a Photo Research PR650 spectral photometer.

Each stimulus had a radially symmetrical gaussian spatial profile (SD = 0.2°) with hue modulation maximum at the centre. The background subtended 22 × 17° at the 100 cm viewing distance. The effects of temporal transients were minimized by presenting the stimulus with a raised cosinusoidal temporal profile so that hue modulation reached a maximum 190 ms after stimulus onset. The stimulus then remained at the set chromatic contrast for a further 190 ms and was then reduced cosinusoidally over the final 190 ms of the presentation.

Procedure

Each chromatic axis was tested in turn starting with $\phi = 0°$, using the following protocol. After 5-min adaptation to the background, isoluminance was determined using heterochromatic flicker photometry. Detection threshold for the chromatic stimulus was then measured using a method of adjustment (MOA) procedure. In a single trial, 32 RTs were recorded to the same stimulus with successive stimuli being randomly presented between 1000 and 3000 ms after the subject's response, or after 5 s if no response was made. The subjects were instructed to respond as fast as possible to the appearance of a stimulus on the screen. Anticipatory responses constituted fewer than 1.5 per cent of the total number of RT measures recorded and did not exhibit any bias to towards any particular chromatic axis. At the completion of a trial the mean and standard error of the RTs were calculated, omitting responses outside the range 150–1200 ms. RT distributions to the rapid onset of visual stimuli are frequently skewed. However, this was not the case in this study, probably owing in some part to the fact that stimulus onset is cosinusoidal rather than square wave, as is more typical of standard RT paradigms. The one-sample Kolmogorov–Smirnov test indicated that the RT distributions obtained were not significantly different from a normal distribution. Furthermore, analysis of RT mean and median data produced the same results.

For each axis, six contrast levels were employed. These levels were evenly spaced on a reciprocal contrast scale that spanned from detection threshold to the maximum modulation possible on the monitor for each particular chromatic axis. Experiments were carried out on three colour-normal subjects (D. McK., N. R. A. P., and I. J. M.) and the main findings were repeated on a fourth naive observer.

Results

Scaling to maximum chromatic excursion

Figure 13.2(a) shows the variation of RT with chromatic axis for subject D. McK., using the maximum chromatic contrast available for each axis. Owing to space constraints, each figure shows only one subject's data. However, all three subjects produced similar

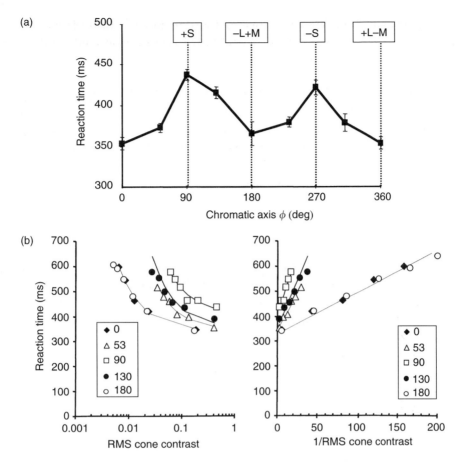

Figure 13.2 (a) Simple RTs plotted as a function of chromatic axis for subject D. McK. The chromatic stimuli in this instance are equated on the basis of their maximum possible excursion from the background for this colour monitor. The stimuli used in this experiment are equivalent to the empty circles shown in Fig. 13.1(a). (b) RTs plotted as a function of RMS cone contrast for five different axes in colour space ($\phi = 0°, 53°, 130°$, and $180°$, subject D. McK). The data on the left hand side have been fitted by the function $RT = RT_0 + k \cdot 1/C$ (see text). On the right hand side the figure also shows the data plotted as a function of 1/RMS cone contrast: the functions exhibit a highly linear relationship for all axes tested.

results in all experiments. There is a statistically significant variation of RT with stimulus chromaticity ($p < 0.05$; ANOVA combined with a Tukey–HSD post hoc test of signi-ficance). The longest RTs occur at $\phi = 90°$ and $270°$, corresponding to the S-varying axis. The shortest RTs were obtained for $0°$ and $180°$ where L- and M-cone activity is maximized. With intermediate axes, RTs in between the two extremes are obtained. The data suggest that RTs to chromatic stimuli are dependent upon the degree of activation

produced in the L/M and S/(L+M) colour opponent pathways. These have been identified as separate processing channels for colour information in the primate pre-cortical
visual pathway (Derrington *et al.* 1984).

Scaling to equal cone contrast

Arguably, a more physiologically meaningful approach to equating chromatic stimuli is
to express their strength in terms of equal magnitudes of cone modulation.

Figure 13.2(b) shows how RT typically varies as a function of RMS cone contrast for
chromatic stimuli along five of the eight axes investigated. For all chromatic axes the RT
versus RMS cone contrast can be described by the following function:

$$RT = RT_0 + k \cdot 1/C \tag{2}$$

where RT $=$ reaction time, $RT_0 =$ the asymptotic (absolute) RT, $k =$ slope and $C =$
RMS cone contrast (Plainis and Murray 2000). Essentially this is a modification of
Piéron's (1952) general equation for RT versus intensity, that is, a power function (here
the exponent is -1). In the same figure the data are also plotted as a function of the
reciprocal RMS cone contrast and for all subjects, the high correlation co-efficient (mean
$r^2 = 0.96$) indicates it is a satisfactory description of the data. All functions obtained
were of this basic form, varying only in slope and y-intercept.

Equation (2) was used to compute RTs for equal RMS cone contrasts along each of the
chromatic axes tested. The results of such computations are shown in Fig. 13.3(a) and
indicate how RT varies as a function of chromatic axis (ϕ) when the stimuli are equated
in terms of the magnitude of cone contrast they produce. As can be observed shortest

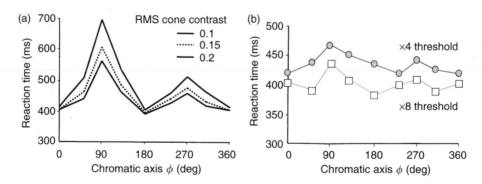

Figure 13.3 (a) RTs produced by chromatic stimuli of varying axis in colour space but each with the
same RMS cone contrast. These iso-contrast functions are computed by extrapolation from the linear
regression analysis of the RT versus 1/contrast functions (see Fig. 13.2(b)). (b) RTs plotted as a
function of chromatic axis for stimuli equated across all chromatic axes in terms of multiples above
detection threshold. Here, RTs measured to stimuli at 4× and 8× above detection threshold are shown
(subject D. McK.).

RTs occur for stimuli that isolate L- and M-cone activity (0° and 180°) and the longest RTs for S-cone isolating stimuli (90° and 270°).

Scaling to multiples of detection threshold

Another method employed to scale the intensity of chromatic stimuli is to set them at equal multiples above MOA detection threshold (Webster and Mollon 1994). We measured RTs at $4\times$ and $8\times$ above detection threshold for each chromatic axis. Figure 13.3(b) shows how RT varies as a function of ϕ for chromatic stimuli scaled in this fashion. There are significant differences in RT as a function of chromatic axis ($p < 0.05$; ANOVA combined with a post hoc Tukey–HSD test). Once again the slowest RTs occur along the S-cone isolating axes, reaching a maximum when $\phi = 90°$.

Discussion

The variation of simple RT with chromaticity would appear to be strongly dependent upon the extent to which the stimulus activates either the L/M or S/(L+M) colour opponent mechanisms. The dominant influence of these two mechanisms suggests that pre-cortical as opposed to cortical colour processing has a strong influence on the RT to chromatic isoluminant stimuli. This conclusion is not qualitatively altered by the three stimulus-scaling methods we compared.

The finding that RTs to tritan stimuli are slowest whilst those for L/M stimuli are fastest is consistent with electrophysiological data that suggest that S-cone mediated signals arrive at the primary visual cortex later than information mediated by the L/M opponent system (Cottaris and DeValois 1998). Primate retinal ganglion cell physiology may provide two explanations. One possibility is that long RTs to tritan (S-cone isolating) stimuli are the result of reduced involvement of magnocellular neurons which have reduced sensitivity to tritan stimuli (Valberg et al. 1992) and have faster conduction velocities than their parvocellular counterparts. Another possibility is that slow RTs to S-cone isolating stimuli may be related to the properties of the koniocellular pathway which is known to mediate S-cone information (see Hendry and Reid 2000 for a review). Neurons in the koniocellular pathway have low synaptic divergence in area V1 and possess more sluggish temporal responses than parvocellular neurons which mediate L- and M-cone information (Irvin et al. 1986; however see Solomon et al. 1999; for a counterview).

In direct opposition to this view of a sluggish S-cone mediated pathway are reports that imply that this pathway is just as fast as the L/M system (McKeefry et al. 2001; Smithson and Mollon 2001 a,b). A common feature of these studies is the recognition that even isoluminant stimuli, particularly L/M-cone isolating stimuli, may elicit responses from non-colour opponent magnocellular neurons. In the studies cited above such unsolicited contributions were counteracted by manipulation of temporal presentation or sophisticated masking strategies. It would appear that isoluminance in itself is not a guarantee of selective stimulation of chromatic pathways. At the heart of the question of whether RT varies as a function of chromaticity or not, may lie the issue as to what extent erstwhile isoluminant stimuli generate residual activation in the magnocellular system. Responses to S-cone isolating stimuli may represent a truer reflection of the performance capabilities of chromatic vision, whilst responses to isoluminant L/M-cone isolating stimuli may be enhanced by contributions from mechanisms that are not purely chromatic.

References

Cottaris, N. P. & DeValois, R. L. (1998). Temporal dynamics of chromatic tuning in macaque primary visual cortex. *Nature*, 395, 896–900.

Derrington, A. M., Krauskopf, J., & Lennie, P. (1984). Chromatic mechanisms in lateral geniculate nucleus of macaque. *Journal of Physiology*, 357, 241–56.

Hendry, S. H. C. & Reid, R. C. (2000). The koniocellular pathway in human vision. *Annual Review of Neuroscience*, 23, 127–53.

Holmes, J. L. (1926). Reaction time to photometrically equal chromatic stimuli. *American Journal of Psychology*, 37, 414–17.

Irvin, G. E., Norton, T. T., Sesma, M. A., & Casagrande, V. A. (1986). W-like response properties of interlaminar zone cells in the lateral geniculate nucleus of a primate (*Galago crassicaudatus*). *Brain Research*, 362, 254–70.

Nissen, M. J. & Pokorny, J. (1977). Wavelength effects on simple reaction time. *Perception & Psychophysics*, 22, 457–62.

Lit, A., Young, R. H., & Schaffer, M. (1971). Simple reaction times as a function of luminance for various wavelengths. *Perception & Psychophysics*, 10, 397–9.

MacLeod, D. I. & Boynton, R. M. (1979). Chromaticity diagram showing cone excitation by stimuli of equal luminance. *Journal of the Optical Society of America*, 69, 1183–6.

McKeefry, D. J., Murray, I. J. M., & Kulikowski, J. J. (2001). Red–green and blue–yellow mechanisms are matched in sensitivity for spatial and temporal modulation. *Vision Research*, 41, 245–55.

Mollon, J. D., & Krauskopf, J. (1973). Reaction time as a measure of the temporal response properties of individual colour mechanisms. *Vision Research*, 13, 27–40.

Parry, N. R. A. (2001). Contrast dependence of reaction times to chromatic gratings. *Color Research and Application*, 26: S161–S164.

Piéron, H. (1932). La sensation chromatique. Données sur la latence proper et l'établissement des sensations de couleur. *Année Psychologique*, 32, 1–29.

Piéron, H. (1952). *The Sensations*. Frederick Muller, London.

Plainis, S. & Murray, I. J. (2000). Neurophysiological interpretation of human visual reaction times: effect of contrast, spatial frequency and luminance. *Neuropsychologia*, 38, 1555–64.

Rabin, J., Switkes, E., Crognale, M., Schneck, M. E., & Adams, A. J. (1994). Visual evoked potentials in three dimensional color space: correlates of spatio-chromatic processing. *Vision Research*, 34, 2657–71.

Schwartz, S. H. & Loop, M. S. (1983). Differences in temporal appearance associated with activity in the chromatic and achromatic systems. *Perception & Psychophysics*, 33, 388–90.

Smith, V. C. & Pokorny, J. (1975). Spectral sensitivity of the foveal cone photopigments between 400 and 500 nm. *Vision Research*, 15, 161–71.

Smithson, H. E. & Mollon, J. D. (2001*a*). Reaction times to brief chromatic stimuli. *Investigative Ophthalmology & Visual Science*, 42, S532.

Smithson, H. E. & Mollon, J. D. (2001*b*). Forward and backward masking with brief chromatic stimuli. *Color Research & Applications*, 26, S165–9.

Solomon, S. G., White, A. J. R., & Martin, P. R. (1999). Temporal contrast sensitivity in the lateral geniculate nucleus of a New World monkey, the marmoset Callithrix jacchus. *Journal of Physiology*, 517, 907–17.

Ueno, T., Pokorny, J., & Smith, V. C. (1985). Reaction times to chromatic stimuli. *Vision Research*, 25, 1623–7.

Valberg, A., Lee, B. B., Kaiser, P. K., & Kremers, J. (1992). Responses of macaque ganglion cells to movement of chromatic borders. *Journal of Physiology*, 458, 579–602.

Webster, M. A. & Mollon, J. D. (1994). The influence of contrast adaptation on color appearance. *Vision Research*, 34, 1993–2020.

CHAPTER 14

INTEGRATION TIMES REVEAL MECHANISMS RESPONDING TO ISOLUMINANT CHROMATIC GRATINGS: A TWO-CENTRE VISUAL EVOKED POTENTIAL STUDY

A. G. ROBSON, J. J. KULIKOWSKI, M. KOROSTENSKAJA, M. M. NEVEU, C. R. HOGG, AND G. E. HOLDER

Introduction

S-cone pathway processing has traditionally been regarded as slower than the L/M colour-opponent system. However, psychophysical and human neurophysiological studies have suggested that additional chromatic-related mechanisms contribute to L/M processing (McKeefry and Kulikowski 1995; McKeefry et al. 2001) and could extend the temporal resolution of responses to L/M stimulation (McKeefry and Kulikowski 1997; Robson and Kulikowski 1998a).

Visual evoked potentials (VEPs) provide an objective technique for monitoring the integrity of the visual pathways and have been used extensively to monitor the activity of post-receptoral chromatic mechanisms (Murray et al. 1987; Berninger et al. 1989a,b; Rabin et al. 1994; Robson and Kulikowski 1995; Suttle and Harding 1999; Davis et al. 2001).

The temporal properties of visual processing may be characterized in terms of VEP integration time, defined as the stimulus duration during which response components are summed to give the highest amplitude VEP. The onset of a luminance-modulated pattern of moderate spatial frequency, elicits the largest VEP when the grating appearance is brief that is, about 40–60 ms (Jeffreys and Axford 1972; Kulikowski 1972; Spekreijse et al. 1973), consistent with predominant activation of transient mechanisms. Likewise, the greatest amplitude chromatic VEPs are obtained with isoluminant coarse L/M gratings when the offset period exceeds the onset duration (Parry et al. 1988; Rabin et al. 1994). The present study compares L/M with tritan integration times by obtaining VEP responses to the onset of 2 cycles per deg gratings of varying onset durations, in order to characterize the temporal response mechanisms contributing to the two chromatic processing streams.

Methods

At Moorfields Eye Hospital (MEH), coarse gratings were generated on a computer graphics system and modulated along two L/M axes (protan and deutan) and a purple/green tritan confusion line (Arden *et al.* 1988). Contrast was defined as a vector in CIE colour space. At UMIST, gratings of identical spatial configuration were generated on a colour monitor and modulated along a similar L/M (protan) axis and subject-specific tritanopic confusion lines, additionally verified according to a minimum distinct border criterion (Robson and Kulikowski 1998a). Contrast was defined as the equivalent Michelson contrast for each component of a bichromatic grating. This value is approximately half that obtained for monochromatic lights of similar wavelength due to the broadband characteristics and overlap of the phosphor emissions (Moreland *et al.* 2001). Isoluminance of gratings was determined for each subject using a minimum flicker paradigm. The degree of chromatic response selectivity was verified and expressed as an index (see insets Fig. 14.1): onset negativity/(onset negativity + onset positivity). Grating onset duration was varied (between 40 and 300 ms) within a fixed temporal cycle (0.96 or 1.9 Hz) and presentations were in random order. All subjects had normal colour vision (Farnsworth–Munsell 100-hue and/or Arden colour contrast sensitivity).

Results and comments

Response selectivity

A small departure from stimulus isoluminance results in VEPs with an additional early positive component which resembles contrast reversal and achromatic VEPs (Murray *et al.* 1987; Berninger *et al.* 1989*b*) and which lowers the index of selectivity (Fig. 14.1, primary axes, large open symbols). At isoluminance, the index approaches 1. At extreme departures from isoluminance the positivity completely dominates the waveform and the ratio approaches zero. The use of identical onset and offset periods (260 ms ON, 260 ms OFF) optimally reveals the existence of achromatic intrusions (Kulikowski *et al.* 1997).

The index of selectivity was used in the current study to assess VEP waveforms illustrated by Suttle and Harding (1999), and Kulikowski and Carden (1989), which were recorded from humans and rhesus monkeys, respectively. Figure 14.1 (primary axes, large filled symbols) shows how chromatic selectivity can be assessed using the index of selectivity described above. This criterion facilitates rapid assessment of response selectivity without the need for recording time-consuming additional controls, and may prove useful in cases where subject cooperation is limited for example, in paediatric or animal studies.

Spatial limitations of selective stimuli

The purity of tritan VEPs is dependent on restricting the spatial size of gratings, and the index of selectivity falls when the circular stimulus field exceeds 3° in diameter (Fig. 14.1, secondary axes, small symbols). L/M VEPs retain an index >0.8 in all three subjects for

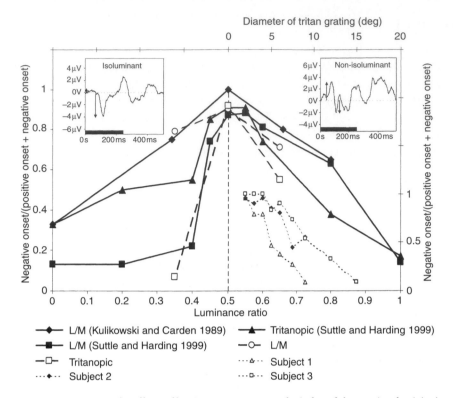

Figure 14.1 Primary axes: the effects of luminance-contrast on the index of chromatic selectivity is reduced for L/M and Tritan VEPs in concordance with retrospective analysis of waveforms published in human (Suttle and Harding 1999) and animal studies (Kulikowski and Carden 1989). Secondary axes: increasing the diameter of tritan gratings reduces the index value of selectivity (three subjects, lightly dotted lines). Insets show how selectivity index was measured for VEPS elicited by L/M gratings (260 ms ON, 260 ms OFF): non-isoluminant stimuli elicit an additional positive wave with a peak at 80 ms.

fields up to 9° in diameter (data not shown). The most likely causes of intrusions associated with tritan VEPs are macular pigmentation (Moreland *et al.* 1998) and chromatic aberration, which is greater for gratings containing shorter wavelengths (Charman 1991). All further experiments described in this study therefore employ stimulus fields less than 3° in diameter.

Integration times

Four subjects were tested at UMIST and four subjects were tested at MEH. One subject was tested in both studies. Figure 14.2 shows representative data recorded from one subject at UMIST and a different subject at MEH.

The Tritan-specific VEP component (time to negative peak 160–200 ms) recorded at UMIST rises in amplitude when the stimulus duration increases up to 200–240 ms

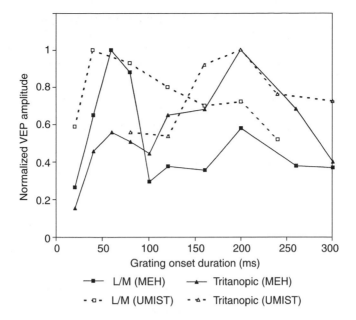

Figure 14.2 Chart showing optimal integration times for VEPs elicited with L/M (square symbols) or tritan gratings (triangular symbols). Recordings were performed at UMIST (broken lines) and on another subject at MEH (solid lines). L/M VEP amplitudes are normalized relative to that attained for 80 ms onset, tritan VEPs are normalized relative to the response obtained when duration is 200 ms. Field size 3°, spatial frequency 2 cycles/deg, temporal frequency 0.96 Hz.

(mean 190 ms, Fig. 14.2). Corresponding stimulation with the L/M gratings elicits the largest VEPs (1st negative peak at about 130 ms) for onset durations of 40–120 ms (mean 85 ms). However, further analysis reveals a secondary maximum in the L/M function, which closely matches the Tritan integration time of ~200 ms.

Gratings of maximum contrast were initially presented monocularly at MEH. Deutan VEPs were similar to protan VEPs in terms of integration times (60–100 ms, mean 63 ms) but differed from tritan VEPs (integration times 100–200 ms, mean 165 ms). Binocular stimulation and reference position (Fz or linked ears) had minimal effect on the results (Table 14.1).

Data obtained from a single subject at both UMIST and MEH were qualitatively similar in terms of different tritan and L/M integration times (Table 14.1), in spite of significant differences in stimuli. Generally, the use of high contrast gratings (MEH) shortened L/M integration times whereas the use of a standard Tritan axis, rather than subject-specific tritan axes (UMIST), had less effect on integration time. This shortening of L/M integration time at high chromatic contrast may reflect activation of magnocellular or transient response mechanisms at high chromatic contrast (discussed below).

If the data from all eight cases are pooled, the mean integration times for L/M VEPs were significantly different compared with Tritan VEPs (Wilcoxon signed rank test,

Table 14.1 Comparison of VEP integration times for a single subject obtained for different stimulus and recording parameters at UMIST and at MEH. When present, onset durations giving secondary maxima are given below the primary integration time. Recording montages were mid-occipital (Oz) referred to linked ears (LE) or mid-frontal (Fz). N/A—not available

	Integration times (ms)		
	Tritan	Protan	Deutan
UMIST	200	120	N/A
Binocular, 0.96 Hz, Oz–LE		160	
MEH	200	80	N/A
Binocular, 0.96 Hz, Oz–LE		200	
MEH	200	60	40
Binocular, 0.96 Hz, Oz–Fz		160	160
MEH	160	80	N/A
Monocular, 0.96 Hz, Oz–LE		160	
MEH	200	60	60
Monocular, 0.96 Hz, Oz–Fz		160	200–260

$p = 0.01$), with mean integration times of 75 and 188 ms, respectively. A secondary peak in the duration-amplitude function of L/M VEPs was present in all eight cases, that closely matched the corresponding integration time for tritan VEPs (no statistical difference).

The increase in L/M and Tritan VEP amplitudes seen for the longer duty cycle (1040 ms) can be explained in terms of the longer offset period which reduces the attenuating effects of chromatic pattern adaptation (Robson and Kulikowski 2001). Shorter L/M integration times presumably reflect the activity of faster, additional response mechanisms which contribute to L/M processing. They are also manifest in the additional negative component associated with L/M onset VEPs at low contrast (Robson and Kulikowski 1998a), and in the band-pass tuning of L/M VEPs (Robson and Kulikowski 1998b; Kulikowski and Robson 1999). Note that in all subjects there is a second peak in the L/M duration-amplitude curves when the presentation period is between 160 and 240 ms, possibly reflecting the activity of a purely sustained colour-specific mechanism, which characterizes the Tritan onset VEPs.

Another possibility is that the double-peaked L/M function reflects interaction between onset and offset VEP components. If the offset wave, following exposure to a long-duration stimulus, is shifted to shorter latencies and summed with the onset component, the effects of interaction between onset and offset components may be simulated (Kulikowski 1972). In the current study, such analysis of chromatic VEPs revealed that electrical cancellation of negative onset and positive offset components may occur for simulated onset durations of less than 80 ms (simulations not shown).

Since it takes 40–50 ms for the afferent volley to reach primary visual cortex it is possible that interaction of L/M VEP onset and offset components may veil a shorter integration time between 50 and 100 ms. Interaction is unlikely to account for the emergence of a second peak in the L/M function at about 160–200 ms.

The isolation of the parvocellular colour-opponent system is confounded by magnocellular neurones responding residually to isoluminant L/M borders (Schiller and Colby 1983; Lee *et al.* 1989), especially at high contrasts (Kulikowski *et al.* 1991, 1997; White *et al.* 1998), and by activation of chromatic-related hybrid mechanisms (Kulikowski 1997; Johnson *et al.* 2001) possibly based on V1 neurones receiving dual parvocellular/magnocelluar inputs (Lund *et al.* 1995; Vidyasagar *et al.* 1998). This could explain increased L/M modulation sensitivity functions and extended L/M spatio-temporal resolution (Granger and Heurtley 1973; Swanson *et al.* 1987; McKeefry and Kulikowski 1997).

When achromatic intrusions due to chromatic aberration and macular pigmentation are minimized, the S-cone-specific VEPs show longer integration times (Fig. 14.2) and low-pass temporal tuning (Robson and Kulikowski 1995, 1998a) reflecting the smaller effect of tritan stimuli on pattern detection; it is considerably more difficult to identify tritan stimuli since their border is not distinct (Tansley and Boynton 1978; Robson and Kulikowski 1998a). Similarly, L/M and Tritan chromatic-opponent contrast sensitivity functions are closely matched in sensitivity and resolution when the transient magnocellular contribution to L/M processing is quantified and subtracted (McKeefry *et al.* 2001), or reduced by spatio-temporal adaptation (Smithson and Mollon 2001). However, evolution of a similar interaction between a transient system and the S-cone pathway, for the benefit of pattern vision, may be unnecessary since chromatic aberration and macular pigmentation disrupts isoluminant camouflage in the natural enviroment.

Conclusions

The selectivity of chromatic stimulation can be quantified using an index derived from the amplitude ratios of early VEP components: onset negativity/(onset negativity + onset positivity).

L/M VEPs have a primary and secondary maximum in terms of integration times. The later maximum matches the single integration time for Tritan VEPs, consistent with activation of a similar, colour-specific mechanism.

References

Arden, G. B., Gunduz, K., & Perry, S. (1988). Colour Vision Testing with a computer graphics system. *Clinical Vision Sciences*, 2(4), 303–20.

Berninger, T. A., Arden, G. B., Hogg, C. R., & Frumkes, T. (1989a). Separable evoked retinal and cortical potentials from each major visual pathway: preliminary results. *British Journal of Ophthalmology*, 73, 502–11.

Berninger, T. A., Arden, G. B., Hogg, C. R., & Frumkes, T. E. (1989b). Colour vision defect diagnosed by evoked potentials. *Investigative Ophthalmology and Vision Science*, 30 (Suppl), 55.

Charman, W. N. (1991). Limits on the visual performance set by eye's optics and the retinal cone mosaic. In: Kulikowski, J.J., Walsh, V., & Murray, I.J. *Limits of Vision* (pp. 81–96). Basingstoke: Macmillan.

Davis, A. R., Neveu, M. M., Hogg, C. R., Fitzke, F. W., Morgan, M. J., Sloper, J. J., & Holder, G. E. (2001). Electrophysiological assessment of magnocellular and parvocellular function in early and late onset strabismic amblyopes. *Investigative Ophthalmology and Visual Science*, 42(4), B265, Abstract No. 292.

Granger, A. M. & Heurtley, J. C. (1973). Visual chromaticity-modulation transfer function. *Journal of the Optical Society of America*, 63, 1173–4.

Jeffreys, D. A. & Axford J. G. (1972). Source locations of pattern-specific components of human visual evoked potentials II. Component of extrastriate cortical origin. *Experimental Brain Research*, 16, 22–40.

Johnson, E. N., Hawken, M. J., & Shapley, R. (2001). The spatial transformation of colour in the primary visual cortex of the macaque monkey. *Nature Neuroscience*, 4, 409–16.

Kulikowski, J. J. (1972). Relation of psychophysics and electrophysiology. *Trace* (Paris), 6, 64–9.

Kulikowski, J. J. (1997). Spatial and temporal properties of chromatic processing: separation of colour from chromatic pattern mechanisms. In: Dickinson, C., Murray, I. J. & Carden, D. *John Dalton's Colour Vision Legacy* (pp. 133–46). London: Taylor and Francis.

Kulikowski, J. J. & Carden, D. (1989). Scalp VEPs to chromatic and achromatic gratings in macaques with ablated visual area 4. In: Kulikowski, J. J., Dickinson, C., & Murray, I. J. (Eds) *Seeing Contour and Colour* (pp. 586–90). Oxford: Pergamon Press.

Kulikowski, J. J., McKeefry, D. J., & Robson, A. G. (1997). Colour selective stimulation: an empirical perspective. *Spatial Vision*, 10, 379–402.

Kulikowski, J. J., Murray, I. J., & Russell, M. H. A. (1991). Effect of stimulus size on chromatic and achromatic VEPs. In: Drum, B., Moreland, J. D. & Serra, A. (Eds) *Colour Vision Deficiencies IX* (pp. 51–6). Dordrecht: Kluwer Academic.

Kulikowski, J. J. & Robson, A. G. (1999). Spatial, temporal and chromatic channels: electrophysiological foundations. *Journal of Optical Technology*, 66(9), 797–808.

Lee, B. B., Martin, P. R., & Valberg, A. (1989). Non-linear summation of M- and L-cone inputs to phasic retinal ganglion cells of the macaque. *Journal of Neuroscience*, 9, 1433–42.

Lund, J. S., Wu, Q., Hardingham, P. T., & Levitt, J. B. (1995). Cells and circuits contributing to functional properties in area V1 of macaque monkey cerebral cortex: bases for neuroanatomically realistic models. *Journal of Anatomy*, 187, 563–81.

McKeefry, D. J. & Kulikowski, J. J. (1995) Psychophysical and occipital responses to *aberration-free* blue/yellow and red/green gratings. In: Drum, B. (Ed.) *Colour Vision Deficiencies XII* (pp. 391–8). Dordrecht: Kluwer Academic.

McKeefry, D. M. & Kulikowski, J. J. (1997). Spatial and temporal sensitivities of colour discrimination mechanisms. In: Dickinson, C., Murray, I. J., & Carden, D. (Eds) *John Dalton's Colour Vision Legacy* (pp. 163–72). London: Taylor and Francis.

McKeefry, D. J., Murray, I. J., & Kulikowski, J. J. (2001). Red–Green and Blue–Yellow mechanisms are matched in sensitivity for temporal and spatial modulation. *Vision Research*, 41, 245–55.

Moreland J. D., Robson A. G., Soto-Leon N., & Kulikowski J. J. (1998). Macular pigment and the colour-specificity of visual evoked potentials. *Vision Research*, 38, 3241–5.

Moreland, J. D., Robson, A. G., & Kulikowski, J. J. (2001). Macular pigment assessment using a colour monitor. *Colour Research and Application*, 26, S261–S263.

Murray, I. J., Parry N. R. A., Carden, D., & Kulikowski, J. J. (1987). Human visual evoked potentials to chromatic and achromatic gratings. *Clinical Vision Sciences*, 1, 231–44.

Parry, N. R. A., Kulikowski, J. J., Murray, I. J., Kranda, K., & Ott, H. (1988). Visual evoked potentials and reaction times to chromatic and achromatic stimulation. In: Hindmarch, I., Aufdembrinke, B., & Ott, H. (Eds). *Psychopharmacology and Reaction Time*, (pp. 155–76). New York, Wiley.

Rabin, J., Switkes, E., Crognale, M., Schneck, M. E., & Adams, A. J. (1994). Visual evoked potentials in three-dimensional colour space: correlates of spatio-chromatic processing. *Vision Research*, 34, 2657–71.

Robson, A. G. & Kulikowski, J. J. (1995). Verification of VEPs elicited by gratings containing tritanopic pairs of hues. *Journal of Physiology*, 475, 22P.

Robson, A. G. & Kulikowski, J. J. (1998a). Objective specification of tritanopic confusion lines using visual evoked potentials. *Vision Research*, 38, 3499–503.

Robson, A. G. & Kulikowski, J. J. (1998b). Relative contributions of parvo and magno inputs to human visual evoked potentials. *European Journal of Neuroscience*, 93(39), 239.

Robson, A. G. & Kulikowski, J. J. (2001). The effect of pattern adaptation on chromatic and achromatic visual evoked potentials. *Colour Research and Applications*, 26, S13–S135.

Schiller, P. H. & Colby, C. L. (1983). The responses of single cells in the LGN of the rhesus monkey to colour and luminance contrast. *Vision Research*, 23, 1631–41.

Smithson, H. E. & Mollon, J. D. (2001). Forward and backward masking with brief chromatic stimuli. *Colour Research and Applications*, 26, S165–9.

Spekreijse, H., Van Der Tweel, L. H., & Zuidema, T. H. (1973). Contrast evoked responses in man. *Vision Research*, 13, 1577–601.

Suttle, C. M. & Harding, G. F. A. (1999). Morphology of transient VEPs to luminance and chromatic pattern onset and offset. *Vision Research*, 39, 1577–84.

Swanson, W. H., Uneo, T., Smith, V. C., & Pokorny, J. (1987). Temporal modulation sensitivity and pulse direction thresholds for chromatic and luminance perturbations. *Journal of the Optical Society of America*, 4, 1992–2005.

Tansley, B. W. & Boynton, R. M. (1978). Chromatic border perception: the role of red- and green-sensitive cones. *Vision Research*, 18, 683–97.

Vidyasagar, T. R., Kulikowski, J. J., Robson, A. G., & Dreher, B. (1998). Responses of V1 cells in primate reveal excitatory convergence of P and M channels. *European Journal of Neuroscience*, 10, S239.

White, A. J. R., Wilder, H. D., Goodchild, A. K., Sefton, J., & Martin, P. R. (1998). Segregation of receptive field properties in the lateral geniculate nucleus of a new-world monkey, the marmoset Callithrix jacchus. *Journal of Neurophysiology*, 80, 2063–76.

CHAPTER 15

TEMPORAL FREQUENCY AND CONTRAST ADAPTATION

ARTHUR G. SHAPIRO, S. MARY HOOD, AND
J. D. MOLLON

Introduction

Chromatic contrast adaptation (i.e. exposure to a field whose chromaticity is temporally modulated along a line in colour space) is a valuable technique for delineating cardinal and higher-order colour mechanisms (Krauskopf *et al.* 1982, 1986; Webster and Mollon 1991). In most studies, contrast adaptation is confined to 1-Hz modulation (Webster and Wilson 2000, being an exception) on the assumption that chromatic mechanisms respond best to low temporal frequencies and that desensitization is proportional to the degree to which the response of the mechanisms is modulated. On the other hand, several studies have suggested that second-order chromatic adaptation may be relatively fast (Zaidi *et al.* 1998; Shapiro *et al.* 2000; Webster and Wilson 2000). Fast adaptation would be favored by computational models that suggest that contrast adaptation improves the internal representation of the stimulus statistics (Zaidi and Shapiro 1993; Zaidi *et al.* 1998).

There have been few parametric investigations into the effects of contrast adaptation, despite its obvious importance. This report gives results for three experiments: the first measures threshold elevation produced by contrast adaptation along the cardinal axes as a function of temporal frequency at two light levels; the second investigates whether the cardinal mechanisms remain independent at these temporal frequencies and light levels; and the third measures the temporal contrast sensitivity of the cardinal mechanisms in conditions similar to those used for the first experiment. We show that contrast adaptation can occur at frequencies greater than 1 Hz; that the cardinal mechanisms remain independent at the temporal frequencies and light levels that we measured; and that contrast adaptation cannot be easily related to the temporal sensitivity of the cardinal mechanisms.

Methods

Specification of colours and equipment

The lights were confined to the axes of the Derrington *et al.* (1984) colour space. We will refer to these axes as the S, the L–M, and the LUM lines. All axes had a mid-point at W with a MacLeod–Boynton chromaticity of 0.66, 0.017, and a luminance of either 5 or 40 cd/m^2. The maximum excursion on the S axis was ± 0.01445, and on the L–M axis, ± 0.055.

Images were generated with a Cambridge Research 2/4 VSG Graphics Board, and were displayed on a Sony 21″ Trinitron monitor running at 120 frames/s. The chromaticity and luminance were measured with a Spectrascan 650 Spectroradiometer. The lights were expressed in terms of S, M, and L photoreceptor luminance (Shapiro *et al.* 1996), with a Judd correction, and then converted into MacLeod–Boynton units.

Observers

The data are from two of the authors, A. G. S. and S. M. H., both colour normal.

Procedure

The procedure follows the general design of the habituation experiment of Krauskopf *et al.* (1982): the observer adapts either to a field with a chromaticity of W (baseline condition) or to a field whose chromaticity is modulated sinusoidally in time along one of the cardinal axes of colour space (temporal contrast adaptation); discrimination thresholds are measured for excursions from W along one of the cardinal axes; threshold elevation is calculated by dividing the discrimination threshold measured following temporal contrast adaptation by the threshold measured following adaptation to a uniform field.

Figure 15.1 shows the spatial configuration and the temporal sequence for the lights used in these experiments. The temporal contrast adaptation was confined to a 3° disk. The chromaticity of the field was modulated along the S, L–M, or luminance cardinal axis at a fixed temporal frequency; for baseline measurements, the chromaticity was set at W. The phase of the modulated field was such that the initial portion of the sine wave was in the +S, +(L–M), and +LUM directions. The surrounding field was dark. Initial adaptation lasted for 2 min.

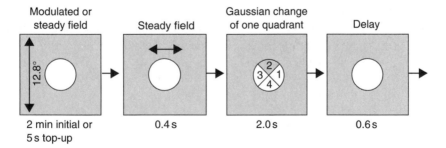

Figure 15.1 Spatial configuration and temporal sequence for Experiments 1 and 2. Discrimination thresholds were measured following W adaptation and following temporal contrast adaptation. The modulation for temporal contrast adaptation was always along the S, L–M or LUM cardinal axis; test lights were in the S, −(L–M), or −LUM cardinal direction. The test light differed from W as a Gaussian with $\mu = 1.0$ and $\sigma = 0.3$.

The test consisted of a 3° disk divided into four quadrants. A dark border served to define the test regions and to mask residual luminance artifacts. The chromaticity of one quadrant changed from W in a Gaussian pattern ($\mu = 1$ s, $\sigma = 0.30$ s) for 2 s; the chromaticity of the other three quadrants remained fixed at W. All quadrants remained at W for 0.6 s after offset of the test. The observer then readapted for a 5-s "top-up" period. The observer's task was to press a button to indicate which quadrant contained the test light. The maximum amplitude of the test light was changed in a 1-up/2-down staircase procedure. Threshold was defined as the mean of 12 reversals from two interleaved staircases. Feedback was provided if the observer responded in the 1.0-s interval following presentation of the test light.

Experiment 1: How is threshold elevation affected by the temporal frequency of the adaptation light?

In the first set of experiments the test and the adapting modulation were along the same axis. We measured threshold elevation as a function of the frequency of the adapting modulation at two luminance levels (5 and 40 cd/m^2). The original Krauskopf et al. (1982) studies were conducted at 50 td against a dark background; in free viewing conditions with standard pupil estimates, this equals a luminance of about 6 cd/m^2.

In each session all variables were fixed except for temporal frequency, which varied in random order. Baseline was measured at the beginning of each set of temporal frequencies and re-measured twice during the set. An observer measured threshold for four to eight temporal frequencies in a sitting, which lasted 1–2 h. At the beginning of each sitting, the observer dark-adapted for at least 10 min. Each set of temporal frequencies was run twice.

Figure 15.2 shows threshold elevations for probes and contrast adaptation along the same cardinal axis for observers S. M. H. and A. G. S. Panels A and C show threshold elevation for adaptation along the L–M axis; panels B and D show threshold elevations for adaptation along the S axis. Circles indicate threshold elevations at 5 cd/m^2; squares, the threshold elevations at 40 cd/m^2. Solid lines are included for visual guidance. Most of the maximal threshold elevations are between 1.9 and 2.5 times the baseline, except for those in panel C, which are elevated by less than 1.5 times the baseline at 5 cd/m^2. Thresholds are elevated at a range of temporal frequencies. At 40 cd/m^2, the thresholds show greater elevation at higher temporal frequencies than at 5 cd/m^2. In panel A the thresholds are still elevated at 15 Hz.

Experiment 2: Are the cardinal directions independent at different temporal frequencies?

The defining feature of the cardinal directions, that contrast adaptation along one of them does not elevate thresholds along the others, has been documented only at 1 Hz. We measured threshold elevations for test directions orthogonal to the adaptation direction at 1, 4, and 8 Hz, in counterbalanced order. The temporal sequence and spatial configuration were as in experiment 1. The results for observers S. M. H. and A. G. S. are shown

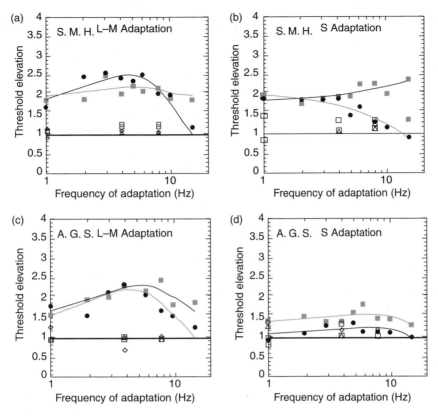

Figure 15.2 Threshold elevations as a function of temporal frequency of the adaptation light for observers S. M. H. and A. G. S. Panels on the left (A and C) show threshold elevations following contrast adaptation along the L–M axis; panels on the right (B and D) show threshold elevations following contrast adaptation along the S axis. The filled symbols indicate tests along the same axis as contrast adaptation: squares, 40 cd/m^2; and circles, 5 cd/m^2. The solid lines are included for visual guidance. The open symbols show threshold elevations following adaptation along orthogonal cardinal axes: squares, 40 cd/m^2 LUM adaptation; circles, 5 cd/m^2 LUM adaptation; triangles, 40 cd/m^2 orthogonal chromatic axis; and diamonds, 5 cd/m^2 orthogonal chromatic axis.

as the open symbols in Fig. 15.2. Thresholds measured for S and L–M tests following LUM adaptation did not show significant elevations (these results are not shown).

For most conditions there is no significant threshold elevation, and so the directions remain independent of each other at these frequencies. A two-tailed independent-groups t-test was performed between the baseline threshold and adaptation threshold. Even with no correction for type I errors, only three out of the 72 conditions had a $p < 0.1$. These conditions were, for observer S. M. H., the 1 Hz LUM and S adaptation for—(L–M) probes; for A. G. S., the condition was 8 Hz L–M adaptation for S-cone probes. In the latter condition, the threshold elevation was nearly as high as elevation following S adaptation.

Experiment 3: How do the temporal contrast sensitivity functions of the cardinal mechanisms compare to the threshold elevation curves?

To test whether the shape of the threshold elevation curves depends upon the temporal sensitivity of the S and L–M systems, we measured the temporal contrast sensitivity functions for lights with the same spatial configuration as the adapting stimuli in experiment 1. We used a two-interval forced-choice procedure: one interval contained a 3° flickering test light; the other, a steady W field. The observer had to identify which interval contained the test light. Each interval lasted for 1 s and was separated from the next by a 0.2 s delay. Threshold was calculated as the average of 10 reversals from a 1-up/3-down staircase.

The temporal contrast sensitivity functions were measured for all conditions used in experiment 1. Figure 15.3 shows thresholds for S and $-(L–M)$ detection at 5 and 40 cd/m^2 for observer S. M. H. These results are typical of other reports in the literature (McKeefry *et al.* 2001). The light level does not create a dramatic change in the shape of the function, nor are the peaks near those of the threshold elevation curves in Fig. 15.2. The shape of observer A. G. S.'s curves did not differ significantly from S. M. H.'s. However, S. M. H. was substantially more sensitive than A. G. S. in the S-cone condition (more so at 40 cd/m^2 than at 5 cd/m^2).

Discussion

One purpose of this study was to lay the groundwork for further investigations into mechanisms of contrast adaptation. Krauskopf *et al.* (1982), Webster and Mollon (1994), Shapiro and Zaidi (1992), and Zaidi and Shapiro (1993) investigated chromatic contrast adaptation at 1 Hz. The practical implication of our first finding is that a 1-Hz adaptation light may not be the optimal stimulus for studying how mechanisms respond to contrast adaptation. It is unlikely that threshold elevations at higher temporal frequencies are the result of luminance detection or of a luminance signal in the adapting light since this would run contrary to the results of Experiment 2.

Threshold elevation at high modulation rates is consistent with a number of studies that have suggested a fast adaptive response. Webster and Wilson (2000) used an asymmetric matching procedure to measure the effects of contrast adaptation at a range of temporal frequencies at 27.5 cd/m^2. They found that exposure to lights modulated up to 17.5 Hz produced a substantial change in saturation and concluded that the range of temporal frequencies that can lead to contrast adaptation is very broad. Zaidi *et al.* (1998) showed that second-order chromatic adaptation can be produced by exposure to static checkerboards, suggesting that contrast adaptation could be caused by miniature eye movements across element boundaries. Additionally, cortical adaptation can take place at the time scale of a single fixation (Muller *et al.* 1999).

The function relating threshold elevation to adapting frequency is of a very different form from the temporal CSF for the same stimulus conditions: although temporal contrast sensitivity is approximately 1 log unit lower at 10 Hz than at 1 Hz (Fig. 15.3), the

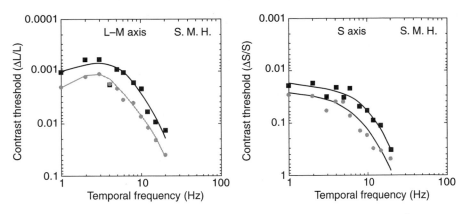

Figure 15.3 Temporal contrast sensitivity function for S and L–M lights: squares, 40 cd/m² and circles, 5 cd/m².

threshold elevations after adaptation at these two frequencies are comparable in most conditions (Fig. 15.2). This result allows us firmly to exclude one class of models of the underlying neural adaptation, models in which the loss of sensitivity is proportional to the magnitude of response of the neural channel during the adaptation period.

What are the alternatives? One possibility is that the change in sensitivity is controlled by mechanisms that are physiologically distinct from those carrying the colour signal that is ultimately detected, and that these external mechanisms have different time constants from the primary channel. The adaptive mechanism could, in theory, exist at any stage in visual processing; however, a retinal locus is consistent with models of retinal processing in which the function of many retinal circuits is to carry out supporting functions (e.g. to provide gain or combat distortion) rather than to transmit signals along the optic nerve (Masland and Raviola 2000).

A second possibility is that adaptation does depend entirely upon changes within the neurons that are transmitting the primary signal, but that the channel's loss of sensitivity depends as much on the frequency with which the channel's response is modulated as it does on the maximal depth of modulation. This could occur in a number of ways: (1) If the adaptive system were controlled by the leading edge of a transient signal, then a fast modulation rate (say, 8 Hz) would generate more relevant adaptation signals than would a slow modulation speed. (2) If along each cardinal axis there were two separate mechanisms sensitive to opposite directions of modulation, then both mechanisms would produce large responses time-locked to one phase of the modulation, but would also be silent in the opposite phase, during which time that mechanism could recover from adaptation. In such a system, a fast modulation rate would reduce the recovery period and therefore be a more effective adapting stimulus. (3) The adaptive system could be controlled by the ac signal; thus a 1 s duration, 10 Hz signal might create nearly the same amount of adaptation as would 1 s of 1 Hz modulation.

References

Brown, S. P. & Masland, R. H. (2001). Spatial scale and cellular substrate of contrast adaptation by retinal ganglion cells. *Nature Neuroscience, 4*, 44–51.

Derrington, A. M., Krauskopf, J., & Lennie, P. (1984). Chromatic mechanisms in lateral geniculate-nucleus of macaque. *Journal of Physiology-London, 357*, 241–65.

Krauskopf, J. (2001). A journey in color space. *Color Research and Application, 26*, S2–S11.

Krauskopf, J., Williams, D. R., & Heeley, D. W. (1982). Cardinal directions of color space. *Vision Research, 22*, 1123–31.

Krauskopf, J., Zaidi, Q., & Mandler, M. B. (1986). Mechanisms of simultaneous color induction. *The Journal of the Optical Society of America A, 3*, 1752–7.

Masland, R. H. & Raviola, E. (2000). Confronting complexity: Strategies for understanding the microcircuitry of the retina. *Annual Review of Neuroscience, 23*, 249–84.

McKeefry, D. J., Murray, I. J., & Kulikowski, J. J. (2001). Red–green and blue–yellow mechanisms are matched in sensitivity for temporal and spatial modulation. *Vision Research, 41*, 245–55.

Muller, J. R., Metha, A. B., Krauskopf, J., & Lennie, P. (1999). Rapid adaptation in visual cortex to the structure of images. *Science, 285*, 1405–8.

Shapiro, A. G., Beere, J. L., & Zaidi, Q. (2000). Time course of higher-order adaptation in the S−(L+M) color system. *Investigative Ophthalmology & Visual Science, 41*, 4292.

Shapiro, A. G., Beere, J. L., & Zaidi, Q. (2001). Time course of adaptation along the RG cardinal axis. *Color Research and Application, 26*, S43–S47.

Shapiro, A. G., Pokorny, J., & Smith, V. C. (1996). Cone-rod receptor spaces with illustrations that use CRT phosphor and light-emitting-diode spectra. *The Journal of the Optical Society of America A, 13*, 2319–28.

Shapiro, A. G. & Zaidi, Q. (1992). The effects of prolonged temporal modulation on the differential response of color mechanisms. *Vision Research, 32*, 2065–75.

Webster, M. A., Miyahara, E., Malkoc, G., & Raker, V. E. (2000). Variations in normal color vision. I. Cone-opponent axes. *The Journal of the Optical Society of America A, 17*, 1535–44.

Webster, M. A. & Mollon, J. D. (1991). Changes in colour appearance following post-receptoral adaptation. *Nature, 349*, 235–8.

Webster, M. A. & Mollon, J. D. (1994). The influence of contrast adaptation on color appearance. *Vision Research, 34*, 1993–2020.

Webster, M. A. & Wilson, J. A. (2000). Interactions between chromatic adaptation and contrast adaptation in color appearance. *Vision Research, 40*, 3801–16.

Zaidi, Q. & Shapiro, A. G. (1993). Adaptive orthogonalization of opponent-color signals. *Biological Cybernetics, 69*, 415–28.

Zaidi, Q., Shapiro, A. G., & Hood, D. (1992). The effects of adaptation on the differential sensitivity of the S-cone color system. *Vision Research, 32*, 1297–318.

Zaidi, Q., Spehar, B., & DeBonet, J. (1998). Adaptation to textured chromatic fields. *The Journal of the Optical Society of America A, 15*, 23–32.

CHAPTER 16

CONTRIBUTION OF ACHROMATIC AND CHROMATIC CONTRAST SIGNALS TO FECHNER–BENHAM SUBJECTIVE COLOURS

J. LE ROHELLEC, H. BRETTEL, AND F. VIÉNOT

Introduction

In a previous chapter, we have argued that mechanisms underlying Benham subjective colours are situated in a neurophysiological site high enough in the visual information processing hierarchy to allow both types of non-spectral-specific signals (e.g. L + M parvo- and magno-systems) to be modulated by the duration of the white phase following the dark half disc and preceding the arc, thus reducing the operation of retinal mechanisms (Le Rohellec and Viénot 2001).

The question arises whether subjective colours are generated through achromatic channels only (Campenhausen *et al.* 1992), or whether a spatio-temporal chromatic contrast contributes to the production of colours. On the one hand, if chromatic channels are involved in the phenomenon, it is worth testing whether a chromatic contrast by itself is sufficient to initiate the subjective colours. On the other hand, the result that an achromatic contrast signal weaker than the chromatic contrast signal allows to differentiate subjective colours could indicate that achromatic mechanisms play a major role in eliciting Benham subjective colours.

Here, we describe an experiment aimed at examining the respective contribution of achromatic contrast and isoluminant chromatic contrasts for generating subjective colours. We compare the efficiency of cone contrasts that we manipulate in an additive mode or in an antagonistic mode to differentiate subjective colours produced by different spatio-temporal stimuli.

Methods

Display and software

The modified Benham disc was produced on a computer-controlled CRT video display. A Java applet was executed through the Internet. The generic version of the software which allows to rotate a regular Benham disc is available at the website http://tsi.enst.fr/~brettel/.

A proprietary version of the software, which is different from the public version available on the web, has been used for this experiment and is described in the next paragraphs.

Construction of the stimulus

The disc is divided into a uniform half surface of colour A and a half surface of colour B in which an arc of colour A is embedded. The arc can be located close to one or the other half diameter (Fig. 16.1(a and b)). The display consists of a periodic sequence of pictures of the disc at angular positions increasing by regular steps. This display produces apparent motion when the angle is increased in small steps or produces a steady flickering percept as in our experiment, where the stimulus consists of a periodic sequence of three pictures, showing the disc at 0°, 120°, and 240° angular position (Fig. 16.1). This spatio-temporal pattern generates a stimulus made of six flickering sectors in fixed position, three of which being spatially uniform, and the three others displaying the arc (Fig. 16.1). Within sectors with arc, every cycle is composed of a uniform image of colour "A", a uniform image of colour "B" and an image with the arc of colour "A" embedded into the background of colour "B". The image with the arc can either immediately follow the uniform surface

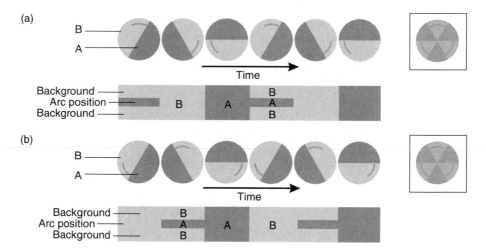

Figure 16.1 (a) Image sequence that is presented on the CRT to produce 2 cycles of a modified Benham disc in which the arc immediately follows surface A, and time course of the light stimulus. (b) Image sequence that is presented on the CRT to produce 2 cycles of a modified Benham disc in which the arc immediately precedes surface A, and time course of the light stimulus. These spatio-temporal patterns generate a stimulus made of six flickering sectors in fixed position, three of which being spatially uniform, and the three others displaying an arc. The position of the arc controls the temporal sequence of the stimulus. The inset shows the spatial appearance of the corresponding display.

"A" or immediately precede it, thus simulating the arcs that are contiguous either to one or the other radius of a classical rotating Benham disc.

Real stimulus used in the experiment

The spatio-temporal pattern used in the real experiment generates a stimulus made of six flickering sectors in fixed position, three of which being spatially uniform, and the three others displaying two arcs at two different eccentricities (diameter of the disc: 5°, thickness of the arc: 10 arc min, radial distance between both arcs: 40 arc min). On each trial, each arc of the modified Benham disc, whether at an external or an internal position, can either precede or follow the uniform surface A. So, the stimulus with the two arcs offers four possible configurations depending on the spatio-temporal pattern selected for each arc (preceding–preceding, following–following, preceding–following, following–preceding) (Fig. 16.2).

The presentation time for each picture of the sequence was about 40 ms, and the resulting fundamental frequency was 8 cycles per second. We controlled the period of

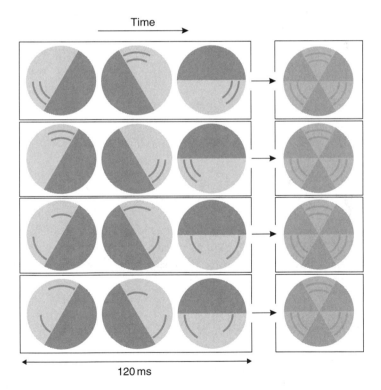

Figure 16.2 Left: Possible disc configurations with 2 arcs at different eccentricities which yield the 4 spatio-temporal configurations that were used in the experiment. Right: Reproduction of the modified Benham disc produced on the CRT as it appears to the observer. In reality, all sectors are flickering with a specific temporal profile.

the temporal sequence using the analog signal output of a photometer (Pritchard model 1980-A from Photo Research) and an oscilloscope, and the average luminance of the disc using a calibrated photometer (LMT L1009), prior to the experiment.

Calibration

The display has been calibrated in terms of L-, M-, and S-cone stimulation. The spectral power distribution (SPD) of the three primaries $E_{Rmax}(\lambda)$, $E_{Gmax}(\lambda)$, $E_{Bmax}(\lambda)$ and the CRT transfer function of each channel were measured with a calibrated spectro-radiometer (Minolta CS-1000). We have used the measured SPD of each CRT primary at its maximum and the $\bar{l}(\lambda)$, $\bar{m}(\lambda)$, $\bar{s}(\lambda)$ normalized cone spectral sensitivities (in linear energy units) proposed by Stockman and Sharpe (2000) to calculate the relative cone excitations produced by each primary. These are expressed in units that are consistent with normalized luminance units.

$$L_{Rmax} = \Sigma E_{Rmax}(\lambda)\bar{l}(\lambda)\Delta\lambda; \quad M_{Rmax} = \Sigma E_{Rmax}(\lambda)\bar{m}(\lambda)\Delta\lambda; \quad S_{Rmax} = \Sigma E_{Rmax}(\lambda)\bar{s}(\lambda)\Delta\lambda$$

$$L_{Gmax} = \Sigma E_{Gmax}(\lambda)\bar{l}(\lambda)\Delta\lambda; \quad M_{Gmax} = \Sigma E_{Gmax}(\lambda)\bar{m}(\lambda)\Delta\lambda; \quad S_{Gmax} = \Sigma E_{Gmax}(\lambda)\bar{s}(\lambda)\Delta\lambda$$

$$L_{Bmax} = \Sigma E_{Bmax}(\lambda)\bar{l}(\lambda)\Delta\lambda; \quad M_{Bmax} = \Sigma E_{Bmax}(\lambda)\bar{m}(\lambda)\Delta\lambda; \quad S_{Bmax} = \Sigma E_{Bmax}(\lambda)\bar{s}(\lambda)\Delta\lambda$$

For each primary, we used the Gain-Offset-Gamma model recommended by CIE (1996) to model the relative luminance R, G, or B, corresponding to any digital count I, J, or K, which writes for the red primary

$$\frac{R}{R_{max}} = \left\{g_r\left(\frac{I}{I_{max}}\right) + (1 - g_r)\right\}^\gamma \quad \text{with } I_{max} = 2^N - 1$$

with $R = 0$, if the formula yields negative values.

Once the calibration had been performed, the experimenter sets the video signals that yield the required L-, M-, or S-cone excitation.

Medium gray (128, 128, 128) is at 16 cd·m^{-2}. The background of the disk is a light gray (192, 192, 192) at 43 cd m^2 behind the display, the wall is illuminated at about 150 cd m^2 over 50°. It provides the permanent light adaptation for the observer necessary to stabilize the subjective colours (Rotgold & Spitzer 1997).

Preliminary experiment on isoluminance

Our hypothesis on the role of the achromatic versus chromatic contrast for eliciting Benham subjective colours imposes a strict control of luminance. Psychophysical evidence of no or very little contribution of S-cones to luminous efficiency has often been reported in the literature, so we assume that the weighted sum of $\bar{l}(\lambda)$ and $\bar{m}(\lambda)$ represents spectral luminous efficiency function

$$V(\lambda) = w_L\bar{l}(\lambda) + w_M\bar{m}(\lambda)$$

where w_L and w_M are weighting constants which do not vary throughout the visible spectrum but do considerably vary from one observer to another.

A typical experiment to estimate w_L and w_M is heterochromatic flicker photometry (HFP) between the red and the green primary of the display. The HFP visual match yields the weight ratio to be input into the software in order to produce isoluminant Benham discs.

In a preliminary experiment, each observer was asked to obtain an HFP match at 12 Hz between the red primary at its maximum $R_{max}(I = 255)$ and the green primary $G(G < G_{max})$ by adjusting the green digital intensity $J(J < 255)$. The average of 100 readings J for each observer has been used to determine the amount of green primary G that can be considered as equiluminous to the red R_{max} for this observer. When the visual luminance match is achieved between red and green, we assume that the sum of the weighted fundamental responses are equal, that is,

$$w_l L_{Rmax} + w_m M_{Rmax} = w_l(G/G_{max})L_{Gmax} + w_m(G/G_{max})M_{Gmax}$$

which yields

$$w_l/w_m = ((G/G_{max})M_{Gmax} - M_{Rmax})/(L_{Rmax} - (G/G_{max})L_{Gmax})$$

Note that as a visual luminance match is not a colour match; so, individual cone contributions are not equal, only the sum of L- and M-cone contributions is equalized in the HFP match.

For each observer, we have built tables that give the digital values to be entered onto the keyboard of the computer in order to vary the (L–M) signal around a medium gray without changing the visual luminance. We have also built tables that give the digital values corresponding to the variation of the S-signal only.

Procedure

Classically, when colour "A" is black and colour "B" is white, the arc of colour "A" appears reddish or bluish depending whether it follows or precedes the surface of colour "A".

In our experiment, six colour patterns have been studied, referring to specific cone contrasts.

"A" : uniform medium gray ($I = J = K = 128$)

"B" : $(L - M) > (L - M)_{gray};\quad S = S_{gray}$

$(L - M) < (L - M)_{gray};\quad S = S_{gray}$

$S > S_{gray};\quad L = L_{gray};\quad M = M_{gray}$

$S < S_{gray};\quad L = L_{gray};\quad M = M_{gray}$

$(L + M + S) > (L + M + S)_{gray}$ by a uniform factor

$(L + M + S) < (L + M + S)_{gray}$ by a uniform factor

For each colour pattern, a limited number of contrast steps was used in order to determine the contrast threshold that elicits a just noticeable difference when the two arcs are different.

The observer's task was to report difference/similarity of appearance between the external and internal arcs that were presented inside the upper sector. Each of the four possible temporal configurations of the two arcs was presented. All the configurations are randomized and numerically balanced within short sessions of 16 trials. One session refers to a specific colour pattern and to a single contrast step. Each observer performed five sessions (80 measurements at every contrast step).

After a few learning sessions, the observer could report any slight colour difference he could see: lightness and/or chromatic difference. Between trials, he (she) could freely look around. At each trial, although he (she) was allowed to scroll around the test, his (her) definitive judgement should be based on the upper sector.

Three observers took part in the experiment (two authors, J. L. R., male, 37 years, F. V., female, 54 years, and one naive observer, E. D. S. C., male, 19 years).

Results

Figure 16.3 shows the discrimination threshold for subjective colours elicited by different temporal patterns versus normalized contrast (80 measurements at every contrast step), for three observers. The star shows the LM contrast, the achromatic contrast or the S-cone contrast which is elicited by a uniform medium gray ($I = J = K = 128$). Note that LM contrast values have been normalized depending upon each observer's isoluminance characterization : 0 corresponds to the isoluminant colour that stimulates M-cones at a maximum, and 1 corresponds to the isoluminant colour that stimulates L-cones at a maximum, within the colour gamut of the CRT. This means that the abscissa of the star depends upon the LM isoluminance characterization of the observer.

For achromatic or isoluminant LM contrast, the score follows U-shaped curves, the minimum of which is at about 50 per cent—which corresponds to a random choice since identical and different patterns were equally presented. The threshold is defined as 75 per cent. The branches of the achromatic contrast curves rise steeply over 75 per cent success, indicating that a change as small as about 0.02 ($\pm 0.038; \pm 0.020$ and ± 0.021 for observers F. V., J. L. R., and E. D. C. S., respectively, from a Weibull adjustment) on the normalized achromatic contrast scale is sufficient to elicit different subjective colours on different temporal patterns. For the isoluminant LM contrast, the curves reach 75 per cent success also, but only for high possible contrast values ($\pm 0.245, \pm 0.134$, and ± 0.133 for observers F. V, J. L. R., and E. D. C. S., respectively). This illustrates that when isoluminance is strictly controlled for the observer, a chromatic contrast cannot generate Benham-like colours as efficiently as a luminance contrast. As far as the S contrast is concerned, the proportion of successful trials hardly attains the threshold assessment, for any contrast value ($+0.58, +0.30$ for observers J. L. R. and E. D. C. S., respectively; the proportion of correct responses has not reached 75 per cent for observer

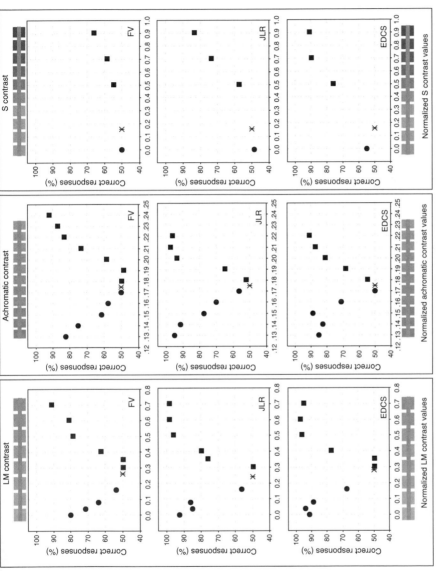

Figure 16.3 See also colour plate section. Discrimination threshold for subjective colours. Abscissas: range of contrast values that can be produced on the CRT, normalized from 0 to 1. The star indicates gray (128, 128, 128). Ordinates: percentage of correct responses for discrimination. Left: Discrimination threshold versus isoluminant chromatic LM contrast. Partial abscissa scale: 0 is the minimum L–M value; 1 would be the maximum L–M value. The scale varies slightly from one observer to the other depending upon the range of colours that can be produced at isoluminance for this individual. Centre: Discrimination threshold versus achromatic contrast (L + M + S). Enlarged abscissas scale: 0 would indicate black; 1 would indicate white. Right: Discrimination threshold versus isoluminant chromatic S contrast. Abscissas: 0, minimum S value; 1, maximum S value. Colour illustrations above and below the graphs show the variation of the stimulus: the central line represents the colour A as defined in Fig. 16.1. (medium gray 128, 128, 128) and the squares represent discrete values of the colour B as defined in Fig. 16.1.

F. V.). Observer E. D. C. S. has produced results with a slight lowering of all contrast thresholds, probably because he was younger.

After every session of 16 trials had been performed, corresponding to a given contrast value/contrast type condition, the observer was presented with two different patterns on the disk and forced to identify their colour. Results confirm the reversal of bluish/reddish subjective colours when LM contrast is substituted for ML contrast which we have described in former publications (Viénot and Le Rohellec 1992).

Conclusion

Our findings demonstrate the prevalence of the achromatic contrast to elicit Benham subjective colours. It seems that isoluminant chromatic contrast needs to be boosted to a very high value to produce subjective colours. Our findings confirm that S-cone signals alone are inefficient to generate Benham colours, a result which we had previously suggested by filtering the light that illuminated a classical Benham top (Le Rohellec and Viénot 2001) and which is in contradiction with the proposal by Schramme (1992).

Of interest is the comparison of high threshold values measured for isoluminant LM contrast and low threshold values measured for achromatic contrast. Let us note that within the colour gamut of the CRT, a high chromatic LM contrast modifies individual L- or M-cone contrast to a small amount only. Then it is possible that isoluminant chromatic contrast cannot generate Benham colours as long as any cone contrast is not large enough.

In conclusion, it seems that subjective colours disappear as soon as only chromatic contrast is present, especially when the luminance balance approaches equilibrium. Clearly, a very large S-cone contrast cannot by itself elicit subjective colours. These observations strengthen previously published results on Benham discs seen under monochrome illumination (Le Rohellec and Viénot 2001) which have led to the conclusion that S-cone signals do not contribute to subjective colours and that an explanation based on the participation of a parvo achromatic mechanism and of a magno achromatic mechanism should be considered.

Acknowledgments

We thank Emmanuel Da Costa Santos for assisting in the experiment. We are grateful to the reviewer for his suggestions.

References

Campenhausen, C. von, Hofstetter, J., Schramme, J., & Tritsch, M. F. (1992). Color induction via non-opponent lateral interactions in the human retina. *Vision Research, 32,* 913–23.

Commission Internationale de l'Eclairage (1996). The relationship between digital and colorimetric data for computer-controlled CRT displays. *CIE 122–1996,* Vienna.

Le Rohellec, J. & **Viénot, F.** (2001). Interaction of luminance and spectral adaptation upon Benham subjective colours. *Color Research and Application, 24,* S174–S179.

Rotgold, G. & **Spitzer, H.** (1997). Role of remote adaptation in perceived subjective colours. *Journal of the Optical Society of America, 14,* 1223–30.

Stockman, A. & **Sharpe, L. T.** (2000). The spectral sensitivities of the middle- and long-wavelength-sensitive cones derived from measurements in observers of known genotype. *Vision Research, 40,* 1711–37.

Schramme, J. (1992). Changes in pattern induced flicker colours are mediated by blue-yellow opponent process. *Vision Research, 32,* 2129–34.

Viénot, F. & **Le Rohellec, J.** (1992). Reversal in the sequence of the Benham colours with a change in the wavelength of illumination. *Vision Research, 32,* 2369–74.

CHAPTER 17

SENSITIVITY TO MOVEMENT OF CONFIGURATIONS OF ACHROMATIC AND CHROMATIC POINTS IN AMBLYOPIC PATIENTS

M. L. F. DE MATTIELLO, M. MANEIRO, AND
S. BUGLIONE

Introduction

The degradation of spatial vision is the principal defining feature of amblyopia (Hess *et al.* 1990). The deficit is greatest for foveal stimuli and stimuli in motion (Westheimer and McKee 1975; Morgan *et al.* 1983; Chung and Levi 1997). Amblyopia is a complex disturbance of visual function that includes disorders of spatial summation, alterations in contrast vision, visual acuity, differential luminance thresholds, dark adaptation, and color vision. The color vision deficiency, when present, resembles that of a normal observer using eccentric fixation. Further information on this subject can be found in the review carried out by Roth in 1968, and the recent work of Kocak-Altintas *et al.* (2000), who, by analyzing the error scores of 67 amblyopic eyes, concluded that this deficit is not related to visual acuity or the type of amblyopia.

Amblyopia has been attributed to a shift in sensitivity of the visual system toward low spatial-frequency filter mechanisms (Chung *et al.* 1996). Currently, there are three prevalent models: (i) a decrease in neuronal spatial sampling density (Levi *et al.* 2000); (ii) spatial uncertainty due to a scrambling or an upward shift in the scale of spatial filter sizes (Watt and Hess 1987; Hess and Field 1994); and (iii) a topographical disorder of the cortical receptive field which is uncalibrated (Hess *et al.* 1978; Watt and Hess 1987; Hess and Field 1994; Field and Hess 1996).

In a previous paper on contrast vision in amblyopic eyes (Lado *et al.* 2000), we identified three similar causes, by simulating the response of the observers with a neural network model. The possible causes were: (i) impairment of the visual channels; (ii) variation of the Gaussian kernels that hampers the integration of the correct signals, and (iii) the variation of the permeability factor that modifies the responses of the neural population.

In the present study, our interest lies in the analysis of the capacity to recognize moving signals and how color can help in this task.

Materials and methods

The stimulus display included a variable quantity (20, 15, or 10) of randomly moving black dots on a gray or colored background (Fig. 17.1(a)). Three different spatial organizations of the coherently moving dots, A, B, and C (Fig. 17.1(b)) were then presented against this background, which acted as a distractor. These samples were in coordinated movement, as shown by horizontal arrows for case A, on the left of Fig. 17.1(a). The experimental situations were grouped into three subgroups. The first employed achromatic test dots and backgrounds. The second group used red or green test dots with colorimetric purities equal to 0.12. The third group had similarly colored test dots but included red or green backgrounds of 0.18 purity, with the red test dots being presented on the green background and vice versa (opponent chromatic backgrounds). See also the caption to Figs 17.2 and 17.3.

The stimuli were presented on a PC monitor with a resolution of 640×350 pixels. They were generated through the Macromedia Flash 4 program. The display was positioned at 110 cm from the observer's eyes, and at this viewing distance the test region subtended $10°$ of visual angle. Each of the experimental trials consisted of four 1-s duration sequences (in terms of the Macromedia Flash 4: 15 frames per second). All the sequences were presented randomly and only one of them included the sample with coherently moving dots. The observer reported after each sample whether coherently moving dots were present. This experimental sequence avoided misleading results produced by the moving dots on the background.

The clinical profiles of the six amblyopic observers are summarized in Table 17.1. The amblyopic and non-amblyopic eyes were tested separately, with the untested eye occluded with a black patch. The observers had no previous experience of tests of motion sensitivity.

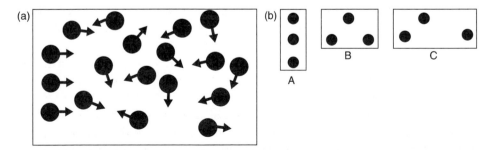

Figure 17.1 Diagram of the stimulus display. (a) Background dots move in random directions, the stimulus dots (the three at the left) all move in the same direction. Presentation time was 1500 ms. (b) The spatial organizations of the coherently moving dots.

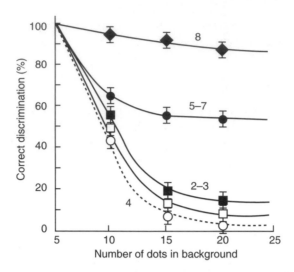

Figure 17.2 Percentage of recognition according to the number of dots in the background. Result obtained with normal observers. The numbers indicate: (4) black stimulus dot configuration A on a gray background; (1) color stimulus dot configuration B on a gray background; color stimulus dot configuration C (2) and B (3) on a gray background; color stimulus dot configuration C (5) and B (6) on a opponent chromatic background and (7) color stimulus dot configuration A on a gray background; (8) color stimulus dot configuration A with opponent chromatic background.

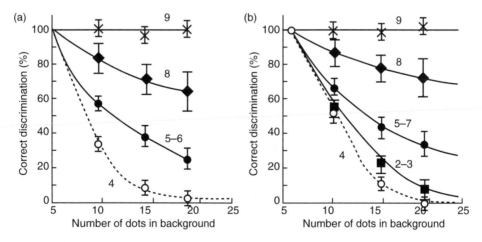

Figure 17.3 Summary of the average of estimations made by the four first patients in Table 17.1: amblyopic eye (a) and non-amblyopic eyes (b). The situation (4) of Fig 17.2 is included for comparison. The curve 9 indicate the situation when intermediate dots were added in both chromatic and achromatic samples B and C. The other stimulus situations are the same as those of Fig. 17.2. Note that the stimuli for experimental conditions 1–4 could not be recognized by any of the amblyopic eyes.

Table 17.1 Clinical data for the amblyopic subject group

Diagnosis	Obs	Age/sex	Eye	Refractive status	Acuity	Fixation of amblyopic eye	Binocularity Fixation
Anisometropic amblyopes	G. P.	50/F	RE	$+1.50/+0.50 \times 80°$	20/20	Unsteady central with central scotoma	Fluctuation high frequency and ampleness 12′
			LE(A)	plano	Less than 20/200		
	S. D.	18/F	RE(A)	plano	Less than 20/200	Unsteady peripheral eccentric 1/2° nasal	Fluctuation high frequency and ampleness 22′
			LE	plano	20/20		
	D. R.	25/F	RE(A)	$-0.75/-6.75 \times 30°$	20/200	Parafoveal eccentric	Fluctuation high frequency and ampleness 15′
			LE	$-0.25/-0.25 \times 75°$	20/20		
	J. R.	25/M	RE(A)	$-17/-3 \times$ T55°	20/100	Unsteady central	Fluctuation high frequency and ampleness 12′
			LE	$+0.50/-0.25 \times 90°$	20/20		
Amblyope by intoxication	E. G.	35/M	RE	$+0.75$	20/50	Unsteady central	Fluctuation high frequency and ampleness 17′ Loss of chromatic vision
			LE(A)	$+1$	20/50		
Strabismic amblyope	F. S.	48/M	RE	$-1.25/-0.75 \times 160°$	20/20	Unsteady peripheral	Fluctuation high frequency and ampleness 25′ constant 10 Δ right exotropia
			LE(A)	$-275/-1 \times 120°$	20/60	Eccentric 2° nasal with scotoma	

Results and discussion

Results from 10 normal observers (Chague *et al.* 2001) are shown in Fig. 17.2. These results reveal that: (i) the increase in the number of dots distributed on the background is inversely related to discrimination; (ii) decreasing the conspicuity of samples A, B, and C (Fig. 17.1(b))—reduces correct identification of the samples; and (iii) the identification is increased by the presence of color.

Based on these results, we made threshold measurements for the amblyopic and non-amblyopic eye of the patients included in Table 17.1. These results show that with their amblyopic eye the observers were unable to recognize achromatic situations as can be seen in Fig. 17.3(a) where cases 1–4 of Fig. 17.2 could not be detected. Please note that we included the situation 4 data of Fig. 17.2 in Fig. 17.3 for reasons of comparison. With respect to the non-amblyopic eyes (Fig. 17.3(b)) observers also could not identify case 1 of Fig. 17.2, and although the rest of the cases were perceived, the level of perfomance was lower.

Continuing with the analysis of the data, we observed that the loss of conspicuity of the stimulus was accentuated when the arrangement of the moving dots was not symmetric with respect to the horizontal meridian (Pointer and Watt 1987), as in arrangement C. Generally, the discrimination failed when the backgrounds included more than 20 dots, but complete recognition was achieved when the number of dots was reduced to 5.

In order to get a better discrimination of the movement, we decided to include a new experimental condition, in which the purity of the samples was increased to 0.18 and the background to 2.3, and, considering the pertinent bibliography, intermediate dots were also inserted in both chromatic and achromatic samples B and C. This new situation, labeled number 9 in Fig. 17.3, led to a noticable improvement in recogntion.

For all four amblyopic eyes analyzed (Fig. 17.3(a)), irrespective of aetiology, the best performance was observed in situation (8) in which the stimulus dots were in configuration A, were colored, and were presented on a color opponent background. The special case, situation 9, in which the stimulus cues were greatly enriched, in all cases resulted in recognition of 100 per cent, with exception of the observer 5 in Table 17.1. He had highly impaired chromatic vision (100 Hue Test error scores of 610 for the right eye and 773 for the left eye) and was not able to discriminate in any situation.

Lastly, patient 6, a typical case of amblyopia with strabismus and central scotoma, could only partially detect situation A, when it presented chromatic opponency between the background and the target and high saturation.

These results show that changes in perceived form or color can cause changes in perceived motion.

References

Chague, M. M., de Mattiello, M., & Buglione, S. (2001) Movement and colour: for independent or complementary channels? *Proceedings AIC 2001*, Rochester, NY (in press).

Chung, S. T. L. & Levi, D. M. (1997) Moving vernier in amblyopic and peripheral vision: greater tolerance to motion blur. *Vision Research, 37,* 2527–33.

Chung, S. T. L., Levi, D. M., & Bedell, H. E. (1996) Vernier in motion: what accounts for the threshold elevation? *Vision Research, 36,* 2395–410.

Field, D. J. & Hess, R. F. (1996). Uncalibrated distortions versus undersampling. *Vision Research, 36,* 2121–4.

Hess, R. F., Campbell, F. W., & Greenhalgh, T. (1978) On the nature of the neural abnormality in human amblyopia: neural aberrations and neural sensitivity loss. *Pflugers Archives, 377,* 201–7.

Hess, R. F. & Field, D. (1994) Is the spatial deficit in strabismic amblyopia due to loss of cells or an uncalibrated disarray of cells? *Vision Research, 34,* 3397–406.

Hess, R. F., Field, D., & Watt, R. J. (1990) The puzzle of amblyopia. In C. Blakemore (Ed.), *Vision: Coding and Efficiency.* Cambridge, UK: Cambridge University Press.

Kocak-Altintas, A. G., Satana, B., Kocak, I., & Dumas, S. (2000) Visual acuity and color vision deficiency in amblyopia. *European Journal of Ophthalmology, 10/1,* 77–81.

Lado, G. & de Mattiello, M., & Tonti, A. (2000) Analysis of acquired contrast vision defects using a network model. *Proceeding of IBERAMIA/SBIA 2000, Workshop on Artificial Intelligence and Computer Vision November 2000,* San Paulo, Brazil, pp. 158–61.

Levi, D. M., Klein, S. A., Sharma, V., & Nguyen, L. (2000) Detecting disorder in spatial vision. *Vision Research, 40,* 2307–27.

Morgan, M. J., Watt, R. J., & McKee, S. P. (1983) Exposure duration affects the sensitivity of vernier acuity to target motion. *Vision Research, 23,* 541–6.

Pointer, J. S. & Watt, R. J. (1987) Shape recognition in amblyopia. *Vision Research, 27,* 651–60.

Roth, A. (1968) Le sens chromatique dans l' amblyopie fonctionelle. *Documenta Ophthalmologia, 24,* 113–200.

Watt, R. J. & Hess, R. F. (1987) Spatial information and uncertainty in anisometropic amblyopia. *Vision Research, 27,* 661–74.

Westheimer, G. & McKee, S. P. (1975) Visual acuity in the presence of retinal image motion. *Journal of the Optical Society of America, 65,* 847–50.

CHAPTER 18

CONVERGENCE AS A FUNCTION OF CHROMATIC CONTRAST: A POSSIBLE CONTRIBUTOR TO DEPTH PERCEPTION?

GALINA V. PARAMEI AND WOLFGANG JASCHINSKI

Introduction

Recently, a growing body of research has investigated whether chromatic features can contribute to depth perception. The problem has traditionally been addressed by measuring stereoscopic performance at equiluminance, when luminance mechanisms are theoretically excluded (for review see Howard and Rogers 1995). Ample evidence for independent chromatic stereopsis mechanisms has been obtained, showing that at sufficient contrast, chromatic mechanisms subserve stereoperception (Simmons and Kingdom 1995, 1997). Until now, studies on binocular vision using chromatic contrast have concentrated upon its role in stereoscopic depth, whereas little is known about its influence on oculomotor functions; in particular, on convergence, which is considered a cue for distance in depth perception (Trotter 1995). Conversely, previous investigations of vergence have focused mainly on achromatic features of fusion stimuli (for review, see Collewijn and Erkelens 1990). In the present study we addressed the question of whether vergence, an oculomotor component of binocular vision, is related to variation of chromatic information in stimuli, thereby contributing to binocular "color-and-depth" perception. In particular, we investigated whether a near-vergence response elicited by a fusion stimulus would change when stimulus chromatic contrast is varied. The results were compared to a reference condition, in which luminance contrast was varied.

Method

Observers

Twelve subjects (six females, six males) aged 19–44 years old (median age 22.5) participated in the experiment. They had normal color vision (as determined by standard pseudoisochromatic plates, Rayleigh matching, and the Farnsworth-Munsell 100-Hue test) and normal stereopsis (stereo acuity ≤30 arc s, as measured with the differential stereotest of the Polatest). The observers were emmetropic, except two who were mildly myopic and wore their non-tinted prescription lenses during the experiment.

Apparatus

For generating stimuli, two Sony GDM-500PST monitors (21 in. display, 800 × 600 pixels, 120 Hz) driven by a Cambridge Research Systems (CRS) Video Board were used. The CIE (x, y) coordinates for the monitors primaries were: red (0.60, 0.34), green (0.28, 0.60), and blue (0.16, 0.06). The maximum outputs of the monitors were calibrated, and the voltage/luminance relationship was linearized, independently for each of the guns using a CRS Gamma Correction System (OptiCal OP200-E). Photometric control was made with a Minolta Chroma Meter CS100.

The monitors were placed to the right and left of an observer at 90° to the gaze direction, so that fixation stimuli presented dichoptically were viewed in mirrors as a fused stimulus at a total distance of 38 cm (Fig. 18.1). (The disparity of dichoptically presented stimuli was corrected individually, contingent on pupil distance.) The observers' head position was stabilized with a chin and forehead rest. The experiment was carried out in a dark room, in which equipment was obscured by a blackout material.

Stimuli

The fixation stimulus was a black cross on a yellow background. The test stimuli were vertical gratings, consisting of a 0.5 cycle/deg sinusoidal variation in color (red/green; equiluminance) or luminance (yellow/black; isochrominance) modulated by a Gaussian (the "envelope"). The spatial parameters were designed to minimize luminance artifacts due to chromatic aberration (Scharff and Geisler 1992). The mean luminance of the fixation and the test stimuli at the eye was approximately 4 cd/m^2.

The gratings were 8° squares, implying a projection onto the retinal area where the relative numbers of L and M cones remain approximately invariant (Nerger and Cicerone 1992). With the stimuli employed, a variation in S-cone excitation was supposedly

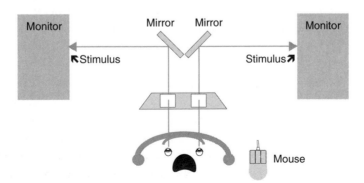

Figure 18.1 Top-view of the experimental set-up.

involved too, since a line intersecting the R and G phosphor chromaticities of the color monitor does not pass through the origin point of the CIE chromaticity diagram. The S-cone input might, however, be considered minimal for the function under study, since the S cones are sparsely distributed in the retina (Williams *et al.* 1981), have low photon catches, and provide vergence accuracy poorer than for the L/M cones conditions (Wilson *et al.* 1988).

For chromatic gratings, equiluminance was obtained using heterochromatic flicker photometry, with the stimuli presented in the same spatial configuration as in the main experiment. Lights produced by the Red and Green guns were alternated at 30 Hz; the relative luminance of the lights was varied, with the sum kept constant. A staircase procedure with five reversals was used. On any trial, the subject identified high and low points to define the range where flicker was either eliminated or minimized, by pressing a button of a mouse. The trial response was the mean of these two extremes, and the mean of the last four settings was taken as the equiluminant point. Individual equiluminance settings, the ratio of Red to overall mean luminance $[R/(R + G)]$, were then incorporated for calculating subject-specific contrasts. Chromatic contrast was generated by modulating Red and Green guns of the monitors in spatial antiphase, and luminance contrast by modulating these guns in spatial phase. The chromatic and luminance contrasts reported here are the Michelson contrasts $[(L_{max}-L_{min})/(L_{max} + L_{min})]$. The luminances, L, were those measured with a photometer. The contrasts were varied in a geometric series, and covered the range between the highest (90 per cent) and zero (0 per cent) values. (A pilot experiment has shown that rather low contrasts could still elicit a near-vergence response.)

Procedure

In the main experiment, a run started with presentation of the fixation fusion stimulus for 2 s, which elicited a baseline vergence of 9°. To stimulate a near-vergence response, the cross was substituted for 300 ms by the test grating—red/green ("chromatic" series) or yellow/black ("luminance" series)—presented as a near-vergence step of 1°. The duration of the test was chosen, taking into account that the vergence response has a latent period of 160–200 ms (Rashbass and Westheimer 1961), and assuming that by 300 ms the disparity vergence would be accomplished. The brief presentation of the test stimulus also helped insure that color/brightness fading during voluntary fixation would be avoided (cf. Gur 1989).

During an additional 100 ms of the test interval, fixation disparity (FD), a vergence error relative to the expected final vergence state of 10°, was measured (Schor 1983). The FD measurement was realized using nonius lines (e.g. Jaschinski 2001). These were presented dichoptically as white vertical bars, subtending 15×6 arc min, above and below the black horizontal meridian and were superimposed on the grating. The subject indicated whether the upper nonius line was seen to the right or left of the lower one by pressing a corresponding mouse button; after this the fixation stimulus reappeared. The interleaving of the test and fixation stimuli was repeated 30 times within the run

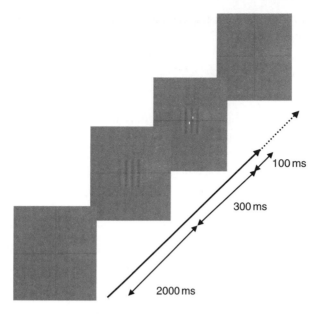

100 ms

300 ms

2000 ms

Figure 18.2 See also colour plate section. Sequence and time course of stimulus presentation for measuring fixation disparity (FD). On the grating, white nonius lines with varying physical offset are shown (for details see the text).

(see Fig. 18.2), with the amount of the nonius offset varied in small steps of 0.66 arc min, using the adaptive psychometric procedure Best-PEST (Lieberman and Pentland 1982).

In a given run, the contrast was kept constant but it was varied between runs. Each session comprised a "chromatic" series with seven runs according to varying contrast levels, as well as a "luminance" series with eight contrast-level runs, the latter including, additionally, a zero-contrast level as a baseline. For each observer, data across four daily sessions were collected, while counterbalancing the order of "chromatic" versus "luminance" and "decreasing" versus "increasing" contrast series.

Data analysis

In a given run, whenever the subject's response changed from "left" to "right" or vice versa (a reversal), the amount of nonius offset was recorded and taken as an estimation of actual FD (for details see Jaschinski 1998). For each observer, the FD for a run was calculated as a median of all "reversal" FDs. For each contrast, FD was a mean and SD of the values in four sessions. The data were also averaged across all observers to obtain FD means and SEs for each contrast level. A negative sign indicates an "exo" FD, when the visual axes converge slightly behind the fixation plane; conversely, a positive sign indicates an "eso" FD, a slight convergence of the axes in front of the plane.

A three-way analysis of variance (ANOVA) was carried out separately for the chromatic–contrast and luminance–contrast data with "contrast level" and "replication" as fixed, within-subject factors, and "subjects" as a random factor. The BMDP Statistical Software was used (Dixon 1992).

Results and discussion

Individual data revealed remarkable interindividual differences. These were confirmed by the ANOVA: for chromatic contrast, the "subject" factor accounted for 61 per cent of variance and for luminance contrast 64 per cent. Figure 18.3 presents vergence error, FD, as a function of chromatic contrast (a) and luminance contrast (b) for three (emmetropic) observers. Their data exemplify the distribution range for the whole subject sample, showing two extreme (about zero for BB; greatest for NP) and medium (for EA) sets of vergence error. Figure 18.3 demonstrates that with decreasing contrast, chromatic and

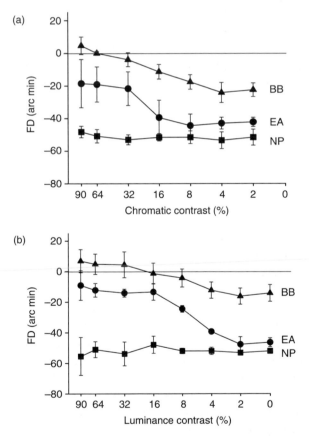

Figure 18.3 Fixation disparity (FD) as a function of (a) chromatic contrast and (b) luminance contrast. Presented are individual data for three subjects, which exemplify extreme (BB versus NP) and medium (EA) sets of FD within the distribution range for the total sample of observers. Bars indicate SDs.

luminance, the vergence error typically increases. It also indicates that at lower contrast levels, there is a tendency for response saturation.

Several features of the data are worth noting. (i) Intraindividually, FD functions for both chromatic and luminance contrast are comparable. At higher contrasts, in particular, the subject-specific vergence error has the same sign and comparable value regardless of the type of the contrast (cf. "eso" FD for BB with "exo" FD for the two other subjects). (ii) Between subjects, there is an appreciable variability, which shows itself in absolute FD values. Also, individual shapes of the contrast-dependent FD function—its slope and level of response saturation—differ dramatically. A function may presumably reflect individual differences in *actual* contrast perception, which varies among observers at nominally equal, defined in percentage, contrast level, and as such steers vergence. Alternatively, parameters of a "vergence plant" (cf. a model of Horng *et al.*, 1998) might be subject-specific and play a role. A way of disentangling the two potential factors may be sought in estimating individual contrast sensitivity functions prior to measuring a vergence response. (iii) As the data for observer NP indicate, when vergence error is remarkably great even at the highest-contrast condition (viz. FD value of (-50)–(-60) arc min), no further change in FD emerges with decreasing contrast. The finding suggests that the vergence system might execute a contrast-sensitive response under the premise that the system's shortfall (at optimal conditions) would be within a certain limit.

Figure 18.4 presents the relationship of vergence error, FD, to chromatic contrast (a), and luminance contrast (b) averaged across the sample of observers. For chromatic contrast, at the highest contrast level, the vergence deviates on average from the perfect response (i.e. at $10°$) by a negative exo FD value of -22 arc min. With decreasing contrast, exo FD further increases, that is, the near response gets worse, indicating that the eyes increasingly converge behind the plane of the target. This is confirmed by the ANOVA, which revealed a highly significant effect of chromatic contrast on vergence error, FD ($F = 14.35$; d.f $= 6/66$; $p < 0.01$ according to Greenhouse-Geisser; $\varepsilon = 0.27$). The lowest effective contrast was at 8 per cent and yielded the sample FD value of -36 arc min, suggesting a saturation constraint of efficacy of chromatic contrast on the vergence function.

A similar change of FD is found contingent on luminance contrast, that is, FD systematically increases with reduced contrast ($F = 14.70$; d.f $= 7/77$; $p < 0.001$ according to Greenhouse-Geisser; $\varepsilon = 0.22$). The vergence error is, however, smaller: for the highest contrast level, FD is -19 arc min, and the range of effective contrasts is greater (up to 2 per cent) than for chromatic contrast. The latter is confirmed by the ANOVA showing that variation of luminance contrast accounted for 9 per cent of variance, as compared with 7 per cent for chromatic contrast. It is notable, however, that at 2 per cent luminance contrast, the vergence error reaches the value of -36 arc min, identical to that at 8 per cent chromatic contrast.

The main finding in this study is that chromatic contrast yields information for a distance cue in dichoptically presented stimuli, as indicated by a systematic increase of

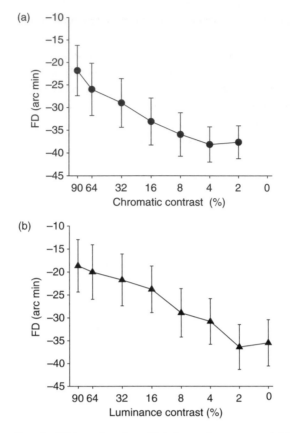

Figure 18.4 Fixation disparity (FD) as a function of (a) chromatic contrast and (b) luminance contrast, averaged for all observers. Bars indicate SEs.

the vergence error with reducing contrast. Similarly, reducing luminance contrast results in increasing vergence error.

While inspecting the difference in absolute FD values in the two functions, it is tempting to consider chromatic contrast less effective than luminance contrast: FD = −22 to −36 arc min versus FD = −19 to −29 arc min, respectively, in the comparable range above response saturation (i.e. 90–8 per cent). This assertion would be, however, premature, for contrasts for the chromatic and achromatic stimuli, expressed in terms of Michelson contrast, are not directly comparable, since the cone contrasts are unlikely to be equivalent for the two types of stimuli. Though Michelson contrast has been used extensively for specification of chromatic modulation in studies of "color-and-depth" perception (e.g. Mullen 1985; Gur and Akri 1992; Simmons and Kingdom 1998), we are aware that a solution of an "apples versus oranges" dilemma (cf. Switkes and Crognale 1999) for the set of present data would require expression of contrast in cone excitation units; this is being examined. Nevertheless, the presently employed contrast measure still demonstrates the dependence of a near-vergence response on variation of stimulus chromatic contrast.

One may be concerned that the obtained effect of chromatic contrast on vergence might be due to an artifact resulting from a residual activation in the "luminance" magnocellular (MC) system, since MC ganglion cells have been shown to be sensitive to red–green temporal chromatic modulation (Lee *et al.* 1989), as well as chromatic-border movement (Valberg *et al.* 1992). However, the light level employed in the present study, $4\,cd/m^2$ (<100 effective trolands, Le Grand 1968) is sufficiently low that the potential of the artifact is minimized (Lee *et al.* 1989).

It is worth noting that even for the highest contrast level, vergence deviated from an ideal, zero-error response. We cannot exclude the possibility that this error may be due to the presentation time course that we used (fixation fusion stimulus for 2 s; test for 300 ms with nonius lines superimposed for another 100 ms etc.), whereby at the moment of the actual FD measurement, the vergence process has not completely developed (cf. Pobuda and Erkelens 1993). This view is also supported by the temporal parameters in a recently developed model for the control of disparity-vergence eye movements: the first 200–300 ms constitute an initial component, or a rapid preprogrammed portion of the vergence response, whereas a highly accurate final position of the eyes, guided by visual feedback control, is reached during a late component (Horng *et al.* 1998).

In addition, the exposure duration employed might be a cause for greater FD with chromatic contrast than with luminance contrast, due to a difference between the time for a pure chromatic signal to establish vergence compared with a luminance signal (a suggestion made by an anonymous reviewer). This issue could be resolved in a more extensive study with varying temporal parameters of stimulus exposure.

A complementary explanation of the imperfect vergence response even at the highest contrast is that the vergence error might be related to blur of the stimuli used, since a "vergence plant", according to neurophysiological findings in monkeys, is "crosslinked" to a "blur controller" (Judge and Cumming 1986). This possibility is supported by the psychophysical findings that blur is additive with contrast in affecting depth perception (O'Shea *et al.* 1997).

The efficacy of contrast on depth perception, demonstrated by the present results, is in line with previous findings of O'Shea *et al.* (1994), who showed that contrast is a cue to depth, namely the lower the contrast of a target, the farther its apparent depth. However, these authors employed stimuli with achromatic contrast and were interested in perceptual measures of relative target depth. As suggested by the authors, achromatic (luminance) contrast exerts its effect primarily at a monocular site.

By the same token, the effect of chromatic contrast may be explained by a monocular color mechanism that makes possible the detection of chromatic contours; it then feeds in chromatic contrast-contingent information at a binocular site. Such an explanation is rooted in compelling evidence for a monocular color mechanism that inputs to a higher site where color and depth are processed together (e.g. Domini *et al.* 2000).

A further interpretation can be in terms of a contrast gain-control along the lines proposed by Shevell and Wei (2000): each contrast edge is coded monocularly by a neural response regulated by a subsequent, central binocular gain-control mechanism, with the gain control depending on chromatic variation over a large area. According to Shevell and Wei, changing the depth separation between the test and its immediately contiguous retinal stimulus is the critical factor that causes a change in color appearance. We suggest that the relationship between depth perception and color appearance is *mutual*; specifically, as a result of a binocular gain-control coding, variation of chromatic contrast ($\sim$ color appearance) could have an effect on perceived depth.

The present study suggests that the stereoscopic mechanism, on which binocular depth perception is primarily based, is supplemented by the oculomotor component—vergence driven by chromatic contrast. Conceivably, chromatic contrast-driven vergence provides information about the absolute distance to a stimulus, and thereby serves as a modulator of disparity sensitivity, the basis of the stereoscopic mechanism (Trotter 1995). Based on neurophysiological studies of the primary visual cortex, a putative site in which retinal and extraretinal signals involved in 3D space perception are integrated, is the human homologue of V1, where "tuned vergence-gated" cells are part of the neural mechanism that favors stereopsis at an early step of the visual pathway (Trotter *et al.* 1992). Recent psychophysical studies (Domini *et al.* 2000), however, provide an indication that the site of combining chromatic and depth information is likely to lie beyond V1.

Acknowledgment

Supported by DFG grant JA 747/2-1. We thank E. Alshuth for computer support, A. Bentler for collecting subject data, and U. Lobisch for preparing the illustrations. We are grateful to J. Pokorny, C. R. Cavonius, and an anonymous referee for helpful suggestions and comments on a previous version of the paper.

References

Collewijn, H. & Erkelens, C. J. (1990). Binocular eye movements and the perception of depth. In E. Kowler (Ed.) *Eye movements and their role in visual and cognitive processes* (pp. 213–261). Amsterdam: Elsevier.

Dixon, W. J. (1992). *BMDP Statistical Software Manual*. Berkeley: University of California Press.

Domini, F., Blaser, E., & Cicerone, C. M. (2000). Color-specific depth mechanisms revealed by a color-contingent depth effect. *Vision Research, 40,* 359–64.

Gur, M. (1989). Color and brightness fade-out in the Ganzfeld is wavelength dependent. *Vision Research, 29,* 1335–41.

Gur, M. & Akri, V. (1992). Isoluminant stimuli may not expose the full contribution of color to visual functioning: Spatial contrast sensitivity measurements indicate interaction between color and luminance processing. *Vision Research, 32,* 1251–62.

Horng, J.-L., Semmlow, J. L., Hung, G. K., & Ciuffreda, K. J. (1998). Initial component control in disparity vergence: A model-based study. *IEEE Transactions on Biomedical Engineering, 45,* 249–57.

Howard, I. P. & Rogers, B. J. (1995). *Binocular vision and stereopsis.* New York: Oxford University Press.

Jaschinski, W. (1998). Fixation disparity at different viewing distances and the preferred viewing distance in a laboratory near-vision task. *Ophthalmic and Physiological Optics, 18,* 30–9.

Jaschinski, W. (2001). Fixation disparity and accommodation for stimuli closer and more distant than oculomotor positions. *Vision Research, 41,* 923–33.

Judge, S. J. & Cumming, B. G. (1986). Neurons in the monkey midbrain with activity related to vergence eye movement and accommodation. *Journal of Neurophysiology, 55,* 915–30.

Le Grand, Y. (1968). *Light, Colour and Vision.* 2nd Edition. London: Chapman and Hall.

Lee, B. B., Martin, P. R., & Valberg, A. (1989). Nonlinear summation of M- and L-cone inputs to phasic retinal ganglion cells in macaque. *Journal of Neuroscience, 9,* 1433–42.

Lieberman, H. R. & Pentland, A. P. (1982). Microcomputer-based estimation of psychophysical thresholds: The Best-PEST. *Behavior Research Methods and Instrumentation, 14,* 21–5.

Mullen, K. T. (1985). The contrast sensitivity of human colour vision to red–green and blue–yellow chromatic gratings. *Journal of Physiology, 359,* 381–400.

Nerger, J. L. & Cicerone, C. M. (1992). The ratio of L to M cones in the human parafoveal retina. *Vision Research, 32,* 879–88.

O'Shea, R. P., Blackburn, S. G. & Ono, H. (1994). Contrast as a depth cue. *Vision Research, 34,* 1595–604.

O'Shea, R. P., Govan, D. G., & Sekuler, R. (1997). Blur and contrast as pictorial depth cues. *Perception, 26,* 599–612.

Pobuda, M. & Erkelens, C. J. (1993). The relationship between absolute disparity and ocular vergence. *Biological Cybernetics, 68,* 221–8.

Rashbass, C. & Westheimer, G. (1961). Disjunctive eye movement. *Journal of Physiology, 159,* 339–60.

Scharff, L. V. & Geisler, W. S. (1992). Stereopsis at isoluminance in the absence of chromatic aberrations. *Journal of the Optical Society of America A, 9,* 868–76.

Schor, C. M. (1983). Fixation disparity and vergence adaptation. In C. M. Schor & K. J. Ciuffreda (Eds.) *Vergence Eye Movements: Basic Clinical Aspects* (pp. 465–516). Boston: Butterworths.

Shevell, S. K. & Wei, J. (2000). A central mechanism of chromatic contrast. *Vision Research, 40,* 3173–80.

Simmons, D. R. & Kingdom, F. A. A. (1995). Differences between stereopsis with isoluminant and isochromatic stimuli. *Journal of the Optical Society of America A, 12,* 2094–104.

Simmons, D. R. & Kingdom, F. A. A. (1997). On the independence of chromatic and achromatic stereopsis mechanisms. *Vision Research, 37,* 1271–80.

Simmons, D. R. & Kingdom, F. A. A. (1998). On the binocular summation of chromatic contrast. *Vision Research, 38,* 1063–71.

Switkes, E. & Crognale, M. A. (1999). Comparison of color and luminance contrast: apples versus oranges? *Vision Research, 39,* 1823–31.

Trotter, Y. (1995). Cortical representation of visual three-dimensional space. *Perception, 24,* 287–98.

Trotter, Y., Celebrini, S., Stricanne, B., Thorpe S., & Imbert, M. (1992). Modulation of neural stereoscopic processing in primate area V1 by the viewing distance. *Science, 257,* 1279–81.

Valberg, A., Lee, B. B., Kaiser, P. K., & Kremers, J. (1992). Responses of macaque ganglion cells to movement of chromatic borders. *Journal of Physiology, 458,* 579–602.

Williams, D. R., MacLeod, D. I. A., & Hayhoe, M. M. (1981). Punctate sensitivity of the blue-sensitive mechanism. *Vision Research, 21,* 1357–75.

Wilson, H. R., Blake, R., & Pokorny, J. (1988). Limits of binocular fusion in the short wave sensitive ("blue") cones. *Vision Research, 28,* 555–62.

RODS AND COLOUR VISION

CHAPTER 19

THE INFLUENCE OF RODS ON COLOUR NAMING DURING DARK ADAPTATION

JANICE L. NERGER, VICKI J. VOLBRECHT, AND
KRISTIN A. HAASE

Introduction

Early studies investigating peripheral colour vision reported differences between foveal and peripheral perceptions (e.g. see Johnson 1986; Moreland 1972). Later, it was shown that peripheral colour vision was comparable to that of the fovea if stimulus size was sufficiently increased, effects of macular pigment density were considered, and rod signals were minimized (e.g. Abramov et al. 1991; van Esch et al. 1984; Nagy and Doyal 1993; Stabell and Stabell 1980, 1996).

One factor that appears crucial to equating peripheral colour perception to foveal colour perception is that the size of the stimuli must equal or exceed the perceptive field sizes for the four elemental hue sensations (i.e. red, blue, green, and yellow). Interestingly, the rate of change in perceptive field size across the horizontal meridian differs for the four hue sensations. While the perceptive field sizes for the four hues are quite similar near the fovea, the perceptive field size for green increases more rapidly with eccentricity than the others—for example, between 10° and 20° retinal eccentricity, the perceptive field size for green is twice as large as the perceptive field sizes for the other three hues (Abramov et al. 1991). This finding suggests that the neural processing mediating colour perception may differ between the fovea and the peripheral retina.

It is well documented that rod input affects peripheral colour perception. Many studies report colours become more desaturated and appear more bluish with rod input (e.g. Abramov et al. 1991; Ambler and Proctor 1976; Gordon and Abramov 1977; Trezona 1970), and Buck et al. (1998) report that rods affect the perception of all four elemental hues. Since physiological studies have demonstrated that rods share a common pathway with short-wavelength-sensitive cones (Daw et al. 1990) and provide input to the red/green parvocellular ganglion cells (Lee et al. 1997), it seems reasonable to expect that rod signals influence all aspects of colour perception. We do not know, however, how these peripheral perceptions develop over time or under what conditions they arise.

Methods

Colour-naming functions were obtained from three colour-normal observers in the fovea and at 8° in the nasal retina. All stimuli were presented in Maxwellian view. Channel 1 produced the monochromatic test field (440, 460, 480, 500, and 520 nm), Channel 2 created the pinhole-sized (5500 K) fixation points, and Channel 3 generated the 20° broadband (5500 K) bleaching field which was calculated to bleach 99 per cent of the rod pigment when viewed for 10 s. Test sizes were selected to fill the largest of the hue perceptive fields (Abramov *et al.* 1991) and measured 1.0° in diameter in the fovea and 1.5° in the peripheral retina. All test stimuli were presented for 500 ms and were equated to 25 photopic trolands.

After 10 min dark adaptation, observers viewed the bleaching stimulus (which was centered over the retinal area being tested). Test stimuli were then presented 1, 3, 8, 12, 18, and 30 min after extinction of the bleaching field. At each time period, one wavelength was randomly selected for presentation. The time periods were chosen in order to obtain measurements prior to and after the rod–cone break, on the cone plateau, and on the rod plateau of the dark-adaptation function. Following each test flash, observers used the "4 + 1" method (Gordon *et al.* 1994) to assign percentages to their perceptions of red, green, yellow, and blue with the restriction that the assigned percentages total 100 per cent. Although the observers were permitted to use any combination of hue terms, there were no instances where any observer described a single stimulus as appearing both red and green or both blue and yellow. Observers were also required to rate the percentage of saturation from 0 to 100 per cent. Four responses for each of the five wavelengths were obtained at each of the six time periods. For all trials, the observers were unaware of the wavelength of the stimulus. Twenty 2-h sessions were required of each observer to complete data collection.

Results and discussion

A general pattern of results emerged for all wavelengths. First, saturation was reduced at 8° as compared to the fovea. Second, in general, the percent assigned to blue was less at 8° nasal retinal eccentricity than in the fovea. Finally, while the foveal data remained essentially constant across time, the nasal data changed, both in saturation and in hue.

Figure 19.1 illustrates the mean results of the three observers for the 480-nm test field in the fovea (left panel) and at 8° in the nasal retina (right panel). Different symbols denote saturation and the different hue terms. Error bars represent ±1 standard error of the means (SEM) across the three observers. Results in Fig. 19.1 were scaled to saturation, that is, the percent hue was adjusted so that the sum of the hue percepts totaled the percent assigned for saturation. Plotted in this manner, comparisons of the total colour experience (achromatic and chromatic) between the fovea and periphery can be directly ascertained.

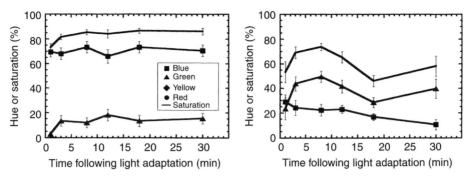

Figure 19.1 Mean colour-naming functions of the three observers obtained in the fovea (left panel) and 8° nasal retinal eccentricity (right panel) are shown for the 480-nm stimulus. Percent saturation and hue are plotted as a function of time in the dark following light adaptation. Different symbols denote saturation and the different hue terms. Error bars denote ±1 SEM across the three observers. Data are scaled to saturation.

As illustrated in the figure, the 480-nm stimulus appeared less saturated in the periphery. In addition, whereas the stimulus was described as greenish-blue when presented to the fovea, it was described as bluish-green when presented to the periphery. Thus, a change in both saturation and hue occurred when the stimulus was seen in the periphery as compared to the fovea. Similarly, although not shown, the 460-nm stimulus was perceived as reddish-blue when presented to the fovea and greenish-blue when presented at 8°. This reduction in blueness and increase in greenness is consistent with studies from our lab, which demonstrated that the locus of unique blue shifts to shorter wavelengths at 8° as compared to the fovea (Nerger *et al.* 1998). A notable feature in the 500 and 520 nm data was a decrease in green and an increase in the perception of yellow at 8°. This result is also in agreement with our study showing unique green in the peripheral retina occurs at shorter wavelengths than in the fovea (Nerger *et al.* 1995).

Figure 19.2 plots the percent saturation (upper panel) and percent blue (lower panel) as a function of wavelength for stimuli presented to the fovea (circles) and peripheral retina (squares). Filled symbols represent data obtained on the cone plateau (8 min post bleach) and unfilled symbols denote data obtained on the rod plateau (30 min post bleach). In this figure, the percent assigned to blue was not scaled to saturation in order to clearly depict only the chromatic content of the observers' percepts.

Stimuli presented in the fovea appeared the same in saturation and blueness regardless of whether measurements were taken on the cone (filled circles) or rod (unfilled circles) plateau. This was expected since the test stimulus was relatively small and the input from rods was minimal. The peripheral data obtained after 30 min post bleach (unfilled squares) showed a marked decline in saturation as compared to measurements made 8 min post bleach (filled squares). We attribute this decrease in saturation seen in the 30 min peripheral data to the influence of rods.

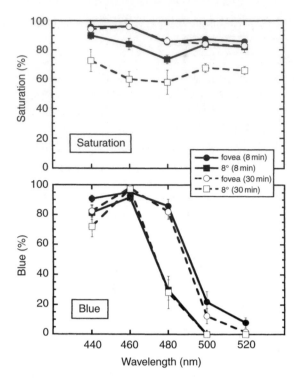

Figure 19.2 Mean percent saturation (upper panel) and mean percent blue (lower panel) are plotted as a function of the wavelength of the test stimuli presented to the fovea (circles) and peripheral retina (squares). Filled symbols represent data obtained on the cone plateau (8 min post bleach) and unfilled symbols represent data obtained on the rod plateau (30 min post bleach). Error bars denote ±1 SEM across the three observers. Data in the lower panel are *not* scaled to saturation.

In examining the percentage assigned to blueness (lower panel), two findings are of interest. First, in general, the percent blue seen in the peripheral stimuli was less than the percent blue reported in the fovea. This was most marked in the 480 and 500 nm stimuli. It should be noted that none of the stimuli in our study were described as being bluer when presented to the peripheral retina. This is contrary to previous studies (e.g. Ambler and Proctor 1976; Trezona 1970) that report an increase in the perception of blueness with rod input. Second, unexpectedly, the percent blue obtained in the peripheral retina at 8 min post bleach (filled squares) did not differ from that obtained at 30 min post bleach (unfilled squares). If the differences in hue perception seen between the fovea and peripheral data were due solely to the rods, then one would expect to see differences in the peripheral data between that obtained on the cone plateau (8 min) versus the rod plateau (30 min). Since no differences were observed between these two time periods, it is likely that the differences observed between the two retinal locations is not due to rod signals alone and may be due to differences in the neural processing of cones in the two locations. Likewise, the peripheral data obtained at 8 min post bleach differed from the foveal data obtained at 8 min post bleach. If our bleaching paradigm was successful in eliminating the rod signals at 8 min, then this finding also suggests that neural processing of colour by the peripheral cones differs from that of the foveal cones.

Various studies have demonstrated that the effects of rods on hue judgments are dependent on the size and intensity of the test stimulus. For example, Stabell and Stabell (1996) found that rods impart a yellow component to colour matches of long- and middle-wavelength stimuli, but that this effect diminishes as stimulus intensity increases. Likewise, our unique hue studies demonstrated more rod influence with smaller stimuli than with larger stimuli (Nerger *et al.* 1995, 1998). Thus, in this study, the differences in hue perception between the fovea and 8° nasal retinal eccentricity may have been minimized if we had either increased the size or the intensity of the stimuli presented to the peripheral retina. In this manner, the cone signals may have increased to the point required to effectively attenuate rod contribution to hue perception. Overall, this line of research may help contribute to an understanding of how the visual system constructs a uniform percept given that it is based upon signals derived from an extremely inhomogeneous receptor mosaic.

Acknowledgement

This research was supported by a National Science Foundation grant (IBN-9603613) to V. J. Volbrecht and J. L. Nerger.

References

Abramov, I., Gordon, J., & Chan, H. (1991). Color appearance in the peripheral retina: effects of stimulus size. *Journal of the Optical Society of America A, 8*, 404–14.

Ambler, B. A. & Proctor, R. W. (1976). Rod involvement in peripheral color processing. *Scandinavian Journal of Psychology, 17*, 142–8.

Buck, S. L., Knight, R., Fowler, G., & Hunt, B. (1998). Rod influence on hue-scaling functions. *Vision Research, 38*, 3259–63.

Daw, N. W., Jensen, R. J., & Brunken, W. J. (1990). Rod pathways in the mammalian retinae. *Trends in Neuroscience, 13*, 110–15.

van Esch, J. A., Koldenhof, E. E., van Doorn, A. J., & Koenderink, J. J. (1984). Spectral sensitivity and wavelength discrimination of the human peripheral visual field. *Journal of the Optical Society of America A, 1*, 443–50.

Gordon, J. & Abramov, I. (1977). Color vision in the peripheral retina. II. Hue and saturation. *Journal of the Optical Society of America, 67*, 202–7.

Gordon, J., Abramov, I., & Chan, H. (1994). Describing color appearance: hue and saturation scaling. *Perception & Psychophysics, 56*, 27–41.

Johnson, M. A. (1986). Color vision in the peripheral retina. *American Journal of Optometry and Physiological Optics, 63*, 97–103.

Lee, B. B., Smith, V. J., Pokorny, J., & Kremers, J. (1997). Rod inputs to macaque ganglion cells. *Vision Research, 37,* 2813–28.

Moreland, J. D. (1972). Peripheral colour vision. In *Handbook of Sensory Physiology, Vol. VII/4, Visual Psychophysics.* In: D. Jameson & L. M. Hurvich (Eds), Springer, New York.

Nagy A. L. & Doyal, J. A. (1993). Red–green color discrimination as a function of stimulus field size in peripheral vision. *Journal of the Optical Society of America A, 10,* 1147–56.

Nerger, J. L., Volbrecht, V. J., & Ayde, C. J. (1995). Unique hue judgments as a function of test size in the fovea and at 20-deg temporal eccentricity. *Journal of the Optical Society of America A, 12,* 1225–32.

Nerger, J. L., Volbrecht, V. J., Ayde, C. J., & Imhoff, S. M. (1998). Effect of the S-cone mosaic and rods on red/green equilibria. *Journal of the Optical Society of America A, 15,* 2816–26.

Stabell, B. & Stabell, U. (1996). Peripheral colour vision: Effects of rod intrusion at different eccentricities. *Vision Research, 36,* 3407–14.

Stabell, U. & Stabell, B. (1980). Variation in density of macular pigmentation and in short-wave cone sensitivity with eccentricity. *Journal of the Optical Society of America, 70,* 706–11.

Trezona, P. W. (1970). Rod participation in the 'blue' mechanism and its effect on color matching. *Vision Research, 10,* 317–32.

CHAPTER 20

STIMULUS DURATION AFFECTS ROD INFLUENCE ON HUE PERCEPTION

STEVEN L. BUCK AND ROGER KNIGHT

Introduction

Signals originating from rod photoreceptors interact with cone signals to affect the balance of all four basic hues and both opponent hue dimensions. These rod influences appear to fall into at least two categories: a "faster", less-light-level dependent enhancement of green relative to red, and a "slower" more-light-level dependent enhancement of blue relative to yellow and short-wavelength red (SW red) relative to green (Buck 2001). We have found good agreement on this set of rod influences across procedures investigating rod effects on the loci of unique and binary hues (Buck Knight and Bechtold 1997, 2000) and the hue scaling of both single test stimuli (Buck *et al.* 1998) and compound probe-flash stimuli (Knight and Buck 2002).

Our prior studies of the time-course of rod influences on hue employed a probe-flash procedure in which observers judged the hue of a 30-ms mesopic test probe presented with different delays after the onset of a scotopic background flash (Knight and Buck 2001). This earlier procedure reveals how prolonged *rod* stimulation (adaptation) drives changes of rod influence on hue but cannot tell us how prolonged *cone* stimulation and chromatic adaptation might affect the various rod influences on hue. Our probe-flash studies showed that the balance of rod influences on hue is altered dramatically over the first second of rod stimulation and only slightly over the remainder of 5 s of rod stimulation (Knight and Buck 2002). The present study explores the effects of simultaneous rod and cone stimulation on rod hue influences over this same time scale. The issue bears on both our understanding of the visual processes mediating rod influences on hue and on the generality of those influences to more natural visual environments with prolonged stimulation of both rods and cones.

Methods

Observers, apparatus, and stimuli

Two experienced and two inexperienced observers (two females and two males, ages 24–43 years) participated in all conditions. All observations were made with a previously described computer-controlled Maxwellian-view apparatus (Buck 1997). The wavelength of the 8°-diameter test probe was varied between 420 and 620 nm in discrete steps of either 10 nm (for 30-ms duration condition) or 20 nm (for 5-s duration condition) by means of a PTR monochromator having a full bandwidth at 50 per cent of peak transmission of less than 2 nm. Uniblitz shutters produced either 30-ms or 5-s presentations of the test stimulus with a 20-s inter-trial interval of darkness. Spectrally calibrated neutral-density filters controlled the illuminance of all stimuli. The monochromator, shutters, and variable neutral-density filters were controlled by computer to provide a random order of presentation of test wavelengths at 1.5 log scotopic trolands for all conditions, a light level shown by Buck *et al.* (1998) to produce significant rod influence on hue appearance. Spectral and illuminance calibrations were performed *in situ* by means of a calibrated Gamma Scientific spectroradiometer system.

A dim, continuously illuminated, 1°-square fixation cross was presented by means of a second channel 7° to the left of center of the probe and background. This placed the stimulus along the horizontal meridian in the nasal retina of the observer's right eye. The 7° eccentricity and 8° test diameter were chosen to maintain comparability with prior work from this laboratory on hue-scaling, scotopic color contrast, and rod influence on unique and binary hue loci.

Hue- and saturation-scaling procedures

We used a hue-scaling procedure similar to that used by others (e.g. Abramov *et al.* 1991). After inspecting the test probe for one or two presentation cycles, the observer first described its appearance with up to two of the four basic hues (red, green, blue, and yellow) and assigned a percentage to the relative strength of each component hue, so that the sum of the percentages equaled 100 per cent. Observers were permitted to use any combination of the four hue names; however they rarely selected the classical opponent combinations on any given trial. Observers then assigned a percentage to the relative strength of saturation of the stimulus that could vary from 0 to 100 per cent. Observers were unaware of the wavelength of the probe and had only their perceptions to guide scaling responses.

One hue judgment and one saturation judgment were made for each wavelength in each of 10 daily sessions. The apparatus computer randomized stimulus presentation order for each session and recorded all responses.

Adaptation conditions

In order to measure the influence of rods on hue and saturation, we compared judgments made to physically identical stimuli under two different conditions of adaptation that maximized and minimized rod contribution, respectively.

Dark-adapted condition

Before beginning an experimental session, observers dark-adapted the right eye for 30 min.

Cone-plateau condition

Rod influence was minimized by making judgments during the cone plateau, 3–8 min following exposure to a xenon flash. The bleaching flash was provided by a Quantum Qflash, model T, which delivers 0.5 joules in a 3.3-ms duration flash. Observers viewed the flash through heat-absorbing glass and fixated the left edge of the flash unit so that the bleached area of retina subtended approximately 17° and extended beyond the area of the probe and background stimuli. Pre-testing confirmed that the flash illuminance was sufficient to produce stable cone-plateau measurements and invisibility of the background stimulus for at least 8 min. Several flash-bleach cycles, with a minimum 15-min interval between bleaches, were required during a single session in order to make a single hue- and saturation scaling judgment for each wavelength.

Results and discussion

Figure 20.1 shows the mean hue-scaling data averaged across the four observers. For clarity, the data are presented in separate panels for red (R) and green (G) or blue (B) and yellow (Y) hue responses but ratings of all hues were made simultaneously. Error bars represent ±1 SE of the individual observer means. Within each panel, Fig. 20.1 compares hue ratings for cone-plateau (open symbols, dashed lines) and dark-adapted (solid symbols and lines) conditions. Rod influences on hue show up as differences between the hue ratings for these two adaptation conditions. Consistent with our prior reports, rod influence affects the distribution of the four basic hues throughout most of the spectrum, for both 30-ms (top panels) and 5-s (bottom panels) test durations.

Some of the specific rod influences on hue are apparent at both test durations. For both 30-ms and 5-s test durations, rods enhance blue relative to yellow, and green relative to long-wavelength red. The rod blue bias results in a shift of the blue–yellow transition (an indirect measure of unique green) by 30–40 nm toward longer wavelengths (right panels) in the dark-adapted condition (solid symbols and lines) compared to the cone-plateau condition (open symbols, dashed lines). This is accompanied by increased blue ratings and decreased yellow ratings in a broad region spanning the transition. (Figure 20.1 shows data averaged across observers but each of the four individual observers showed the rod blue bias at both test durations. For all four observers, rods extended blue to longer wavelengths in the 30-ms condition than in the 5-s condition.)

The rod green bias results in a shift of the long-wavelength green–red transition (an indirect measure of unique yellow) by about 10 nm, as shown in the left panels of Fig. 20.1. (Three of the four observers showed the rod green bias at long wavelengths at both test durations, although two showed somewhat less at 5 s than at 30 ms. One observer showed no rod effect on long-wavelength red–green balance at either duration.)

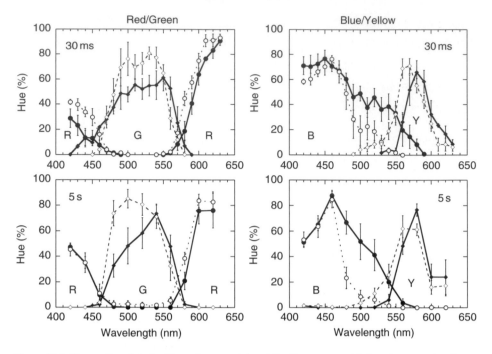

Figure 20.1 Hue scaling data for 30-ms (top panels) and 5-s (bottom panels) duration test stimuli. Each panel compares hue-scaling values assigned to the same physical stimuli under dark-adapted (filled symbols, solid lines) and cone-plateau (open symbols, dashed lines) conditions. Each data point shows the mean of four observers. Error bars represent ±1 SE of the observer means in all figures.

The magnitudes of both of these rod hue biases are within the ranges found in our prior studies, although the present rod blue bias is on the high side, while the present rod green bias is on the low side.

The major difference in rod influence on the two test durations is found at short wavelengths. Figure 20.1 (left panels) shows that the rod enhancement of green relative to red is found at short wavelengths only for the 30-ms test duration. For this condition, the rod green bias shifts the short-wavelength red–green transition corresponding to unique blue to shorter wavelengths by 15–25 nm, while increasing ratings of green and decreasing ratings of red below 470 nm. (All four individual observers showed this short-wavelength rod green bias for the 30-ms test duration.) For the 5-s stimuli, there is no net rod influence on the short-wavelength red–green transition or the ratings of red or green below 470 nm.

Figure 20.1 also shows that, for both test durations, there is a reduction of green ratings in mid-spectrum (ca. 480 nm to at least 520 nm) under dark-adapted compared to cone-plateau conditions. This likely reflects a relative reduction of green by the strong rod blue bias described above, and not a change in the strength of green relative to red. Recall that an observer's hue ratings were constrained to sum to 100 per cent at each

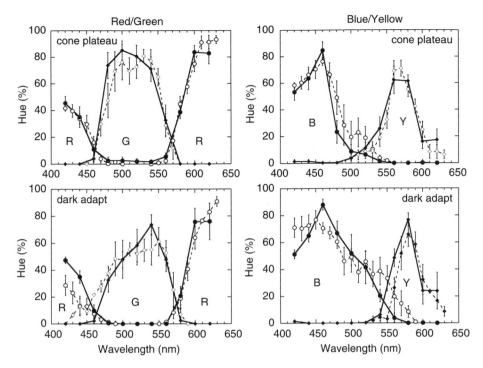

Figure 20.2 Hue scaling data for cone-plateau (top panels) and dark-adapted (bottom panels) conditions. Each panel compares hue-scaling values for 5-s duration (filled symbols, solid lines) and 30-ms duration (open symbols, dashed lines) test stimuli. Each data point shows the mean of four observers. Error bars represent ±1 SE of the observer means in all figures.

wavelength, so an increase of blue in this portion of the spectrum necessitates a reduced rating of green.

We infer that a "slow" rod enhancement of short-wavelength red relative to green shifts the short-wavelength red–green transition back toward longer wavelengths in the 5-s conditions. This short-wavelength rod red bias can be seen explicitly in Fig. 20.2, which shows that under dark-adapted conditions (lower left panel), the short-wavelength red–green transition shifts toward longer wavelengths in 5-s conditions (solid symbols and lines) compared to 30-ms conditions (open symbols, dashed lines). (All four individual observers showed this short-wavelength rod red bias.) No such shift is seen under cone-plateau conditions (upper left panel).

There are two lines of evidence to support the emergence of a rod red bias, as opposed to a decay of the rod green bias. First, the rod green bias continues at long wavelengths for both test durations, suggesting that different rod influences operate at the two ends of the spectrum for the 5-s condition. Second, although the present 5-s duration data show no net red or green rod hue bias at short wavelengths, other data sets have shown a net rod red bias at short wavelengths for stimuli providing rod stimulation for 1 s or longer (Buck *et al.* 1997, 1998, 2000; Knight and Buck 2002). No net rod red bias has been observed at long-wavelengths in any of our studies.

In addition to affecting rod hue biases, test duration also affects the balance of hues determined purely by cones, as can be seen by comparing the cone-plateau conditions (open symbols, dashed lines) in corresponding upper and lower panels. There is no apparent change of red–green balance with test duration but blue is enhanced relative to yellow and green between about 460 and 540 nm for the 30-ms test duration. This cone-mediated blue enhancement results in a 20-nm shift toward longer wavelengths of the blue–yellow transition (corresponding to unique green) for the 30-ms test and mirrors previous reports of mid-spectral blueness of small or brief peripheral targets (Gordon and Abramov 1977; Weitzman and Kinney 1969) and other phenomena that have been interpreted as showing M-cone contributions to blueness (Drum 1989; Ingling 1977). This phenomena has been dubbed "tritan blue" by Abramov *et al.* (1991) because blueness spreads up to about 570 nm, the tritanopic confusion point.

The present data show that "tritan" blueness can be produced solely by cone stimulation but can also be enhanced by rod stimulation. Inspection of the right-hand panels of Fig. 20.1 reveals that rod signals can enhance both the blueness commonly attributed to S cones (5-s conditions, lower right panel, 520 nm and below) and that attributed to "tritan" blue (30-ms conditions, upper right panel, 520–570 nm). It is also clear that the S-cone rod blue enhancement and the "tritan" rod blue enhancement have different time courses: Rod blue enhancement below 520 nm is greater for the longer test duration, while rod blue enhancement above 520 nm is greater for the shorter test duration. Whether this demonstrates a new "fast" rod blue bias, in addition to the "slow" rod blue bias previously described, and whether the "fast" effect is mediated by S-cone or M-cone pathways, remains to be determined.

A comparison of the present results with those of our probe-flash studies (Knight and Buck 2002) makes three points. First, the effects of prolonged cone stimulation (chromatic adaptation) on rod hue biases are small or negligible. Changes over time in the effects of rod stimulation on hue are similar when only rods are stimulated (probe-flash) and when both rods and cones are stimulated (variable test duration) for up to 5 s. However, one possible cone-mediated effect is attenuation of the short-wavelength rod red bias that is slightly more pronounced in the probe-flash studies. Second, stimulation of rods in the area of the test spot is sufficient to produce all of the immediate and delayed rod effects on hue observed in either study. The same rod hue effects were driven by rod stimulation from the smaller, brighter test stimulus as from the larger, dimmer background. Third, both procedures showed a slight reduction over time in the magnitude of the rod green bias at long wavelengths. This increases our confidence in the reliability and generality of this decrease.

Figure 20.3 shows observers' mean scaling of the degree of perceived saturation of 30-ms and 5-s test-stimulus durations for dark-adapted (solid symbols) and cone-plateau (open symbols) conditions. Both panels show that rods desaturate the stimulus throughout the spectrum, although less so for the 5-s condition and also least at longer

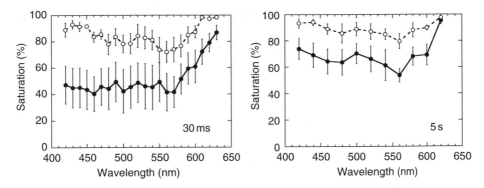

Figure 20.3 Comparison of saturation scaling between dark-adapted (solid lines and symbols) and cone-plateau (open symbols, dashed lines) conditions for 30-ms (left panel) and 5-s (right panel) test stimulus durations. Each data point shows the mean of four observers.

wavelengths where the ratio of cone to rod excitation is greatest. Thus, in contrast to the meager and uncertain effect of prolonged cone stimulation on rod hue influences, these data are consistent with data from other labs in showing a clear effect of prolonged cone stimulation on rod desaturation effects. While prolonged cone stimulation reduces the desaturating effect of rods, our prior work showed that prolonged rod stimulation alone (up to 5 s) does not (Knight and Buck 2002). Because the rod hue biases were so similar in both sets of studies, it seems unlikely that the rod hue biases are directly related to changes of desaturation in a manner similar to the cone-based Abney effect (Burns *et al.* 1984; Kurtenbach *et al.* 1984).

In conclusion, the present study reveals the same three rod hue biases seen in our past work and shows that the balance among them varies with test-stimulus duration. There appears to be little effect of prolonged cone stimulation on the balance of rod hue biases, which instead appears to be primarily controlled by the duration of rod stimulation. We speculate that the "faster" rod green bias is determined by a differential rod influence on M- versus L-cone pathways. The "slower" red and blue rod hue biases could result from rod signals having the same sign of influence as S-cone signals in chromatic pathways. The present results raise the possibility of an additional "fast" rod blue bias and raise the question of its mediation by S-cone or M-cone pathways.

Acknowledgement

Supported by NIH grant EY03221.

References

Abramov, I., Gordon, J., & Chan, H. (1991). Color appearance in the peripheral retina: effects of stimulus size. *Journal of the Optical Society of America A, 8*, 404–14.

Buck, S. (1997). Influence of rod signals on hue perception: evidence from successive scotopic color contrast. *Vision Research, 37,* 1295–301.

Buck, S. (2001). What is the hue of rod vision? *Color Research & Application, 26 Suppl.,* S57–S59.

Buck, S., Knight, R., & Bechtold, J. (1997). Effect of rod stimulation on unique and binary hue judgments. *IS&T/OSA Optics in the Information Age* (pp. 11–15). Springfield, VA: IS&T.

Buck, S., Knight, R., & Bechtold, J. (2000). Opponent-color models and the influence of rod signals on the loci of unique hues. *Vision Research, 40,* 3333–44.

Buck, S., Knight, R., Fowler, G., & Hunt, B. (1998) Rod influence on hue-scaling functions. *Vision Research, 38,* 3259–63.

Burns, S. A., Elsner, A. E., Pokorny, J., & Smith, V. C. (1984). The Abney Effect: Chromaticity coordinates of unique and other constant hues. *Vision Research, 24,* 479–89.

Drum, B. (1989). Hue signals from short- and middle-wavelength-sensitive cones. *Journal of the Optical Society of America A, 6,* 153–7.

Gordon, J. & Abramov, I. (1977). Color vision in the peripheral retina II. Hue and saturation. *Journal of the Optical Society of America, 67,* 202–7.

Ingling C. R. Jr. (1977). The spectral sensitivity of the opponent-color channels. *Vision Research, 17,* 1083–9.

Knight, R. & Buck, S. (2001). Rod influence on the hue perception: effect of background light level. *Color Research & Application, 26 Suppl.,* S60–S64.

Knight, R. & Buck, S. (2002). Time-dependent changes of rod influence on hue. *Vision Research, 42,* 1651–62.

Kurtenbach, W., Sternheim, C. E., & Spillmann, L. (1984). Change in hue of spectral colors by dilution with white light (Abney effect). *Journal of the Optical Society of America A, 1,* 365–72.

Weitzman, D. O. & Kinney, J. A. S. (1969). Effect of stimulus size, duration, and retinal location upon the appearance of color. *Journal of the Optical Society of America, 59,* 640–3.

NATURAL SCENES AND COLOUR CONSTANCY

CHAPTER 21

COLOUR DISCRIMINATION, COLOUR CONSTANCY AND NATURAL SCENE STATISTICS*

DONALD I. A. MACLEOD

Introduction

This year in Cambridge we remember Thomas Young (Mollon, "Thomas Young and the development of the trichromatic theory", Introduction to this volume), but in this particular college, Peterhouse, we also remember James Clerk Maxwell, who so admirably filled out Thomas Young's sketch of the trichromatic theory while still an undergraduate here and at Trinity (Sherman 1981). I think of Maxwell as a kind of prototype for all of us, because he combined a nice appreciation for the phenomena of colour with a penchant for quantitative analysis and mechanistic modelling. Although, as Goethe complained, all theory is gray, treatments of colour vision ever since Maxwell's time have tended to involve quantitative models, and the present one is no exception. My discussion also typifies a much more recent theoretical trend: I will attempt to relate the processes of colour vision to the characteristics of the natural environment. The reference to natural scene statistics is the main connection between the two parts of the chapter—the following five sections concerned with colour discrimination, and the seventh section concerned with colour appearance and its transformation or constancy under changes of illumination. Also central to both discussions is the indispensable and now familiar intellectual device that we owe to Maxwell: cone excitation space, the alpha and omega of colour spaces, where the three Cartesian co-ordinates specify the colour stimulus through the rates of isomerization of the three visual pigments of normal trichromatic colour vision.

Discrimination and the distribution of natural colours

Following von der Twer and MacLeod (2001), colour discrimination is here considered as a slicing of cone excitation space into distinguishable cells, and the questions considered are: What is the distribution of naturally occurring stimuli in cone excitation space? Is the slicing pattern that is revealed in psychophysical measures of colour discrimination well adapted for representing colours from that distribution? And how is the slicing pattern related to the neural representation of colour within the visual system?

....

* The Verriest Lecture. Delivered at Peterhouse, Cambridge, 16 July, 2001

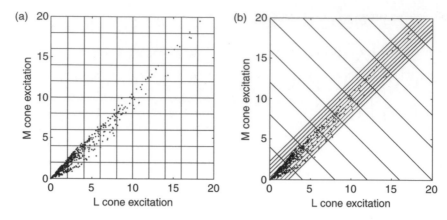

Figure 21.1 Distribution of Brown's haphazard sample of natural colours in the (L, M) plane of cone excitation space. Linear co-ordinates show a clustering near the origin. Slicing pattern at left achievable by independent L and M cone signals (for which the constant responses are vertical and horizontal lines, respectively). Slicing pattern at right uses a luminance signal (lines of negative slope) and a red–green opponent (L–M) signals (lines of positive slope).

The key idea to be developed is that it is advantageous to slice cone excitation space more finely in regions where natural colour stimuli are most densely concentrated. Imagine that successive, reliably different, levels of each neural signal define bins or slices into which our visual system can reliably divide colour stimuli (e.g. in Fig. 21.1 at left, separate signals originating from the L and M cones slice the shown plane of the space horizontally and vertically with 10 distinguishable levels each). The total number of these slices is fixed for a given signal by the range of output signal strength, going from zero to some maximum firing rate, and also varies reciprocally with the degree of intrinsic randomness or noise present in the neural signal. It has been clear since the time of Fechner and Helmholtz that the visual system slices cone excitation space in a distinctly non-uniform manner. In some respects at least the non-uniformity takes the form of finer slicing where natural stimuli are most frequent. For example: the first characteristic of the slicing pattern to be recognized (Helmholtz 1896) was that equal percentage changes in the linear cone excitations are roughly equally detectable, as if the excitation differences seen by each cone are divided by the mean excitation, a scenario supported by psychophysical (He and MacLeod 1997; MacLeod *et al.* 1992) and physiological evidence (Dacey *et al.* 1996). Since equal percentage changes correspond to equal intervals in the logarithm, a log-cone-excitation space in which each cone excitation is logarithmically compressed is more uniformly sliced than the linear one. The approximately logarithmic slicing pattern is efficient for representing natural surface colours, since natural stimuli are more symmetrically distributed in the logarithmic cone excitation space (Ruderman *et al.* 1998), without the concentration of dark colours near the origin seen in the linear space of Fig. 21.1.

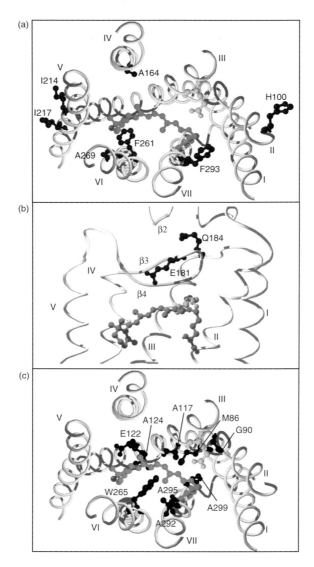

Figure 1.1 Views of an atomic model of bovine rhodopsin. Helices are labelled: I is helix I etc. The 11-*cis*-retinal chromophore is in green, and the counterion (Glu113) is in cyan. (a) Atomic model of rhodopsin viewed from the extracellular side of the membrane. Extracellular and cytoplasmic loops have been removed from this view, to allow the retinal-binding pocket to be viewed more easily. Residues implicated in a red-shift are shown in red, and are labelled (Ala164, Phe261, and Ala269—Chan *et al.* 1992; His100, Ile214, Ile217, and Phe293—Asenjo *et al.* 1994). (b): Side view of the retinal-binding pocket, with the extracellular surface at the top of the figure. Helix VI to the C terminus has been removed to expose the retinal-binding site. The β-sheet regions contributing to part of the extracellular "plug" are shown in yellow. β3 and β4 are in the second extracellular loop. The residues Glu181 and Gln184 are shown in red. The corresponding residues in the red and green cone pigments are thought to form a chloride ion-binding site, which red-shifts these visual pigments compared to rhodopsin (Wang *et al.* 1993). (c): Atomic model of rhodopsin viewed from the extracellular side of the membrane. Extracellular and cytoplasmic loops have been removed from this view, to allow the retinal-binding pocket to be viewed more easily. Residues whose mutation results in a blue-shift in the "blue-rhodopsin" mutant are shown in blue, and are labelled (Met86, Gly90, Ala117, Glu122, Ala124, Trp265, Ala292, Ala295, and Ala299—Lin *et al.* 1998). These images were created in Swiss-Pdb viewer, and rendered in POV-Ray (Guex and Peitsch 1997).

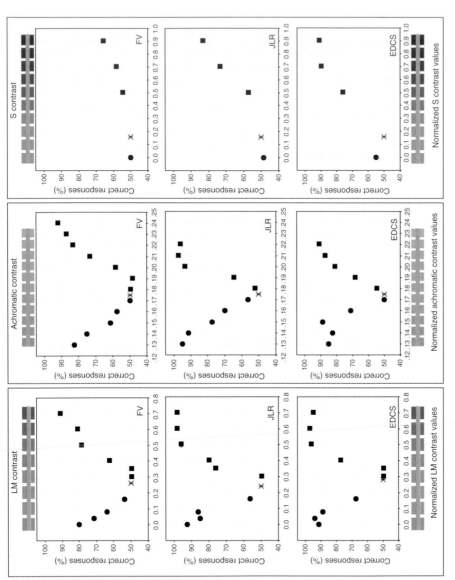

Figure 16.3 Discrimination threshold for subjective colours. Abscissas: range of contrast values that can be produced on the CRT, normalized from 0 to 1. The star indicates gray (128, 128, 128). Ordinates: percentage of correct responses for discrimination. Left: Discrimination threshold versus isoluminant chromatic LM contrast. Partial abscissa scale: 0 is the minimum L–M value; 1 would be the maximum L–M value. The scale varies slightly from one observer to the other depending upon the range of colours that can be produced at isoluminance for this individual. Centre: Discrimination threshold versus achromatic contrast (L + M + S). Enlarged abscissas scale: 0 would indicate black; 1 would indicate white. Right: Discrimination threshold versus isoluminant chromatic S contrast. Abscissas: 0, minimum S value; 1, maximum S value. Colour illustrations above and below the graphs show the variation of the stimulus: the central line represents the colour A as defined in Fig. 16.1 (medium gray 128, 128, 128) and the squares represent discrete values of the colour B as defined in Fig. 16.1.

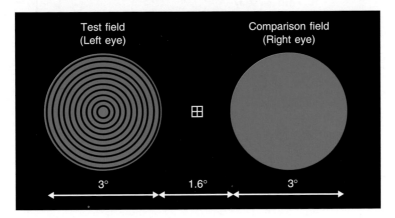

Figure 12.1 Schematic of haploscopically presented test and comparison fields. Observers set the uniform comparison field to match the appearance of the test background. The comparison field and test background shown here are physically identical.

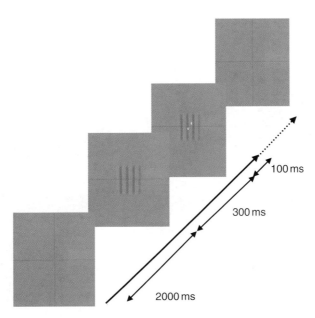

Figure 18.2 Sequence and time course of stimulus presentation for measuring fixation disparity (FD). On the grating, white nonius lines with varying physical offset are shown (for details see the text).

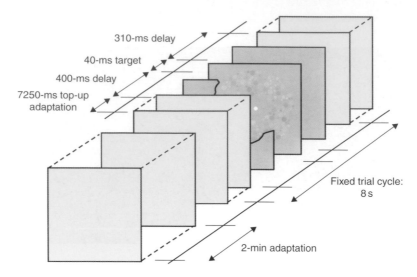

Figure 29.2 A schematic diagram showing the sequence of events in a trial. The initial two minute adaptation is followed by a repeated trial-cycle comprising a period of top-up adaptation followed, after 400 ms, by a 40-ms test array. The test arrays resemble Ishihara plates in that spatial luminance noise is used to mask luminance artefacts. The chromatic target formed a 90° arc that was presented in any one of 4 quadrants chosen at random. Ten different probe chromaticity vectors were tested as candidates for the tritan line. In Experiment 1 we compared three different adapting chromaticities. In Experiment 2 we increased the viewing distance, from 1 to 4 m, to determine whether the tritan axis rotated when the eccentricity of the target was reduced from 3 to 0.75 degrees of visual angle.

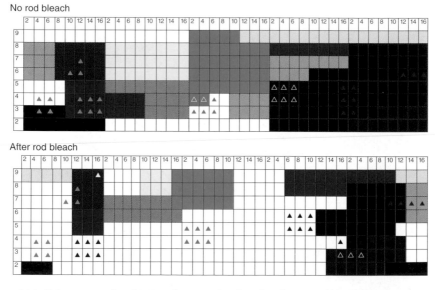

Figure 39.1 Colour categories of J. N. and a control with and without a rod bleach. The array represents the palette of Munsell chips varying in lightness and chroma. Cell colours indicate the range of chips that subject J. N. chose for each colour term before (top) and after (bottom) rod bleach. Filled triangles indicate the corresponding range for a control subject. White-△, pink-▲, orange-▲, yellow-▴, red-▲, brown-▲, black-▲, green-▲, blue-▲, purple-▲, gray-▴; Open triangles indicate agreement between J. N. and the control.

But two main features of the distribution of natural colours are not well dealt with by independent compression of the cone excitations. First, the stimulus distribution is centrally peaked: near-grays of moderate reflectance are relatively common, and the margins of cone excitation space, even in its logarithmic form, are only sparsely populated. Accordingly, fine discrimination is less important in the margins of colour space than in the centre, near white, where natural colour stimuli are most densely packed. Much psychophysical evidence on colour discrimination has indeed indicated a slicing pattern with best discrimination near white (or more precisely, near the stimulus to which the visual system is adapted) and a progressive deterioration as the saturation of the reference stimulus increases (Friele 1961; LeGrand 1949; Mollon 1982; Pugh and Mollon 1979). Superior discrimination for the naturally abundant near-neutral colours cannot be explained by independent compression of the three cone excitations, but requires a comparable compressive nonlinearity in the neural code at the colour-opponent level, where it is the differences between cone excitations that are represented (Friele 1961). The requirement for finer slicing near white thus yields a rationale for colour opponent encoding.

Second, the distribution of natural colours in cone excitation space is highly anisotropic, with much less dispersion in the red–green direction (the negative diagonal in Fig. 21.1, right) than in the luminance direction (the positive diagonal) or in the blue–yellow direction. Correspondingly, colour discrimination thresholds in the red–green direction, expressed in terms of cone contrast, are an order of magnitude lower than they are in the achromatic or luminance direction (Chaparro et al. 1993), implying finer "slicing" of log-cone-excitation space in that direction than in the luminance direction. This anisotropic slicing pattern also calls for colour-opponent signals. In the nonlinear analysis to be developed here, it is the reduced dispersion of natural inputs in the red–green direction that makes such a slicing pattern feasible and advantageous. Indeed, according to von der Twer and MacLeod (2001), only a nonlinear analysis can properly justify this obviously appropriate choice of slicing directions, although the principle of "decorrelation" within a linear framework dictates a similar choice (Buchsbaum and Gottschalk 1983; Fukurotani 1982; Zaidi 1997).

von der Twer and I considered quantitatively how the visual system's distribution of discriminative capacity over cone excitation space ought, in principle, to depend on the distribution of natural colour stimuli as represented in two data sets (Brown 1994; Ruderman et al. 1998). For 574 haphazard samples of natural colours measured in San Diego by Richard O. Brown, the correlation between L and M cone excitation is 0.985. These samples were not selected in such a way as to be representative in any sense, and they may have included a disproportionate number of highly chromatic surfaces since these would more readily have caught the investigator's eye. Ruderman et al. (1998) obtained spectral reflectance estimates, pixel by 3 min arc pixel, for 12 entire views of natural environments. For this data set comprising nearly 200,000 pixels, the correlation between L and M cone excitation is even higher at 0.9983. In that sense, the L and M cones measure almost the same thing—luminance—when used in natural environments. Surface luminance is given simply by the summed excitations of L and M cones, which we denote here simply by L and M (Eisner and MacLeod 1980; Lennie *et al.* 1993). The SD of $\log 10(L + M)$ in Brown's data set is 0.46, which corresponds to a factor of three in luminance; for Ruderman *et al.*'s data the value is 0.24, a little less than a factor of 2. A convenient measure of the red/green dimension of colour is the L cone excitation per unit luminance, $r = L/(L + M)$. As the high LM correlation implies, the SD of r is strikingly smaller than that for luminance: only 7.5 per cent, or 0.03 in the decimal logarithm for Brown's data, and only 1 per cent for the entire scenes of Ruderman *et al.* For the remaining chromatic axis, we adopt the luminance-normalized S cone excitation, $b = S/(L + M)$, which is low for yellows and very high for violets. The SD of b is an order of magnitude greater than for r, though still lower than the one for luminance: 0.39 in $\log 10(b)$ or a factor of about 2.5 in b for Brown's data, and 0.114 in $\log 10(b)$ or 30 per cent in b for the data of Ruderman *et al.* (crosses in Fig. 21.2 show the histogram for $\log 10(b)$). In both these data sets, the average of the natural stimuli is near to, but slightly yellower than, the equal energy white, which plots at a horizontal coordinate of zero in Fig. 21.2.

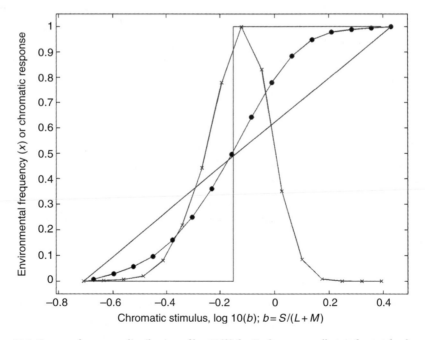

Figure 21.2 Crosses: frequency distribution of $\log 10(b)$ for Ruderman *et al.*'s set of natural colours; b specifies S cone excitation per unit luminance, that is, $b = S/(L + M)$. Whites and greens are near the middle of the distribution, with equal energy white at $\log 10(b) = 0$. To the right of that lie bluish colours; to the left, generally yellowish or reddish ones. Candidate input–outputs functions: pleistochrome (circles), compared with linear (squares) and stepwise alternatives.

We can now ask: what arrangement of slice thicknesses could provide the most precise representation, averaged over all cases, of natural colours conforming to the given distribution? This criterion allows determination of an optimum nonlinear code, subject to the constraint of a limited output range. As will be seen in the next section, on optimal nonlinearity, the optimal code with a single neuron per stimulus dimension is a sigmoid. For two neurons per dimension, it is a split range code employing rectifying opponent cells (fourth section on the benefit of split range coding). In the fifth section on Pleistochrome comparison, this theoretically optimal behaviour is compared with psychophysical results on the one hand and with physiological data on nonlinearity of the postreceptoral neural code on the other.

Optimal nonlinearity: the pleistochrome

The optic nerve constitutes an informational bottleneck for vision, where the number of nerve fibres is relatively limited, and the number of nerve impulses is much less than the number of absorbed photons at daylight light levels (Barlow 1965). Hence relatively large errors are introduced by random fluctuations in the optic nerve impulse counts (Bialek and Rieke 1992, Lee *et al.* 1993). So initially we assume, for simplicity, that variability originating at the retinal output predominates over sources of error at earlier stages.

When discrimination is limited by noise introduced into an output signal, good discrimination around any input value can be achieved by making the gradient of the input–output function at the relevant point as steep as necessary. But the limited total available range in firing rate means that an increase in gradient at one point has to be paid for by a decrease at other points within the input range, and hence by reduced discrimination at those points. By suitable choice of a nonlinear response function, relative discriminative precision can be distributed in any desired way over the range of input values. But which choice is best? For example, what input–output function gives the smallest RMS error in the estimated input, averaged over all naturally occurring cases?

Clearly it would be inefficient to make the code linear (with constant gradient and constant discrimination) over an input range greater than what is naturally encountered, as in the straight line in Fig. 21.2, where the crosses represent the natural distribution of $\log 10(b)$ from the data of Ruderman *et al.* This sacrifices discrimination among frequently occurring stimuli in order to preserve discrimination in ranges where it is never needed. Also inefficient is the opposite extreme, a response function that steps abruptly from minimum to maximum firing rate at the peak of the distribution of natural colours (step function, Fig. 21.2). This provides only categorical colour perception, with exquisite discrimination between bluish and yellowish colours, but no distinction among blues or among yellows. The best choice will be an intermediate one (circles, Fig. 21.2): a gently curving sigmoid, which retains some discrimination in the tails while slicing colour space most finely at the peak. More specifically, the optimal response function has a gradient matched to the cube root of the probability density function of the input distribution, and generates discrimination thresholds inversely proportional to that gradient.

Denote the input by x (which might be, for instance, some weighted sum of cone excitations), and the noisy output (e.g. a retinal ganglion cell firing rate) by a random variable y^*, with mean $y = g(x)$, a generally nonlinear function of x, and with a SD $\sigma(y^*)$ due to the addition of a random noise term, $y^* - y$. With the simplifying assumption that $g(x)$ can be treated as linear over the limited range of confusion, the input x^* that would elicit y^* in the absence of noise is

$$x^* = g^{-1}(y^*) = x + (y^* - y)/g'(y)$$

Since the mean of $(y^* - y)$ is zero, the mean of x^* is simply the true input x, and the mean squared error for input x is the variance of x^*, which we denote $\sigma^2(x^*)$. This is proportional to the output variance $\sigma^2(y^*)$, which we initially assume to be fixed and independent of y:

$$MSE(x) = \sigma^2(x^*) = \frac{\sigma^2(y^*)}{(g'(x))^2} \tag{1}$$

The constant of proportionality is the inverse square of $g'(x)$, the gradient of the input-output function $y = g(x)$ at x : where $g(x)$ is steep, a smaller range of inputs suffices to span the range of the noise that is added at the output.

Denote the environmental probability distribution of x (for all stimuli encountered, or of interest) by $p(x)$. The mean squared error to be minimized is the average of $\sigma^2(x^*)$ for all inputs, or its probability-weighted integral over x:

$$MSE = \int p(x)\sigma^2(x^*)\, dx$$

To see how this can be minimized, consider the effect of small variations in the response gradient or incremental gain $g'(x)$ around its optimal value. An increase in $g'(x)$ at one value of x has to be paid for with an equal decrease at other values of x, and in the optimal condition the effects of such complementary changes must cancel, that is, $p(x)d(\sigma^2(x^*))/dg'(x)$ must be independent of x. Thus

$$d(\sigma^2(x^*))/d(g'(x)) = \alpha/p(x) \tag{2}$$

with a constant α.

Since from (1)

$$d(\sigma^2(x^*))/d(g'(x)) = -2(\sigma^2(y^*))/(g'(x))^3$$

the optimal condition occurs when the gradient is matched to the cube root of the pdf:

$$g'(x) = \beta p(x))^{1/3} \tag{3}$$

The scaling factor β absorbs the factor equal to the output variance. It serves only to define units of measurement for y and can be set to 1 if those units are not defined independently. Hence

$$g(x) = \int_{-\infty}^{x} \beta(p(u))^{1/3} du \qquad (4)$$

Here the input quantity can be any function of the cone excitations (e.g. the log, in this example.) The optimum response gradient just has to be matched to the cube root of the probability distribution of the input quantity for which error is to be minimized.

von der Twer and I refer to this optimal response function, illustrated by the circles in Fig. 21.2, as the *pleistochrome*, from the Greek *pleistos* meaning 'most'. As Fig. 21.2 shows, the pleistochrome is roughly similar to the cumulative distribution of environmental stimulus values dictated by the principle of histogram equalization and suggested by Simon Laughlin, the first person to consider these issues quantitatively (Laughlin 1983). With histogram equalization all of the "slices" are equally populated. But the pleistochrome is wider than the histogram-equalization sigmoid by a factor of about $\sqrt{3}$, allowing much better discrimination in the margins of colour space.

The benefit of split range coding

Our discussion has not yet yielded any rationale for the familiar colour-opponent codes (Derrington *et al.* 1984; DeValois and DeValois 1975). On the contrary, the sigmoidal nature of the pleistochrome is incompatible with a null response to white. But when more than one neuron is available to represent a single stimulus dimension, new opportunities for coding are introduced. The non-opponent pleistochrome that optimizes encoding by a single neuron has an opponent counterpart when the encoding is done by a pair of neurons. Two rectifying neurons, one red-excitatory and the other green-excitatory, and each with a purely compressive nonlinearity, can represent opposite halves of the red–green stimulus continuum with positive firing rates, but with little or no response to greenish or to reddish stimuli, respectively. Such a representation is almost equivalent to that produced by a single neuron with sigmoidal nonlinearity (Marr 1974). The responses of two such neurons correspond to the two halves of the single-neuron pleistochrome sigmoid, but with the left half flipped up so that the response gradients for the neuron responding in the left half of the stimulus range are simply reversed. This, however, uses only the upper half the output range of each neuron. If the appropriate segment of the input range elicits the maximum possible response range from each neuron, the gradients of the response functions are doubled everywhere.

By using two neurons in this way the visual system can therefore double the precision in its representation of the input in the presence of output noise. If, alternatively, the two neurons had each been endowed with the same sigmoidal nonlinearity that is optimal for single neurons, then averaging of their signals (on the generous assumption of independent noise) would have reduced average error by only the $\sqrt{2}$. Thus the net benefit of adopting the 'split range' code (as opposed to the alternative of similar neurons operating in parallel with optimal nonlinearity) is a square root of two reduction of average error.

Location of white

If the split-range colour opponent code is designed for optimal characterization of natural colours in the least-average-error sense, and if the null stimulus for the colour-opponent neurons is the subjectively achromatic white, typical natural colours should be nearly white. This is of course roughly correct, but the prediction is not fulfilled exactly. Typical natural colours, at least in the chosen environments, where vegetation tends to be predominant, are greenish and yellowish. There are a number of more or less plausible post hoc rationalizations for the somewhat unexpected placement of the white point (and of the optimum point for colour discrimination). First, although most natural surfaces are yellowish, the sky is bluish. If equilibrium hue loci are adaptively fixed by the average input, the blue of the sky might act as a massive low-r and high-b counterweight to shift the environmental mean substantially from the mean of surface colours. Second, the location of the white point could be a compromise between optimizing discrimination for the most frequent surface colours (which, if the images of Ruderman *et al.* are typical, would put it in the part of colour space we actually identify as yellow–green) and preserving some discrimination for saturated blue and red surfaces. Even if this choice is not optimal by the unweighted least-squared-error criterion, it could be appropriate if saturated colours (other than the greens) tend to have greater than average biological importance. Osorio and Bossomaier (1992) suggest that discrimination among the greens of vegetation is not important or even desirable, whereas discrimination of reddish fruits from vegetation is important. A null point, with optimal discrimination, near white might usefully promote those discriminations at the expense of the less important ones. Such considerations are the focus of much recent discussion (Regan *et al.* 2001).

Comparison of the pleistochrome with psychophysical and electrophysiological data

Testing the cube root rule

The proposal that visual nonlinearity is optimized for discrimination among natural colours in the presence of output noise leads to a simple prediction: *the average error in visual discrimination or matching should be inversely proportional to $g'(x)$ in eqn (4), and hence to the cube root of the natural probability density function $p(x)$.* This prediction holds even for non-uniform output noise, provided that the nonlinearity $g(x)$ is appropriately optimized in each case (von der Twer and MacLeod 2001).

Psychophysical data for evaluating this prediction are available. For achromatic intensity differences between comparison and standard stimulus patches, set in a common grey background, comparison error is doubled for standards that create a contrast of about

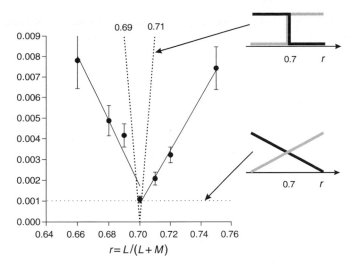

Figure 21.3 Circles, with straight lines fit, show Δr, the difference in $r = L/(L+M)$ just sufficient for 84 per cent correct discrimination between isoluminant, non-adjacent test and standard stimuli, embedded in a common white surround, as a function of value of r for the standard stimulus. The surround was an equal energy white, for which $r = 0.70$; hence abscissa values of 0.707 and 0.693 correspond to a 1 per cent L cone contrast between standard and background. Dashed lines show predictions for the extreme cases of linear encoding (horizontal dashed line: threshold is independent of reference colour) and step function encoding (steep dashed line: discrimination is only categorical). The inset illustrates these encoding schemes.

20 per cent with the background. For isoluminant yellow–blue differences the cone contrast (for S cones in this case) at which error is doubled is again about 20 per cent. But in the case of red–green isoluminant stimuli a standard L cone contrast of only 2 per cent is enough to double the mean comparison error (Fig. 21.3; Leonova and MacLeod, in preparation).[1]

If the visual system adopts the encoding principle of the pleistochrome, we would therefore expect to find the probability density function $p(r)$ for natural colours dropping to 1/8 of its peak value at r values that give a contrast of 2 per cent with white, with half-heights at around 20 per cent contrast for the other axes. This prediction is in

1 The implicit assumption here that contrasts along the three axes of colour space are perceptually related by simple scaling factors is consistent with contrast matching results of Switkes and Crognale (1999). Switkes and Crognale, however, found greater relative sensitivity to achromatic contrast. Their parafoveal grating stimulus may have been high enough in spatial frequency to place the chromatic mechanisms at a disadvantage. The spatial frequency dependence of the relative sensitivities for difference directions in colour space (Parraga *et al.* 1998) is indeed not fully consistent with the statistics of natural scenes, a fact that complicates the simple correspondence noted in this section and limits the generality of the cube root rule.

Table 21.1 L cone contrasts for luminance and for isoluminant red–green direction and S cone contrast for isoluminant blue–yellow direction

"Half-gradient" Contrasts (%)	Psychophysical (Leonova and MacLeod)	Neural (Lee et al. 1993)
Luminance	20	5 for contrast (M)
Blue/yellow	20	??
Red/green	2	10–20 for contrast (P)

Colour discrimination thresholds are doubled ("Psychophysical") column. "Neural" column shows rough estimates from physiological data of the contrast at which the gradient contrast-response function relevant neurons falls to half-maximum.

one respect roughly upheld, since as we saw in the second section on the distribution of environmental colours, the ranges for luminance and for b are indeed wider than for r, by an order of magnitude or so. In that sense the operating ranges of the various relevant neurons are fairly well matched to the very diverse distributions of environmental inputs that they have to represent. Webster and Mollon (1997) likewise noted that the mean contrast of their images along each of these axes was very approximately a constant multiple of the visual contrast threshold. In fact, however, the environmental distributions of b and (especially) of luminous reflectance are somewhat broader than would be expected for strict consistency with the pleistochrome principle (Table 21.1). Why should the operating range of the visual system be narrower than 'optimal' in this way?

Importance of contrast

One answer appeals to visual adaptation. Since retinally stabilized images fade, vision is evidently sustained by the temporal transients that are generated when small eye movements scan spatial gradients in the image. It is therefore relevant to consider the distribution of the spatial *differences* in cone excitation in natural images. In the images of Ruderman *et al.*, the differences in luminance, in b, and in r between adjacent 3 min arc pixels, have SDs of only 30 per cent, 13 per cent, and 0.6 per cent, respectively. The pdfs drop to 1/8 (where optimal differential sensitivity is halved) at about twice these values. These distributions are naturally somewhat tighter than those for the absolute values, owing to correlated variation in the values across the scene. The visual system can therefore advantageously employ an adaptively roving null point for the colour-opponent code (Krauskopf and Gegenfurtner 1992; Thornton and Pugh 1983), if its objective is the precise representation of local contrast (from which a metric representation of local brightness and colour can then be resurrected, perhaps in the way discussed by Land and Marr (Land 1959; Marr 1974)). With a roving null point, the range of input values spanned by the neural response functions need only be wide enough to capture the relatively small *deviations* in the stimulus values from their time and space varying adapting levels—and the precision with which those values can be represented then becomes correspondingly greater. Local-contrast pleistochromes—contrast-response functions that lead to least error in the representation of pixel-wise spatial differences in the images of Ruderman *et al.*—are narrow enough to be fairly consistent with the cited psychophysical results in the case of the chromatic variables. (Table 21.1)

This analysis implies, in agreement with observation (Leonova *et al.*, Chapter 11, this volume) that the very sharp optimum in colour discrimination is observed only when test and reference field are embedded in a common uniform surround that sets the adaptation state.

When light adaptation provides accurately reciprocal sensitivity adjustments in each cone (Dacey *et al.* 1996; He and MacLeod 1997; MacLeod *et al.* 1992), postreceptoral signals become functions of contrast. In the classical bipartite field for which the MacAdam ellipses (MacAdam 1942) were measured, the contrast between the two halves of the field is nearly zero. Postreceptoral neurons sensitive to contrast then operate at a fixed point on their response function for all colours to which the observer is well adapted; the margins of colour space no longer need be disadvantaged. On this view, all the MacAdam ellipses are really the same ellipse, but measured with different cone sensitivities. As noted, Le Grand (1949) showed that this view is too simple: MacAdam's discrimination thresholds do increase somewhat with increasing saturation of the reference colour. But that increase is far less precipitous than what is found with a common uniform surround for reference and test (Fig. 21.3; Smith *et al.* Chapter 11, this volume). In view of the effort that has been lavished on the refinement of colour difference formulas to account well for MacAdam's data, it is important to remember that when test and reference fields are non-adjacent, the pattern of results is very different. Colour difference formulas for that situation have yet to be worked out.

Discrepancies for luminance

For luminance, the contrast operating range implicit in the discrimination results is narrower by a factor of about three than the theoretically optimal pleistochrome. A second limitation in our initial framework, also connected with the role of adaptation, may underlie this remaining discrepancy. We have taken for granted that the purpose of colour and lightness vision is to represent colours and lightnesses with the least possible error and allow these attributes of a surface to be estimated as precisely as possible. But of course, differences in lightness and colour are also indispensable for the detection of spatial features (Boynton 1980; Morgan *et al.* 1992). For spatial vision, local contrasts should be detected with the greatest possible sensitivity wherever they are present in the image. For this purpose, an all-or-none or categorical encoding scheme, with a step function nonlinearity at a small threshold offset from the adapting background stimulus is ideal (since the large, all-or-none spatial contrast signal resists obliteration by fluctuations in the output), and the graded response of the pleistochrome is not needed.

Visual nonlinearity more step-like than the pleistochrome could therefore reflect a compromise in design between the conflicting requirements of surface identification and characterization on the one hand, and of detection of spatial features on the other. This is supported by the electrophysiological data considered below.

Comparison with physiological results

We next apply a Fechnerian construction (Fechner 1860) to derive nonlinear opponent codes for lightness and colour from discrimination data such as those of Fig. 21.3 and to compare the result with physiological data on the response functions of single neurons in the optic nerve.

In Fig. 21.3, predictions for the two extreme cases that were introduced in Fig. 21.2 are illustrated for comparison with the data. A linear code predicts uniform precision of discrimination (horizontal dashed line). An all-or-none response, that distinguishes sharply between reddish and greenish colours but makes no distinction among the colours of each category, permits standards of any redness to be distinguished only from greenish tests, and vice versa; hence the threshold $\Delta r = |r - r^*|$, where r^* is the colour category boundary. In Fig. 21.3 the steep dashed V illustrates this prediction, assuming a category boundary at $r^* = 0.7$ (the value for white). Neither of these extreme models describes the data well; the condition for discrimination is neither constant nor as abruptly standard-dependent as the step nonlinearity would require. Instead, the linear increase in threshold on each side of the white point suggests, by a straightforward extension of Fechner's argument to the colour domain, a logarithmic compression of each of the two colour-opponent neural signals that form the split range code. The linear variation of the discrimination threshold with r on each side of the null point $r = 0.7$ in Fig. 21.3, with an abscissa intercept at r_o, leads to a response-intensity function of the form

$$N = ln|(r - r_o)| \tag{5}$$

where r_o has a value of about 0.714 for the 'green' response (applicable for $r < 0.7$) and 0.68 for the 'red' response (applicable for $r > 0.7$) . The value obtained by reflecting r_o around the null point, $r = 0.7 + (0.7 - r_o)$, is the value of r associated with a doubling of threshold, or a halving of differential sensitivity. This condition occurs at an L cone contrast of about 2 per cent with respect to the null white stimulus in each case.

By reversing the argument that led to eqn (4), one can then ask: for what distribution of environmental inputs is the Weber Law discrimination function—and the logarithmic response nonlinearity of eqn (5)—optimal? The answer is $p(x) = p_{max}/(1 + |(x/x_0)|)^3$. This function does fit tolerably well the central core of the distribution of local contrast in the images of Ruderman et al. Whether we accept Fechner's integration or not, the need to perceptually reconstruct values distributed in this way adds a new functional rationale for Weber's Law for contrast.

The nonlinearity implied by the reviewed psychophysical data is quite severe. The gradient of the red–green response function, assumed in eqn (4) to be directly proportional to differential sensitivity, is halved at an L cone contrast of roughly 2 per cent. No physiological data suggest so severely compressed a response function for responses to chromatic stimuli: half-saturation L cone chromatic contrasts of around 10 per cent appear to be more typical, for the red–green sensitive P cells of the parvo-cellular stream (Lee *et al.* 1990). Thus although the psychophysically estimated visual operating range along the red-green axis is efficiently matched to the range of environmental inputs, the physiological one apparently is not. Elsewhere (MacLeod and von der Twer, in preparation) we consider reasons for this. These include the possibility that output noise inceases with mean firing rate (as in a Poisson process), which makes the optimum physiological nonlinearity a more gentle one.

Along the achromatic axis of colour space, both the psychophysical operating range in cone contrast and the dispersion of the environmental inputs are (as noted above) at least tenfold greater than along the red/green one. The M cells of the magnocellular pathway are a plausible substrate for achromatic discrimination (Livingstone and Hubel 1987). These cells, however saturate at very *low* achromatic cone contrasts, with half-saturation values of around 5 per cent (Kaplan 1986; Lee *et al.* 1990; Wachtler 1996). The M cells thus deviate by an order of magnitude from the optimal behaviour embodied in the pleistochrome. They could not support the observed keen discrimination between test patches with relatively high achromatic contrast relative to their surrounds.

It is therefore likely that the M cells are not responsible for representing the achromatic attributes of surfaces in a continuous fashion, but serve instead as all-or-none detectors of spatial contrast and of change over time. Thus, although responses of P cells to red/green contrast incorporate a degree of nonlinearity only slightly less pronounced than that of the M cells for achromatic contrast, comparison with natural scene statistics actually suggests different functions for these two systems. The red/green nonlinearity of the P cells is roughly appropriate for a metric representation of their natural inputs, but the nonlinearity of the M cells is not. This is consistent with the common view that the luminance system (sometimes tentatively, though questionably, identified with the magnocellular pathway) is more concerned with form and with detection of spatial structure than are the chromatic ones (Boynton *et al.* 1977; Gregory and Heard 1979; Livingstone and Hubel 1987). The metric representation of the achromatic axis as well as the chromatic axes could be the job of the P cells (Allman and Zucker 1990; Pokorny and Smith 1997), which have an almost linear response to achromatic contrast.

Is the nonlinearity optimized developmentally?
Anomalous observers as a test case

Leaving aside the discrepancies noted above, we have seen that the operating ranges of postreceptoral neurons, or the ones implicit in psychophysical discrimination performance, are very roughly appropriate to the range of inputs they receive from natural environments. But is the appropriate form of the neural nonlinearity genetically determ-ined (and specified via natural selection during evolution), or is it shaped during development? In anomalous trichromats, nature has provided a test case that may decide this point. Here our theoretical concerns finally make contact with the work of Guy Verriest, by providing a new perspective on deficiencies of trichromatic colour vision.

Previous treatments of colour discrimination by anomalous observers have impli-citly neglected output noise, supposing that colour discrimination thresholds will, like the cone contrasts, vary inversely with the separation between the L and M pigment absorption curves. This expectation is not generally upheld: although there is some disagreement about the interpretation of the finding (Pokorny and Smith 1977), dis-crimination and pigment spectra (assessed from colour matching measures) vary almost independently among anomalous observers (Hurvich 1972; Pickford 1958; Pokorny *et al.* 1979; Verriest 1960; Willis and Farnsworth 1952).

Consideration of output noise can resolve this paradox. If discrimination is limited by noise added to the colour opponent signal, discrimination around any given point in colour space can be improved, in principle without limit, by increasing the gain of the stage relating the colour opponent signal to the receptor signals. The total number of just-noticeable differences, or slices, along any chromatic continuum is then fixed by the output noise amplitude and output signal range, not by the photoreceptor inputs. With a plastic nonlinearity optimized to the range of photoreceptor excitations generated by the natural environment, the entire available range of output signals can be mapped onto the range of inputs made available by any particular trichromat's photoreceptors. The range of signals might in this way "expand to fill the neural space available" (Regan and Mollon 1997). Discrimination thresholds for trichromats can therefore in principle be completely independent of the (non-zero) separation between the pigment sensitivities![2]

Thus the existence of strongly anomalous observers who violate the naively expected relation between pigment spectra and discrimination by showing near-normal col-our discrimination at all chromatic contrasts can be explained by—and taken as circumstantial evidence for—both the importance of output noise, and plasticity of colour-opponent nonlinearity. I myself may be such a case. I am deuteranomalous, with

---

2   Alternatively, if the nonlinearity is genetically fixed, or for any reason fails to be shaped appropriately by input during development, the impoverished cone contrasts provided by the anomalous observer's photoreceptors will fail to span the full range of the colour opponent signal, and discrimination will then be impaired just as if noise were added at the input (e.g. to the photoreceptor excitations themselves). In this case, the colour opponent signals of anomalous trichromats, being smaller than those of normal observers, will undergo less nonlinear compression, with the interesting consequence that the anomalous observer will have relatively good (conceivably even super-normal) discrimination in situations where the compared stimuli each have high chromatic contrast relative to their common background. Inferior sensitivity at low chromatic contrast will be accompanied by relatively good sensitivity at high chromatic contrast.

a very deviant match point (Nagel $\log_{10}$ (AQ) = 0.56). The implication that my anomalous M photoreceptor spectral sensitivity is close to my normal L sensitivity is supported by dichromat-like behaviour under selective adaptation or selective bleaching: these manipulations alter my relative sensitivity for red and green by less than 10 per cent, as opposed to the tenfold change possible in normals (Eisner and Macleod 1981).

Yet in the experiment of Figure 21.3, my thresholds were only about twice the shown values (which are typical of practiced normal observers). More significantly, this held approximately for all tested chromatic contrasts of test and reference relative to the white surround, with no clear trend toward improved performance at high contrast. This preliminary evidence suggests that my colour-opponent neurons were overloaded to about the same degree as those of normal observers by these coloured stimuli, just as expected if colour-opponent nonlinearity is shaped during development.

Similar theoretical possibilities exist for acquired deficiencies, if these have the effect of reducing chromatic signal strength in the retina before noise is added to the signal at the retinal output. But since plasticity is generally thought to decrease with age it is less likely that neural nonlinearity can be optimized in response to an acquired deficit.

Instead of long-term plasticity, one could alternatively invoke short-term adaptation (Webster and Mollon 1997) and gamut compression/expansion by context (Brown and MacLeod 1997) as the means for "tuning" the nonlinearity of colour-deficient observers to suit their diet of impoverished chromatic contrast. On this view, acquired colour deficiencies and congenital ones should behave alike.

Plasticity of colour appearance

There is reason to believe that the null points of the colour opponent code, as well as the operating range, may be plastic. First, normal observers and anomalous observers show close agreement when asked to identify the unique phenomenally pure spectral yellow or blue that they consider to be neither reddish nor greenish, an agreement possible only if individual variation in the cone spectral sensitivities is in some way compensated postreceptorally; moreover, the slight differences between normal and anomalous unique yellow settings are roughly consistent with the idea that some postreceptoral adaptation to the history of photoreceptor signals sets the opponent null appropriately in relation to the near-white average of environmental stimuli. (Pokorny and Smith 1977). Second, among normal observers the variation in unique yellow has been found to be relatively small despite large variation in the relative contribution of L and M cones to spectral sensitivity (Brainard et al. 2000, Pokorny and Smith 1977). Paul Wise and I have obtained further evidence on this point. Twenty-four normal male observers made flicker photometric matches and unique yellow settings using CRT stimuli. The mean decimal logarithm of the relative M cone weight derived from the flicker photometric settings was 0.045 (where agreement with the standard luminosity curve would imply a zero value), but the values for different observers differed widely, with a true standard deviation of 0.35 (after deduction of experimental variance, assessed from variability in the settings of each observer across sessions). For unique yellow settings, however, the standard deviation among observers was only 0.023, sixteen-fold less (around a mean of 0.429). The yellow setting showed no clear correlation with the observer's spectral sensitivity. The post-receptoral compensation hypothesis is consistent with such lack of correlation, but substantial correlations that it predicts between spectral yellow and other measures are not always found (Mollon and Jordan 1997; Webster *et al.* 2000).

Any such compensation could not only promote uniformity in perception across observers (perhaps a questionable benefit), but could also improve stability in perception over the life span (Werner 1998). It could also minimize differences between sensations from the two eyes, or different regions in the same eye. Donders (Donders 1884; Mollon and Jordan 1997) reports the case of a certain Dr Sulzer, whose two eyes gave different impressions for spectral lights but were in agreement for more natural, broadband stimuli. In a more extreme instance, Peter Lennie and I (MacLeod and Lennie 1976) studied a unilateral deuteranope, RH. Using his dichromatic eye RH saw colours ranging from orange at long wavelengths, through desaturated green, to a slightly reddish blue at short wavelengths. This is qualitatively consistent with expectation for a system designed to minimize, for each deuteranopic chromaticity, the average disagreement with the trichromatic eye. A similar suggestion was made for unilateral tritanopia by Alpern, Kitahara and Krantz (Alpern *et al.* 1983). I have tried (MacLeod and Lennie 1976) to demonstrate a monocular compensation process experimentally by wearing goggles with a red filter over one eye and a green filter over the other, but this failed to produce an obvious perceptual asymmetry. Recent binocular experiments are more encouraging (Yamauchi *et al.* 2001). Perhaps the adaptation process has difficulty treating the two eyes independently. Monet's reaction to unilateral cataract surgery (Werner 1998) is relevant: with the operated eye things appeared too blue, with the other eye too yellow.

Colour constancy: the "anchoring problem" for natural scenes

Ambiguity of mean chromaticity the anchoring problem

The cone excitations associated with a reflecting surface depend both on the surface spectral reflectance function and on the spectral power distribution of the illuminant. The effects of the illuminant are determined by the interplay between lights and surfaces in the natural environment. If vision is to achieve constancy of apparent surface colour under changing illumination, those effects must be allowed for, by a kind of reciprocal mapping from cone excitations to colour appearance.

Fechner and Helmholtz recognized that logarithmic compression of the cone excitations—or, equivalently, sensitivity changes associated with adaptation—could play a key role in making surface colours independent of the illumination despite changes in the retinal stimulus. Fechner (1860) noted that when the sun comes out from behind a cloud, all the logs of the cone excitations go up by the same amount and the differences of the logs are invariant change. A reciprocal adjustment of sensitivity in each cone type, a kind of von Kries normalization, will effectively subtract the same number from all the logs. This yields a representation of the scene that's invariant with illuminant intensity (Cornsweet 1970). But in principle, the effects of changes of illuminant colour need not be removable in this simple way—a point made in many modern discussions (e.g. Brill 1978; Worthey and Brill 1986). The difficulty is that in general, a change of illumination scales the cone excitations by different factors for different surfaces. Conveniently, though, as noted by Foster and Nascimento (1994) the cone excitations for natural surfaces are scaled by approximately the same factor with a change of illumination, and this would allow the effect of varying illumination to be simply corrected by reciprocal adjustments of sensitivity in the different cone types. Jürgen Golz and I (in preparation) have found that in the natural scenes of Ruderman *et al.* (1992) the log shift principle does apply quite well in the three dimensions of cone excitation space. So von Kries normalization for each cone type separately could in principle achieve good constancy.

But this leaves us with a problem, one that Alan Gilchrist (e.g. Gilchrist *et al.* 1999) has called the anchoring problem: Although the resulting representation is invariant with illumination as desired, it also shows a less welcome invariance: it fails to reflect the overall chromatic cast of a scene, rendering each scene as (on average) indeterminate in colour. How, then, do we know what to normalize by? One idea, sometimes termed the "gray world assumption" is that the average chromaticity of the retinal image might be attributed entirely to the illuminant, and not to a predominant colouration of the viewed surfaces themselves (Buchsbaum 1980). If this assumption were operative, the space-average colour of any scene would be perceptually normalized to gray. But constancy is generally not complete: neutral surfaces appear to take on a faint tint of the illuminant colour. Such "under-constancy" is an aspect of the visual system's response to the anchoring problem. Consideration of the statistical variation among natural illuminants and scenes will show that under-constancy is actually not a failure of constancy, but an appropriate best guess about illuminant colour, appropriately based on knowledge of relevant environmental statistics.

An ecological rationale for under-constancy

Under-constancy would not be expected if the gray world assumption were strictly applied. But it may instead reflect commitment to a weaker but more justifiable probabilistic version of that assumption—an assumption that the overall chromatic cast of an individual scene is most likely to be neutral, but that exceptions are frequent enough that deviations from overall neutrality of the retinal image can most plausibly be ascribed to a combination of a chromatic illuminant with a similar chromatic bias inherent in the scene itself. The statistics of natural scenes and illuminants determine what particular apportionment of image colour to the illuminant is most statistically justifiable.

Consider a set of images generated by randomly sampled natural scenes and illuminants. For each image with mean chromaticity r_{image}, let r_{scene} be the mean surface chromaticity (the mean of r) for that external scene when observed under neutral illumination, and r_{source} be the illuminant chromaticity. Let dr_{scene}, dr_{source} and dr_{image} represent the deviations of r_{scene}, r_{source} and r_{image} from the mean chromaticity for all naturally occurring scenes, illuminants and images, respectively. The distributions of dr_{scene} and dr_{source} will be independent; if we assume they are approximately Gaussian, then the joint distribution is bivariate Gaussian, and contours of constant likelihood in $(dr_{scene}, dr_{source})$ are origin-centred ellipses oriented along either the dr_{scene} or the dr_{source} axis (Fig. 21.4). The loci of constant mean image chromaticity (dr_{image}) in $(dr_{scene}, dr_{source})$ will be approximately the negative diagonals, reflecting the equal contributions of illuminant and mean scene chromaticity to the image mean chromaticity: $dr_{image} = dr_{scene} + dr_{source}$. (There is no exact and general relation between image, source and overall scene chromaticities, but the simulations of Fig. 21.6 below support this intuitively plausible and simple relationship as an approximation for natural conditions). Consequently, for a given value of dr_{image}, the corresponding negative diagonal defines the various possible origins (or interpretations) of the image in terms of average surface chromaticity dr_{scene} and illuminant chromaticity dr_{source}.

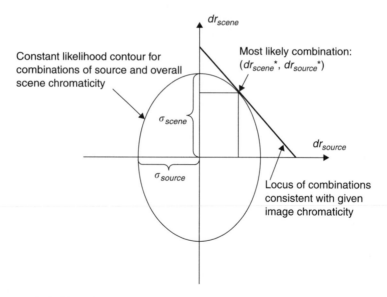

Figure 21.4 Ecological basis for underconstancy. The horizontal axis represents illuminant redness and the vertical axis represents the scene-averaged inherent redness of illuminated surfaces, each expressed as a deviation from its average for natural environments (dr_{source}, horizontal axis and dr_{scene}, vertical axis). If these have approximately Gaussian and independent distributions, the contours of constant likelihood in their joint distribution will be approximately ellipses, as shown. A given reddish image is consistent with the various pairings of scene and illuminant redness traced out by the indicated line of slope −1. The most likely interpretation of the image is that both scene and illuminant are slightly reddish rather than that the redness originates in either one alone.

If the image chromaticity is attributed entirely to the illuminant and the scene is assumed neutral—the gray world assumption—the inferred values of dr_{scene} and dr_{source} become simply 0 and dr_{image} respectively, and this is what is regarded as "full constancy". But other combinations of illuminant and scene characteristics dr_{scene} and dr_{source} are actually more likely. The most likely combination is specified by the point $(dr_{scene}{}^{*}, dr_{source}{}^{*})$ where the negative diagonal

$$dr_{scene} + dr_{source} = dr_{image}$$

is tangent to some constant-likelihood ellipse (Fig. 21.4). At other points on the diagonal, a lower likelihood will prevail, since likelihood decreases monotonically with distance from the origin along any radius. To determine $dr_{scene}{}^{*}$ and $dr_{source}{}^{*}$, note that any ellipse of constant likelihood has an equation of the form

$$(dr_{scene}/\sigma_{scene})^2 + (dr_{source}/\sigma_{source})^2 = \text{constant}$$

where σ_{scene} and σ_{source} are the standard deviations of r_{scene} across scenes and of r_{source} across illuminants. The slope of such an ellipse is $(dr_{scene}/dr_{source})(\sigma_{source}/\sigma_{scene})^2$. Hence the tangent point satisfies the equation

$$dr_{scene}/dr_{source} = (\sigma_{scene}/\sigma_{source})^2$$

Combining the last two equations, the relation between r_{image} and the parameters $(dr_{scene}{}^{*}, dr_{source}{}^{*})$ that give the most likely interpretation of the image is

$$dr_{scene}{}^{*} = (dr_{image})(\sigma_{scene})^2/(\sigma_{scene}{}^2 + \sigma_{source}{}^2)$$
$$dr_{source}{}^{*} = (dr_{image})(\sigma_{source})^2/(\sigma_{scene}{}^2 + \sigma_{source}{}^2)$$

Equivalently,

$$dr_{source}{}^{*}/dr_{image} = (\sigma_{source})^2/(\sigma_{scene}{}^2 + \sigma_{source}{}^2)$$

This last equation gives the ecologically optimal degree of "underconstancy". It expresses the maximum likelihood estimate of the illuminant chromaticity as a fraction of the "gray world" estimate that attributes the image chromaticity entirely to the illuminant. That fraction is about 0.5 for the case of equality between σ_{scene} and σ_{source}.

For the Ruderman et al. scenes and the Judd–MacAdam–Wyszecki daylight distribution (Wyszecki and Stiles 1982), σ_{scene} tends to be less than σ_{source} but comparable in magnitude; for Krinov's spectral data for the space-averages of natural terrains, scene variation is greater and may exceed illuminant variation (Brown, in press).

Environmental statistics therefore call for a considerable degree of "under-constancy". Observers who show moderate under-constancy are closer to a statistically optimal partitioning of scene colour into illuminant and surface colour components than those who show full constancy. In this sense the nearly complete constancy typically found in natural conditions (Kraft and Brainard 1999), or suggested by colour appearance judgements even in severely reduced situations (Thornton and Pugh 1983), is excessive. This conclusion has relevance for a fundamental and long-debated question about the mechanistic basis of constancy. Full or nearly full constancy is to be expected if constancy corrections are shaped by reciprocal sensitivity regulation in the retina. A sophisticated and statistically informed interpretation of the available cues would lead to less complete constancy than is observed. It is possible, however, that nearly complete constancy under natural conditions is supported in part by cues other than space-average colour of the image (Kraft and Brainard 1999). One source of such cues, considered next, is the distribution (in colour space) of the component elements of the scene.

Possible disambiguating cues from other image statistics

We have seen that the anchoring problem originates from an ambiguity: the overall chromatic cast of the retinal image could reflect the predominant colour of the surfaces, or the colour of the illuminant. This ambiguity can be expressed as a problem of discrimination: a reddish scene under white light can produce the same mean stimulation as a neutral scene in red light. How can we tell those two apart? Various potential cues that have been identified and studied, for example, mutual illumination (e.g. Bloj *et al.* 1999) and specular reflections (Lee 1986) turn out to be at best weakly effective.

Jürgen Golz and I have found that higher order statistics of the cone excitation distribution for the surfaces within a natural scene provide a possible basis for solving the anchoring problem—even if the mean redness of a neutral scene under red light and a red room under neutral light are the same, the higher order statistics will generally be different—and we found evidence that the visual system is sensitive to that information and may use it appropriately to achieve colour constancy. In particular, the correlation between surface chromaticity and intensity within an image appears to be a useful and effective cue for constancy.

Reddish surfaces have the colour that they do because they reflect a larger proportion of long-wavelength than of short-wavelength light. This suggests that in the room lit by reddish (predominantly long-wavelength) light, the reddish surfaces will be more luminous relative to other colours within the scene owing to the greater overlap of their spectral reflectances with the spectral range in which the illuminant has its highest power. As a result, the reddish light cast on the predominantly neutral scene will not only shift the mean image chromaticity toward red but, will create a correlation between redness and luminance among the elements of the retinal image—a correlation which will be absent (or less positive) in the case of the reddish scene under neutral illumination. This intuition is confirmed by an analysis of natural images. Thus, a high luminance–redness correlation within the image is evidence that the illuminant is reddish, no matter what the mean chromaticity. By evaluating both mean and correlation, two independent quantities, an observer can estimate two unknowns—the predominant colour (in this case, the degree of redness) inherent in the objects making up the scene, and the redness of the light source that illuminates the scene. In this way, statistics of the distribution

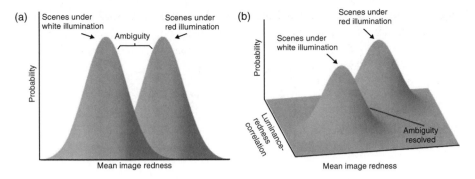

Figure 21.5 (a) The ambiguity of the mean image chromaticity for estimating the illuminant and how it could be resolved by higher order statistics. A given mean image chromaticity could result either from a reddish scene under white illumination or from a white scene under reddish illumination. (b) Taking higher order statistics into account can resolve this ambiguity.

of luminance and chromaticity within the retinal image might resolve the ambiguity encountered in considering mean chromaticity alone (Fig. 21.5).

Simulation using natural scene data

To check how well chromatic statistics in images of natural scenes can support inferences about illuminant colour, we used the hyperspectral data for the scenes of Ruderman *et al.* (1998). To these 12 scenes four CIE daylight illuminations (Wyszecki and Stiles 1982, pp. 142–6) were applied (correlated colour temperatures 4000 K, 5500 K, 8500 K, 20,000 K; with increasing correlated colour temperature the illuminants become less reddish (lower r-values) and more bluish (higher b-values)). For each illuminated scene several statistics (mean, variance, correlation, skewness) of the luminance and chromaticity values were calculated. Somewhat discouragingly at first, all statistics we evaluated except the means were almost independent of illumination. Although within each of the 12 scenes individually, the reddish surfaces became relatively more luminous when the illumination became more reddish, this increase in luminance for reddish surfaces was too weak to introduce consistently higher luminance–redness correlations for images under more reddish illumination. The correlations were indeed almost independent of illumination.

It turns out, however, that the correlation measure can nevertheless resolve the ambiguity inherent in the mean image chromaticity, because when used together with the mean image chromaticity it separates the clusters of images from different illuminations (the four diagonally oriented clusters in Fig. 21.6) and permits the estimation of illumination colour. Thus an image with a mean r value of 0.7 could be a slightly reddish scene under neutral light or a neutral scene under reddish light (Fig. 21.3). But if the visual system takes into account the correlation between redness and luminance, it can distinguish between illumination redness and scene redness. The more

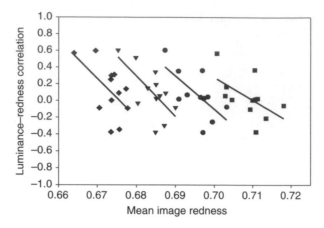

Figure 21.6 Luminance-redness correlation and mean redness for images formed by natural scenes viewed under 4 different illuminations. The vertical coordinate of each data point represents the correlation between pixel redness (r) and pixel luminance within an image of a particular scene under a particular illuminant. This correlation is plotted here against space average image redness (the mean of r averaged over the entire image). The four clusters each show data for 12 natural scenes under one of four different CIE daylight illuminants (■: colour temperature 4,000 K, O: 5,500 K, ▼: 8,500 K, ◇: 20,000 K). For a given scene, the luminance-redness correlation is almost independent of illumination, but within each illuminant cluster the correlation is more negative for the redder scenes, as shown by the negatively sloped regression lines. Thus correlation and mean together separate the distributions of images resulting from different illuminants and make it possible to distinguish scene redness from illuminant redness in a way that is not possible using mean image redness alone.

positive the correlation, the greater the evidence for redness of the illumination. In the above example image A belongs with high probability to the cluster of the reddish 4000 K illuminant whereas image B is a reddish scene under more neutral 5500 K illumination.

The reason why the luminance-redness correlation can resolve the ambiguity inherent in the mean is that scene redness and illuminant redness affect the correlation differently. Under "neutral" lighting, the eye's spectral sensitivity may favour the neutral or comparatively reddish pixels within a neutral or greenish scene, but the eye's diminishing sensitivity at long wavelengths will discriminate against the most reddish pixels of a reddish scene, and these will therefore tend to be of low luminance. The luminance–redness correlation thus becomes more negative the more reddish the scene, as the sloped regression lines in Fig. 21.6 show. No comparable effect occurs if it is not the scene, but the light that is reddish. In this case, the low luminosity of reds is counterbalanced by the illuminant's greater energy at long wavelengths. Reddish scenes, but not reddish illuminants, generate images with negative luminance–redness correlations. The ambiguity inherent in mean image chromaticity can thus be resolved.

Is this cue exploited? experimental tests

To find out whether human vision exploits scene statistics in this way, we used stimuli of a type introduced by R. Mausfeld and J. Andres (Mausfeld 1998; Mausfeld and Andres 1999) which make it possible to vary independently various statistics (means, variances, and correlations) of the distribution of colour and lightness within the display. A circular test field was surrounded by random patterns of overlapping circles; these were of a fixed diameter but varied in colour and luminance to a degree typical of the natural scenes of Ruderman *et al.* We asked subjects to adjust the colour of the test field so that it appeared neutral grey.

In our main experiment we varied the luminance–redness correlation for the elements surrounding the test field (by introducing a linear dependence between log(r) and log (luminance)) independently of other statistics (means and variances). For a given condition, the chromaticity and luminance values for the circles in the surround were chosen to achieve a certain correlation value (-1.0, -0.8, 0.0, 0.8, or 1.0). If the perceived colour of the centre test spot was not influenced by the varied correlation, then the settings to make the test spot neutral grey should be the same for all five conditions, since the space-averaged chromaticities of the surrounds were the same. The surrounds would then be functionally equivalent with respect to the perceived colour of the centre test spot.

For conditions with higher correlation between redness and luminance, a more reddish chromaticity was required to make the test field subjectively achromatic (Fig. 21.7). The data for eight of ten subjects tested were quantitatively similar and individually statistically significant ($p < 0.001$, linear trend test). When the correlation between

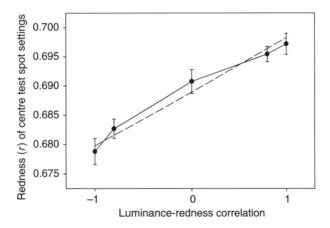

Figure 21.7 Dependence of centre test spot settings on the luminance-redness correlation within the surround. Average results for all subjects (circles), together with the best fitting straight line. Error bars for the experimental results are ±1 SE for variability between subjects (subject sampling error); variability of individual subjects settings is much smaller.

redness and luminance was positive, subjects selected a physically more reddish (higher r) test field as neutral grey. Since higher r values are associated with redder illumination of a physically neutral surface, this is the result expected if the observer infers a more reddish illumination in the case of positive luminance–redness correlation, and perceives neutral grey when a correspondingly reddish light stimulus is received from the test field. Though small, the effect of the luminance–redness correlation is not inconsequential; for comparison, a just noticeable difference in r is only about 0.001 (Fig. 21.3).

These results are consistent with other recent work showing that the correction subserving colour constancy is not governed merely by the space-averaged chromaticity (Bäuml 1994; Brown and MacLeod 1997; Jenness and Shevell 1995; Kraft and Brainard 1999; Mausfeld and Andres 1999; Webster and Mollon 1997); some current colour constancy algorithms provide general frameworks for effects of this sort (Brainard and Freeman 1997; D'Zmura 1995; Forsyth 1990).

Is the luminance–chromaticity correlation cue given appropriate weight?

How much weight should a smart visual system give to the correlation between redness and luminance in estimating the illumination? To answer this question for our simulated world of natural scenes under different illuminations, we calculated a maximum likelihood estimate for the chromaticity of the illumination given the mean and correlation value of an image. An optimal observer, adopting this maximum likelihood estimate, would have reacted to the stimuli of our experiment much as our observers did, giving only about 30 per cent more weight to the correlation cue than is implied by the straight line fit to the data of Fig. 21.7. The size of the observed effect of this statistic on colour perception is therefore roughly consistent with optimal computation.

Acknowledgements

Much of the material was developed during the author's participation in the project, "Perception and the Role of Evolutionary Internalized Regularities of the Physical World." organized by R. Mausfeld, D. Heyer and H. Hecht at the Zentrum für interdisziplinäre Forschung, Bielefeld, 1995–96. Thanks are due to all participants in that project, including collaborators Tassilo von der Twer (Physics, Wuppertal) and Richard O. Brown (Exploratorium, San Francisco), and also to my other collaborators in this work, Anya Leonova (now at Chicago) and Jürgen Golz (Kiel). Dan Ruderman kindly made available the hyperspectral data of Ruderman, Cronin, and Chiao on natural scenes. Barry Lee, John Mollon and Mike Webster provided helpful comments. Jürgen Golz's work at UCSD was supported by the German-American Fulbright Commission. All the work was supported by NIH Grant EY01711.

References

Allman, J., & Zucker, S. (1990). Cytochrome oxidase and functional coding in primate striate cortex: a hypothesis. *Cold Spring Harbour Symposium Quantitative Biology, 55,* 979–82.

Alpern, M., Kitahara, K., & Krantz, D. H. (1983). Perception of colour in unilateral tritanopia. *Journal of Physiology, 335,* 683–97.

Barlow, H. B. (1965). Optic nerve impulses and Weber's law. *Cold Spring Harbor Symposium on Quantitative Biology, 30,* 539–46.

Bäuml, K.-H. (1994). Color appearance: effects of illuminant changes under different surface collections. *Journal of the Optical Society of America A, 11*(2), 531–42.

Bialek, W., & Rieke, F. (1992). Reliability and information transmission in spiking neurons. *Trends in Neuroscience, 15*(11), 428–34.

Bloj, M., Kersten, D., & Hurlbert, A. C. (1999). Perception of three-dimensional shape influences colour perception through mutual illumination. *Nature, 402,* 877–9.

Boynton, R. M. (1980). Design for an Eye. In: D. McFadden (Ed.), *Neural Mechanisms in Behavior.* Berlin: Springer-Verlag.

Boynton, R. M., Hayhoe, M. M., & MacLeod, D. I. A. (1977). The gap effect: chromatic and achromatic visual discrimination as affected by field separation. *Optica Acta, 24,* 159–77.

Brainard, D. H., & Freeman, W. T. (1997). Bayesian color constancy. *Journal of the Optical Society of America A. Optics Image Science and Vision, 14*(7), 1393–411.

Brainard, D. H., Roorda, A., Yamauchi, Y., Calderone, J. B., Metha, A., Neitz, M., Neitz, J., Williams, D. R., & Jacobs, G. H. (2000). Functional consequences of the relative numbers of L and M cones. *Journal of the Optical Society of America A. Optics Image Science and Vision, 17*(3), 607–14.

Brill, M. H. (1978). A device performing illuminant-invariant assessment of chromatic relations. *Journal of Theoretical Biology, 71*(3), 473–8.

Brown, R. O. (1994). The world is not grey. *Investigative Opthalmology and Vision Science (Suppl.), 35/4,* 2165.

Brown, R. O. (in press). Backgrounds and illuminants: the yin and yang of color constancy. In: R. Mausfeld (Ed.) *Colour Perception: From Light to Object.* Oxford: Oxford University Press.

Brown, R. O., & MacLeod, D. I. A. (1997). Color appearance depends on the variance of surround colors. *Current Biology, 7*(11), 844–9.

Buchsbaum, G. (1980). A Spatial Processor Model for Object Colour Perception. *Journal of The Franklin Institute, 310*(1), 1–26.

Buchsbaum, G., & Gottschalk, A. (1983). Trichromacy, opponent colours coding and optimum colour information transmission in the retina. *Proceedings of the Royal Society of London Series B, 220,* 89–113.

Chaparro, A., Stromeyer, C. F., Huang, E. P., Kronauer, R. E., & Eskew, R. T. J. (1993). Colour is what the eye sees best. *Nature, 361,* 348–50.

Cornsweet, T. N. (1970). *Visual Perception.* (pp. xiii, 475). New York: Academic Press.

Dacey, D. M., Lee, B. B., Stafford, D. K., Pokorny, J., & Smith, V. C. (1996). Horizontal cells of the primate retina: cone specificity without spectral opponency. *Science, 271,* 656–9.

Derrington, A. M., Krauskopf, J., & Lennie, P. (1984). Chromatic mechanisms in lateral geniculate nucleus of macaque. *Journal of Physiology (London), 357*, 241–65.

DeValois, R. L., & DeValois, K. K. (1975). Neural coding of color. In: E. D. Carterette, & M. P. Friedman (Eds), *Handbook of Perception*, 5 (pp. 117–66). New York: Academic Press.

Donders, F. C. (1884). Farbengleichungen. *Archiv fur Anatomie und Physiologie. Physiologische Abt. Leipzig, 8*, 518–52.

D'Zmura, M., Iverson, G., & Singer, B. (1995). Probabilistic Color Constancy. In: D. Luce, M. D'Zmura, D. Hoffman, G. Iverson, & A. Romney (Eds), *Geometric Representations of Perceptual Phenomena*. Mahwah: Lawrence Erlbaum Associates.

Eisner, A., & Macleod, D. I. A. (1981). Flicker photometric study of chromatic adaptation: selective suppression of cone inputs by colored backgrounds. *Journal of the Optical Society of America, 71*(6), 705–17.

Eisner, A., & MacLeod, D. I. A. (1980). Blue-sensitive cones do not contribute to luminance. *Journal of the Optical Society of America, 70*, 121–2.

Fechner, G. T. (1860). Elemente der Psychophysik. Leipzig: Breitkopf und Härtel.

Forsyth, D. A. (1990). A Novel Algorithm for Color Constancy. *International Journal of Computer Vision, 5*(1), 5–36.

Foster, D. H., & Nascimento, S. M. (1994). Relational colour constancy from invariant cone-excitation ratios. *Proceedings of the Royal Society of London. Series B: Biological Sciences, 257*(1349), 115–21.

Friele, L. F. C. (1961). Analysis of the Brown and Brown-MacAdam colour discrimination data. *Farbe, 10*, 193–224.

Fukurotani, K. (1982). Color information coding of horizontal cell responses in fish retina. *Colour Research Applications, 7*, 146–8.

Gilchrist, A. L., Kossyfidis, C., Bonato, F., Agostini, T., Cataliotti, J., Li, X., Spehar, B., Annan, V., & Economou, E. (1999). An anchoring theory of lightness perception. *Psychological Reviews, 106*, 795–834.

Gregory, R. L., & Heard, P. (1979). Border locking and the Cafe Wall illusion. *Perception, 8*, 365–80.

He, S., & MacLeod, D. I. A. (1997). Contrast-modulation flicker: dynamics and spatial resolution of the light adaptation process. *Vision Research, 38*, 985–1000.

Helmholtz, H. v. (1896). Handbuch der Physiologischen Optik. Hamburg: Voss.

Hurvich, L. M. (1972). Color vision deficiencies. In: *Handbook of Sensory Physiology*, VII/4 (pp. 582–624). Berlin: Springer-Verlag.

Jenness, J. W., & Shevell, S. K. (1995). Color appearance with sparse chromatic context. *Vision Research, 35*(6), 797–805.

Kaplan, E., & Shapley, R. M. (1986). The primate retina contains two types of ganglion cells, with high and low contrast sensitivity. *Proceedings of the National Academy of Sciences, USA, 83*, 2755–7.

Kraft, J. M., & Brainard, D. H. (1999). Mechanisms of color constancy under nearly natural viewing. *Proceedings of the National Academy of Sciences, USA, 96*(1), 307–12.

Krauskopf, J., & **Gegenfurtner, K.** (1992). Color discrimination and adaptation. *Vision Research,* *32*(11), 2165–75.

Land, E. H. (1959). Experiments in color vision. *Scientific American, 200,* 84.

Laughlin, S. B. (1983). Matching coding to scenes to enhance efficiency. In: O. J. Braddick, & A. C. Sleigh (Eds), *Biological processing of images* (pp. 42–52). Berlin: Springer Verlag.

Lee, B. B., Pokorny, J., Smith, V. C., Martin, P. R., & **Valberg, A.** (1990). Luminance and chromatic modulation sensitivity of macaque ganglion cells and human observers. *Journal of the Optical Society of America A, 7*(12), 2223–36.

Lee, B. B., Wehrhahn, C., Westheimer, G., & **Kremers, J.** (1993). Macaque ganglion cell responses to stimuli that elicit hyperacuity in man: detection of small displacements. *Journal of Neuroscience, 13*(3), 1001–09.

Lee, H. C. (1986). Method for computing the scene-illuminant chromaticity from specular highlights. *Journal of the Optical Society of America A. Optics Image Science and Vision, 3*(10), 1694–9.

Le Grand, Y. (1949). Les seuils différentiels de couleur dans la théorie de Young. *Revue d'Optique, 28,* 261–78.

Lennie, P., Pokorny, J., & **Smith, V. C.** (1993). Luminance. *Journal of the Optical Society of America A, 10,* 1283–93.

Livingstone, M. S., & **Hubel, D. H.** (1987). Psychophysical evidence for separate channels for the perception of form, color, movement, and depth. *Journal of Neuroscience, 7*(11), 3416–68.

MacAdam, D. L. (1942). Visual sensitivities to color differences in daylight. *Journal of the Optical Society of America, 32,* 247–73.

MacLeod, D. I., & **Lennie, P.** (1976). Red-green blindness confined to one eye. *Vision Research, 16*(7), 691–702.

MacLeod, D. I. A., Williams, D. R., & **Makous, W.** (1992). A visual nonlinearity fed by single cones. *Vision Research, 32,* 347–63.

Marr, D. (1974). The computation of lightness by the primate retina. *Vision Research, 14*(12), 1377–88.

Mausfeld, R. (1998). Color Perception: From Grassmann Codes to a Dual Code for Object and Illumination Colors. In: W. Backhaus, R. Kliegel, & J. Werner (Eds), *Color Vision* (pp. 219–50). Berlin/New York: De Gruyter.

Mausfeld, R., & **Andres, J.** (1999). Detecting the presence of a 'non-normal' illumination: cues based on second-order statistics of colour codes. *Perception, 27(Suppl.),* 31–2.

Mollon, J. D. (1982). Color vision. *Annual Review of Psychology, 33*(2), 41–85.

Mollon, J. D., & **Jordan, G.** (1997). On the nature of unique hues. In: D. Carden (Ed.), *John Dalton's Colour Vision Legacy* (pp. 381–92). London: Taylor and Francis.

Morgan, M. J., Adam, A., & **Mollon, J. D.** (1992). Dichromats detect colour-camouflaged objects that are not detected by trichromats. *Proceedings of the Royal Society of London Series B, 248,* 291–5.

Osorio, D., & **Bossomaier, T. R. J.** (1992). Human Cone-Pigment Spectral Sensitivities and the Reflectances of Natural Surfaces. *Biological Cybernetics, 67*(3), 217–22.

Párraga, C. A., Brelstaff, G., Troscianko, T., & Moorehead, I. R. (1998). Color and luminance information in natural scenes. *Journal of the Optical Society of America A Optical Image Science and Vision, 15*(3), 563–9.

Pickford, R. W. (1958). A review of some problems of colour vision and colour blindness. *Advancement of Science, 15,* 104–17.

Pokorny, J., & Smith, V. C. (1977). Evaluation of single-pigment shift model of anomalous trichromacy. *Journal of the Optical Society of America, 67*(9), 1196–209.

Pokorny, J., & Smith, V. C. (1997). Psychophysical signatures associated with magnocellular and parvocellular pathway contrast gain. *Journal of the Optical Society of America A, 14*(9), 2477–86.

Pokorny, J., Smith, V. C., & Verriest, G. (1979). Congenital Color Defects. In: J. Pokorny, V. C. Smith, G. Verriest, & A. J. Pinckers (Eds), *Congenital and Acquired Color Vision Defects* (pp. 183–241). New York: Grune and Stratton.

Pugh, E. N., Jr., & Mollon, J. D. (1979). A theory of the pi1 and pi3 color mechanisms of Stiles. *Vision Res, 19*(3), 293–312.

Regan, B. C., Julliot, C., Simmen, B., Viénot, F., Charles-Dominique, P., & Mollon, J. D. (2001). Fruits, foliage and the evolution of primate colour vision. *Philosophical Transactions of the Royal Society of London B Biological Sciences, 356,* 229–83.

Regan, B. C., & Mollon, J. D. (1997). The relative salience of the cardinal axes of colour space in normal and anomalous trichromats. In: C. R. Cavonius (Ed.), *Colour Vision Deficiencies XIII* (pp. 261–70). Dordrecht: Kluwer.

Ruderman, D. L., Cronin, T. W., & Chiao, C. C. (1998). Statistics of cone responses to natural images: implications for visual coding. *Journal of the Optical Society of America A, 15,* 2036–45.

Sherman, P. D. (1981). Colour Vision in the Nineteenth Century. Bristol: Adam Hilger.

Switkes, E., & Crognale, M. A. (1999). Comparison of color and luminance contrast: apples versus oranges? *Vision Research, 39,* 1823–31.

Thornton, J. E., & Pugh, E. N., Jr. (1983). Red/Green color opponency at detection threshold. *Science, 219*(4581), 191–3.

Verriest, G. (1960). Contribution a l'étude de la correlation entre la quotient d'anomalie et l'étendue des confusions colorimétriques dans les systèmes trichromatiques anormaux. *Revue d'Optique, 39,* 467–71.

von der Twer, T., & MacLeod, D. I. A. (2001). Optimal nonlinear codes for the perception of natural colours. *Network: Computation in Neural Systems, 12,* 395–407.

Wachtler, T., Wehrhahn, C., & Lee, B. B. (1996). A simple model of human foveal ganglion cell responses to hyperacuity stimuli. *Journal of Computational Neuroscience, 3*(1), 73–82.

Webster, M. A., Miyahara, E., Malkoc, G., & Raker, V. E. (2000). Variations in normal color vision. I. Cone-opponent axes. *Journal of the Optical Society of America A Optical Image Science and Vision, 17*(9), 1535–44.

Webster, M. A., & Mollon, J. D. (1997). Adaptation and the color statistics of natural images. *Vision Research, 37*(23), 3283–98.

Werner, J. S. (1998). Aging through the Eyes of Monet. In: W. Backhaus, R. Kliegel, & J. Werner (Eds), *Color Vision* (pp. 1–41). Berlin/New York: De Gruyter.

Willis, M. P., & **Farnsworth, D.** (1952). *Comparative Evaluation of Anomaloscopes.* Bureau of Medicine and Surgery, U.S. Navy.

Worthey, J. A., & **Brill, M. H.** (1986). Heuristic analysis of von Kries color constancy. *Journal of the Optical Society of America A. Optics and Image Science, 3*(10), 1708–12.

Wyszecki, G., & **Stiles, W. S.** (1982). Color science: concepts and methods, quantitative data and formulae. New York: John Wiley & Sons.

Yamauchi, Y., Williams, D. R., Carroll, J., Neitz, J., & **Neitz, M.** (2001). Chromatic adaptation can cause long term shifts in color appearance that arise in binocular visual pathways. *Investigative Ophthalmology and Visual Science, 42 (Suppl.),* #3873.

Zaidi, Q. (1997). Decorrelation of L- and M-cone signals. *Journal of the Optical Society of America A,* 3430–1.

CHAPTER 22

TRITANOPIC COLOUR CONSTANCY UNDER DAYLIGHT CHANGES?

DAVID H. FOSTER, KINJIRO AMANO, AND
SÉRGIO M. C. NASCIMENTO

Introduction

Thomas Young (1807) encapsulated the phenomenon of illuminant colour constancy by observing that a piece of writing paper retained its whiteness in a room illuminated either by the yellow light of a candle or by the red light of a fire. In the natural environment, the most common illuminant changes on surfaces are due to changes in daylight. How, then, do colour-constancy judgements vary under daylight changes?

To address this question, an experiment was performed to estimate the distributional properties of colour-constancy judgements. An operational approach was adopted in which observers were required to distinguish illuminant changes on a scene from changes in the reflecting properties of the surfaces comprising it (Craven and Foster 1992; cf. Rüttiger *et al.* 2001)[1]. Thus, observers with normal colour vision were presented with computer simulations of a Mondrian-like pattern undergoing a change in daylight illuminant, and, at the same time as this illuminant change, the reflectance spectrum of the centre patch of the pattern also changed, its magnitude and colour direction varying from trial to trial. The frequency of "illuminant-change" responses was plotted against an equivalent illuminant change in the CIE 1976 (u', v') chromaticity diagram (cf. Bramwell and Hurlbert 1996). To determine whether an anisotropy in this distribution was related to a diminished contribution from short-wavelength-sensitive cones, the same measurements were undertaken by two tritan observers, and, to provide a theoretical reference, performance of both colour-normal and tritan observers was modelled computationally using the information available from long-, medium-, and short-wavelength-sensitive cones.

---

1   Making these discriminations is equivalent to partitioning colour signals—the cone inputs from each surface in the scene—into classes that correspond one-to-one with constant colour percepts (Foster and Nascimento 1994, appendix I).

Methods

Stimuli and apparatus

The stimulus patterns were square, of side 7° visual angle, and comprised an array of 49 (7 × 7) square Lambertian coloured surfaces of side 1° visual angle, drawn randomly from 1269 samples in the Munsell Book of Color (Munsell Color Corporation 1976). The random sampling producing each pattern was repeated, if necessary, to eliminate any accidental similarities between pairs of surfaces. Fresh random samples were drawn in each trial. Patterns were presented in a dark surround and were viewed binocularly at 100 cm.

One pattern was presented under a fixed, spatially uniform daylight of correlated colour temperature 25000 K and luminance 50 cd/m^2; the other pattern was made of the same materials and was presented under a fixed, spatially uniform daylight of correlated colour temperature 6700 K and luminance 50 cd/m^2, except for the centre square where the 6700 K daylight was replaced by a spatially uniform local illuminant constructed from a linear combination of the daylight spectral basis functions due to Judd et al. (1964). The chromaticity of this local illuminant was sampled randomly in each trial from a large convex gamut in the (u', v') diagram comprising 56 points (shown by the small solid points in Fig. 22.2). Its luminance was sampled randomly from three values: 41, 50, and 59 cd/m^2. Varying the chromaticity and luminance of this local illuminant is closely related (but not equivalent) to varying the chromaticity and luminance of the centre patch, but this parameterization in terms of an illuminant had the advantage that it was independent of the spectral reflectance of the centre surface (Foster et al. 2001).

Stimuli were generated on the screen of a 20-in., 1024 × 768 pixels, RGB colour display monitor (Trinitron, model GDM-20SE2T5; Sony, Tokyo, Japan), controlled by a computer with a raster-graphics card (VSG2/3F; Cambridge Research Systems, Rochester, UK) providing a nominal 15-bit intensity resolution per gun. Only the central 11 cm (4 in.) of the screen was used for stimuli. The screen refresh rate was approx. 100 Hz. A telespectroradiometer (PhotoReseach Inc., SpectraColorimeter PR-650, Chatsworth, CA, USA), calibrated by the National Physical Laboratory, was used for regular calibration of the display system. Calibration was performed sufficiently frequently that errors in the displayed CIE (x, y, Y) coordinates of a white test patch were <0.005 in (x, y) and <3 per cent in Y (<5 per cent at low light levels).

Procedure

In each trial, the two patterns appeared sequentially in the same position, each for 1 s, with no interval. The task of the observer was to decide whether the surfaces in the successive patterns were the same, that is, whether the change was a pure illuminant change. Responses were made on a joypad connected to the computer. Fresh patterns were generated in each trial. Each observer performed in all about 20 trials at each of the 168 (56 × 3) sample points of the local illuminant, but in random order; that is, in each trial, each combination of chromaticity and luminance of the local illuminant was drawn randomly without replacement from about 3360 values.

Subjects

Colour vision was classified with clinical methods, e.g. Ishihara pseudo-isochromatic plates, Farnsworth-Munsell 100-Hue test, Rayleigh and Moreland anomaloscopy (Interzeag Color Vision Meter 712, Schlieren, Switzerland), and luminance matching and increment thresholds on a white background. All observers had normal visual acuity in each eye, verified optometrically. There were 20 observers with normal colour vision, 9 male and 11 female, aged 21–36 years; and two tritanopic observers, both male and aged 52 and 56 years. Although these two observers' colour deficiency was consistent with it being inherited, the possibility cannot be excluded that they may have possessed short-wavelength-sensitive cones that were undetected in the present measurements. As shown later, however, their discriminations of illuminant changes from reflectance changes were not better than expected from predictions of model based on their having no short-wavelength-sensitive cones.

Results and discussion

The frequency of "illuminant-change" responses was calculated as a function of the chromaticity of the local illuminant in the (u', v') chromaticity diagram collapsed over luminance levels of the local illuminant. A three-dimensional perspective plot of the distribution is shown in Fig. 22.1 for pooled data from the 20 observers with normal colour vision. Each plot point was based on 1650 trials.

Despite the approximate uniformity of the (u', v') chromaticity diagram in this region of the colour space, the distribution of responses was anisotropic: observers were less able to detect spectral reflectance changes in one direction than in another (an analogous result was obtained by Rüttiger et al. (2001) in an achromatic matching task). The long axis of the distribution is shown more clearly in the contour plot of Fig. 22.2(a), where the darker the contour, the higher the frequency of "illuminant-change" responses. Also shown in the figure are the points corresponding to the first and second illuminants (open square and circle, respectively), the curve corresponding to the daylight locus (L), and the protanopic, deuteranopic, and tritanopic confusion lines $(P, D,$ and $T,$ respectively) passing through the chromaticity coordinates of the second illuminant. If perfect colour constancy had obtained, then the response contours would have been centred on the coordinates of the second illuminant, but the peak of the distribution is shifted towards the first illuminant (open square) (Bramwell and Hurlbert 1996; Foster et al. 2001).

The long axis of the distribution is close to the tritanopic confusion line (T), although biased towards the daylight locus (L) (Rüttiger et al. 2001). Is the anisotropy therefore a consequence of the failure of short-wavelength-sensitive cones to contribute fully towards the discrimination task? Some support for this hypothesis comes from an experiment

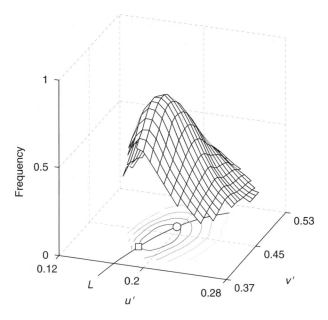

Figure 22.1 Detectability of changes in surface colour during illuminant changes for observers with normal colour vision. The three-dimensional perspective plot based on the 1976 CIE (u', v') chromaticity diagram shows the frequency of "illuminant-change" responses as a function of the colour of the local illuminant (simulating a reflectance change) on the centre patch of a Mondrian-like pattern. The daylight locus is indicated (L).

where observers viewed images in which the ratios of cone-specific excitations arising from light reflected from pairs of surfaces were altered (Nascimento and Foster 1997). In that experiment, observers had to discriminate between a natural illuminant change on a pattern in which ratios were almost but not exactly preserved (Foster and Nascimento 1994) and the same illuminant change in which the image was corrected so that ratios were preserved exactly. Sensitivity to deviations in these ratios was found to be almost absent for short-wavelength-sensitive cones. Other measurements based on asymmetric colour matching have also pointed to failures in colour constancy associated with short-wavelength-sensitive cones (Bäuml 1999).

To test this hypothesis here, the distribution of the detectability of reflectance changes (Fig. 22.1) was determined for two tritan observers. If short-wavelength-sensitive cones contribute little to the task, then the distribution of responses should be similar to that for normal controls. The pooled contour plot for tritan observers is shown in Fig. 22.2(b). Although based on fewer trials per point (120 versus 1650 in Fig. 22.2(a)), the distribution is more elongated than for normal controls, and its long axis, defined more clearly at lower response frequencies, is close to the tritanopic confusion line (T), although, rather as with normal observers, biased slightly towards the daylight locus (L).

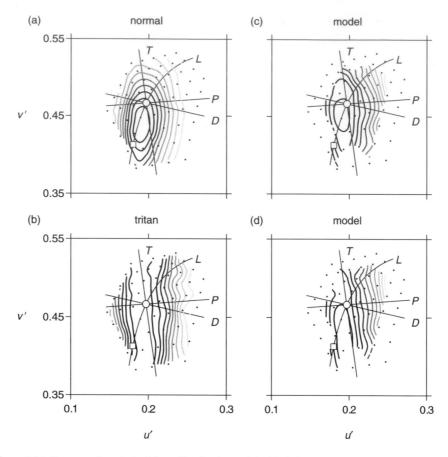

Figure 22.2 Contour plots derived from distributions of the kind shown in Fig. 22.1. Each contour represents a constant frequency of "illuminant-change" responses: the darker the contour, the higher the frequency. Data in (a) and (b) are for normal and tritan observers, respectively, and in (c) and (d) for the corresponding simulations based on deviations in spatial cone-excitation ratios. The open squares and circles show, respectively, the chromaticity coordinates of the first and the second illuminants on the pattern. The daylight locus and the protanopic, deuteranopic, and tritanopic confusion lines are indicated (L, P, D, and T, respectively).

The different anisotropies for normal and tritan observers suggests that short-wavelength-sensitive cones may indeed make a contribution to the normal detection of reflectance changes under changes in daylight, particularly when deviations in spatial cone-excitation ratios are extreme (the lower parts of the contours in Fig. 22.2(a)). To provide an alternative, theoretical reference for these data, the performance of normal and tritanopic observers was modelled computationally under the assumption that the discriminatory cue was generated by deviations in spatial cone-excitation ratios, as described in a previous analysis of relational colour constancy in isoluminant and achromatic images (Nascimento and Foster 2000). No attempt was made to model the discriminatory process in detail, and responses were again collapsed over lumin-ance levels. With contributions from long-, medium-, and short-wavelength-sensitive cones weighted according to their approximate average proportions in the normal eye of $2:1:0.2$ (Curcio *et al.* 1991; Carroll *et al.* 2000; Kremers *et al.* 2000), the predicted response distributions for normal controls showed little anisotropy, but reducing the contribution of short-wavelength-sensitive cones to about one sixth, giving weights of $2:1:0.03$, proved more successful. For tritanopic observers, the contribution of short-wavelength-sensitive cones was assumed to be zero. Changing the balance of the contributions from long- and medium-wavelength-sensitive cones had relatively little effect. Figure 22.2(c) shows the normal model contour plot. It reproduces the aniso-tropy in the observed response distribution, although not exactly its location or the direction of the long axis, consistent with the degree of colour constancy being limited by a bias towards the first illuminant, as noted earlier. Figure 22.2(d) shows the trit-anopic model contour plot. The direction of the long axis is similar to that observed, although the extent of the anisotropy is not correctly reproduced (the fact that some discrimination contours intersect the tritanopic confusion line is not inconsistent with tritanopia: although the direction of the illuminant shift may be along the confusion line, the direction of the product of illuminant and reflection spectra need not). For nor-mal observers, it may be that the apparent failure of short-wavelength-sensitive cones to contribute fully is due to other factors, for example, the size of the cue in relation to the size of the mean illuminant shift. Nevertheless, short-wavelength-sensitive cones seem to make a disproportionately small contribution to the detection of colour-constancy failures under daylight changes.

Acknowledgements

We thank I. J. Murray for assistance and J. K. Bowmaker and J. D. Moreland for advice. This work was supported by the BBSRC, EPSRC, and Wellcome Trust.

References

Bäuml, K.-H. (1999). Simultaneous color constancy: how surface color perception varies with the illuminant. *Vision Research, 39,* 1531–50.

Bramwell, D. I. & Hurlbert, A. C. (1996). Measurements of colour constancy by using a forced-choice matching technique. *Perception, 25,* 229–41.

Carroll, J., McMahon, C., Neitz, M., & Neitz, J. (2000). Flicker-photometric electroretinogram estimates of L:M cone photoreceptor ratio in men with photopigment spectra derived from genetics. *Journal of the Optical Society of America A—Optics Image Science and Vision, 17,* 499–509.

Craven, B. J. & Foster, D. H. (1992). An operational approach to colour constancy. *Vision Research, 32,* 1359–66.

Curcio, C. A., Allen, K. A., Sloan, K. R., Lerea, C. L., Hurley, J. B., Klock, I. B., & Milam, A. H. (1991). Distribution and morphology of human cone photoreceptors stained with anti-blue opsin. *Journal of Comparative Neurology, 312*, 610–24.

Foster, D. H. & Nascimento, S. M. C. (1994). Relational colour constancy from invariant cone-excitation ratios. *Proceedings of the Royal Society of London, Series B, 257*, 115–21.

Foster, D. H., Amano, K., & Nascimento, S. M. C. (2001). Colour constancy from temporal cues: better matches with less variability under fast illuminant changes. *Vision Research, 41*, 285–93.

Judd, D. B., MacAdam, D. L., & Wyszecki, G. (1964). Spectral distribution of typical daylight as a function of correlated color temperature. *Journal of the Optical Society of America, 54*, 1031–40.

Kremers, J., Scholl, H. P. N., Knau, H., Berendschot, T. T. J. M., Usui, T., & Sharpe, L. T. (2000). L/M cone ratios in human trichromats assessed by psychophysics, electroretinography, and retinal densitometry. *Journal of the Optical Society of America A—Optics Image Science and Vision, 17*, 517–26.

Munsell Color Corporation (1976). *Munsell Book of Color–Matte Finish Collection.* Baltimore, MD: Munsell Color Corporation.

Nascimento, S. M. C. & Foster, D. H. (1997). Detecting natural changes of cone-excitation ratios in simple and complex coloured images. *Proceedings of the Royal Society of London, Series B, 264*, 1395–402.

Nascimento, S. M. C. & Foster, D. H. (2000). Relational color constancy in achromatic and isoluminant images. *Journal of the Optical Society of America A—Optics Image Science and Vision, 17*, 225–31.

Rüttiger, L., Mayser, H., Sérey, L., & Sharpe, L. T. (2001). The color constancy of the red-green color blind. *Color Research and Application, 26 (suppl.)*, S209–S213.

Young, T. (1807). *A Course of Lectures on Natural Philosophy and the Mechanical Arts, Volume I, Lecture XXXVIII.* London: Joseph Johnson.

RED–GREEN COLOUR DEFICIENCY AND COLOUR CONSTANCY UNDER ORTHOGONAL-DAYLIGHT CHANGES

KINJIRO AMANO, DAVID H. FOSTER, AND
SÉRGIO M. C. NASCIMENTO

Introduction

Several distinct processing stages are thought to underlie the constant perception of surface colour under change in illuminant (Kraft and Brainard 1999; Walsh 1999). Colour constancy depends, in particular, on preserving spatial ratios of cone-specific excitations arising from light reflected from pairs of surfaces in a scene (Foster and Nascimento 1994; Nascimento and Foster 1997), and deviations in these ratios may account for the rapid, parallel detection of violations in colour constancy (Foster et al. 2001). If such detection involves comparisons of activity within cone classes, then the loss of one cone class might have little effect, providing that there was no significant reduction in coverage of the spectrum and that the remaining cone classes were sensitive to the underlying changes in the colour signal.

This hypothesis was tested operationally in a previous study with computer-simulated surfaces and illuminants (Foster and Linnell 1995). Under illuminants drawn from the daylight locus, red–green dichromats were able to detect simultaneous changes in surface spectral reflectance whose colour directions were along the daylight locus. Their levels of performance were about as good as those for observers with normal colour vision. Under illuminants with chromaticities lying along a line approximately perpendicular to the daylight locus, a deuteranope was still able to perform the corresponding task, but a protanope performed more poorly. In an achromatic-matching task (Rüttiger et al. 2001), red–green dichromats also obtained levels of performance close to those of normal controls for illuminant changes along the daylight locus, but performed more poorly in the approximately orthogonal direction.

In an attempt to further explore the limits on surface-colour perception in red–green colour deficiency, an analogue of the experiment described in Foster et al. (Chapter 22, this volume) was performed to estimate the distributional properties of these discriminations in affected individuals (cf. Rüttiger et al. 2001). Several protan and deutan observers were presented with computer-simulations of a Mondrian-like pattern undergoing a change in illuminant. This illuminant change was constructed so that in the CIE 1976 (u', v') chromaticity diagram it defined an axis that was approximately perpendicular to the daylight locus and therefore close to a red–green dichromatic confusion line. At the same time as the illuminant change, the reflectance spectrum of the centre patch of the pattern also changed, its magnitude and colour direction varying from trial to trial. The detectability of this spectral reflectance change was plotted against an equivalent illuminant change in the (u', v') chromaticity diagram. To provide a theoretical reference, performance of colour-normal, protanopic, and deuteranopic observers was modelled computationally using the information available from long-, medium-, and short-wavelength-sensitive cones.

Methods

Stimuli and apparatus

The stimulus patterns were square, of side 7° visual angle, and comprised an array of 49 (7 × 7) square Lambertian coloured surfaces of side 1° visual angle, drawn randomly from 1269 samples in the Munsell Book of Color (Munsell Color Corporation 1976). The random sampling producing each pattern was repeated, if necessary, to eliminate any accidental similarities between pairs of surfaces. Fresh random samples were drawn in each trial. Patterns were presented in a dark surround and were viewed binocularly at 100 cm.

As in Foster *et al.* (Chapter 22, this volume), the patterns were presented under two successive illuminants. The first illuminant was a fixed, spatially uniform, artificial daylight composed of a linear combination of the daylight spectral basis functions of Judd *et al.* (1964) so that in (u', v') space its chromaticity coordinates were located on the perpendicular to the tangent to the daylight locus at the chromaticity coordinates of the second illuminant, a fixed, spatially uniform daylight of correlated colour temperature 6700 K. The (u', v') coordinates of the first and second illuminants were (0.143, 0.484) and (0.197, 0.467), respectively. Their common luminance was 50 cd/m². On the centre square of the pattern, the 6700 K daylight was replaced by a spatially uniform local illuminant also constructed from a linear combination of the daylight spectral basis functions of Judd *et al.* (1964). Its chromaticity was sampled randomly in each trial from a large convex gamut in the (u', v') diagram comprising 57 points shown by the small solid points in Fig. 23.1. Its luminance was sampled randomly from three values: 41, 50, and 59 cd/m².

Stimuli were generated on the screen of a 20-in., 1024 × 768 pixels, RGB colour display monitor (Trinitron, model GDM-20SE2T5; Sony, Tokyo, Japan), controlled by a computer with a raster-graphics card (VSG2/3F; Cambridge Research Systems, Rochester, UK) providing a nominal 15-bit intensity resolution per gun. Only the central 11 cm (4 in.) of the screen was used for stimuli. The screen refresh rate was approx. 100 Hz. A telespectroradiometer (PhotoReseach Inc., SpectraColorimeter PR-650, Chatsworth,

CA, USA), calibrated by the National Physical Laboratory, was used for regular calibration of the display system. Calibration was performed sufficiently frequently that errors in the displayed CIE (x, y, Y) coordinates of a white test patch were <0.005 in (x, y) and <3 per cent in Y (<5 per cent at low light levels).

Procedure

In each trial, the two patterns appeared sequentially in the same position, each for 1 s, with no interval. The task of the observer was to decide whether the surfaces in the successive patterns were the same, that is, whether the change was a pure illuminant change. Responses were made on a joypad connected to the computer. Fresh patterns were generated in each trial. Each observer performed, in all, 10–20 trials at each of the 171 (57×3) sample points of the local illuminant, but in random order; that is, in each trial, each combination of chromaticity and luminance of the local illuminant was drawn randomly without replacement from at least 1710 values.

Subjects

Colour vision was classified with clinical methods, e.g. Ishihara pseudo-isochromatic plates, Farnsworth–Munsell 100-Hue test, Rayleigh and Moreland anomaloscopy (Interzeag Color Vision Meter 712, Schlieren, Switzerland), and luminance matching. All observers had normal visual acuity in each eye, verified optometrically. There were 10 observers with normal colour vision, 4 male and 6 female, aged 21–36 years; and five red–green colour-deficient observers, all male, comprising two protanopes and one protanomalous trichromat, aged 21–35 years, and two deuteranopes, aged 25 and 26 years.

Results and discussion

The frequency of "illuminant-change" responses was plotted against the chromaticity of the local illuminant in the (u', v') chromaticity diagram collapsed over luminance levels of the local illuminant (as in Foster *et al.*, Chapter 22, this volume). The distribution of responses for the 10 observers with normal colour vision is summarized in the contour plot of Fig. 23.1(a), where the darker the contour, the higher the frequency of "illuminant-change" responses. Also shown in the figure are the points corresponding to the first and second illuminants (open square and circle, respectively), the curve corresponding to the daylight locus (L), and the protanopic, deuteranopic, and tritanopic confusion lines (P, D, and T, respectively) passing through the chromaticity coordinates of the second illuminant. If perfect colour constancy had been obtained, then all the response contours would have been centred on the coordinates of the second illuminant (open circle), but the peak of the distribution is shifted towards the first illuminant (open square) (cf. Bramwell and Hurlbert 1996; Foster *et al.* 2001). Unlike the normal response distribution for illuminant changes along the daylight locus (Foster *et al.*, Chapter 22, this volume), here the distribution was almost isotropic.

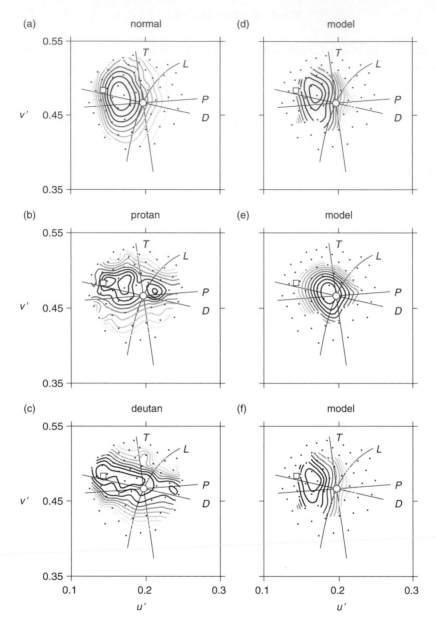

Figure 23.1 Detectability of changes in surface colour during orthogonal-daylight illuminant changes for observers with normal and red–green colour deficiency. Each contour represents a constant frequency of "illuminant-change" responses in the 1976 CIE (u', v') chromaticity diagram. Data in (a), (b), and (c) are for normal, protan, and deutan observers, respectively, and in (d), (e), and (f) for the corresponding simulations based on deviations in spatial cone-excitation ratios. The open squares and circles show, respectively, the chromaticity coordinates of the first and the second illuminants on the pattern. The daylight locus and the protanopic, deuteranopic, and tritanopic confusion lines are indicated (L, P, D, and T, respectively).

Figure 23.1 (b and c) shows the corresponding contour plots for the protan and deutan observers, respectively. As anticipated from Rüttiger *et al.* (2001), these observers' distributions were more elongated than for normal controls in the directions of their confusion lines, suggesting that information about deviations in spatial cone-excitation ratios in the remaining medium-to-long-wavelength-sensitive cone class was not used as effectively as it might be. As with tritan observers (Foster *et al.*, Chapter 22, this volume), the fact that the discrimination contours cut the protanopic and deuteranopic confusion lines is not inconsistent with observers having the corresponding deficiencies: although the direction of the illuminant shift may be along the confusion line, the direction of the product of illuminant and reflection spectra need not.

To provide a theoretical reference for these data, the performance of normal, protanopic, and deuteranopic observers was modelled computationally under the assumption that the discriminatory cue was generated by deviations in spatial cone-excitation ratios, as in Nascimento and Foster (2000) and Foster *et al.* (Chapter 22, this volume). Again, no attempt was made to model the discriminatory process in detail. The contributions from long-, medium-, and short-wavelength-sensitive cones were weighted according to their approximate average proportions in the normal eye (Curcio *et al.* 1991; Carroll *et al.* 2000; Kremers *et al.* 2000) but with the contribution from short-wavelength-sensitive cones reduced to one-sixth, as in Foster *et al.* (Chapter 22, this volume), that is, $2:1:0.03$. For protanopes and deuteranopes, the respective contributions of long- and medium-wavelength-sensitive cones were assumed to be zero. The model contour plots for normal, protanopic, and deuteranopic observers are shown, respectively, in Fig. 23.1 (d, e, and f).

Although the plot for normal controls is similar to that observed, the large anisotropies found with the sample of protan and deutan observers were not reproduced by the corresponding dichromatic models, confirming that information about deviations in spatial cone-excitation ratios in the remaining medium-to-long-wavelength-sensitive cone class was indeed not used effectively.

Acknowledgements

We thank E. K. Oxtoby for assistance and J. K. Bowmaker and J. D. Moreland for advice. This work was supported by the BBSRC, EPSRC, and Wellcome Trust.

References

Bramwell, D. I. & Hurlbert, A. C. (1996). Measurements of colour constancy by using a forced-choice matching technique. *Perception*, 25, 229–41.

Carroll, J., McMahon, C., Neitz, M., & Neitz, J. (2000). Flicker-photometric electroretinogram estimates of L : M cone photoreceptor ratio in men with photopigment spectra derived from genetics. *Journal of the Optical Society of America A—Optics Image Science and Vision*, 17, 499–509.

Curcio, C. A., Allen, K. A., Sloan, K. R., Lerea, C. L., Hurley, J. B., Klock, I. B., & Milam, A. H. (1991). Distribution and morphology of human cone photoreceptors stained with anti-blue opsin. *Journal of Comparative Neurology, 312*, 610–24.

Foster, D. H., Amano, K., & Nascimento, S. M. C. (2001). Colour constancy from temporal cues: better matches with less variability under fast illuminant changes. *Vision Research, 41*, 285–93.

Foster, D. H. & Linnell, K. J. (1995). Evidence for relational colour constancy in red–green colour-deficient human observers. *Journal of Physiology, 485.P*, 23P–24P.

Foster, D. H. & Nascimento, S. M. C. (1994). Relational colour constancy from invariant cone-excitation ratios. *Proceedings of the Royal Society of London, Series B, 257*, 115–21.

Foster, D. H., Nascimento, S. M. C., Amano, K., Arend, L., Linnell, K. J., Nieves, J. L., Plet, S., & Foster, J. S. (2001). Parallel detection of violations of color constancy. *Proceedings of the National Academy of Sciences, USA, 98*, 8151–56.

Judd, D. B., MacAdam, D. L., & Wyszecki, G. (1964). Spectral distribution of typical daylight as a function of correlated color temperature. *Journal of the Optical Society of America, 54*, 1031–40.

Kraft, J. M. & Brainard, D. H. (1999). Mechanisms of color constancy under nearly natural viewing. *Proceedings of the National Academy of Sciences, USA, 96*, 307–12.

Kremers, J., Scholl, H. P. N., Knau, H., Berendschot, T. J. M, Usui, T., & Sharpe, L. T. (2000). L/M cone ratios in human trichromats assessed by psychophysics, electroretinography, and retinal densitometry. *Journal of the Optical Society of America A—Optics Image Science and Vision, 17*, 517–26.

Munsell Color Corporation (1976). *Munsell book of color–matte finish collection.* Baltimore, MD: Munsell Color Corporation.

Nascimento, S. M. C. & Foster, D. H. (1997). Detecting natural changes of cone-excitation ratios in simple and complex coloured images. *Proceedings of the Royal Society of London, Series B, 264*, 1395–402.

Nascimento, S. M. C. & Foster, D. H. (2000). Relational color constancy in achromatic and isoluminant images. *Journal of the Optical Society of America A—Optics Image Science and Vision, 17*, 225–31.

Rüttiger, L., Mayser, H., Sérey, L., & Sharpe, L. T. (2001). The color constancy of the red–green color blind. *Color Research and Application, 26 (Suppl.)*, S209–S213.

Walsh, V. (1999). How does the cortex construct color? *Proceedings of the National Academy of Sciences, USA, 96*, 13594–96.

CHAPTER 24

CALCULATING APPEARANCES IN COMPLEX AND SIMPLE IMAGES

JOHN J. MCCANN

Introduction

In real scenes and in complex Mondrians the appearance of two identical colored papers in different locations is remarkably constant. Changing the position, and hence the surround, does not usually alter appearance. In simple displays, grays vary in lightness with surround. The spatial arrangement of the surround can make appearance more similar to (assimilation), or different from (contrast) the surround. A model that converts real image radiances to calculated sensations exhibits contrast, but not assimilation (McCann 1999). In order to expand the model to also exhibit assimilation, it is necessary to process the image in parallel, keeping separate the outputs of different spatial frequency channels (McCann 2001a). This paper studies the visual effects of segmented surrounds to understand the transition from contrast to assimilation. Shevell and colleagues have measured the effect of checkerboard backgrounds on color chromatic displays (Shevell and Wei 1998; Barnes *et al.* 1999; Shevell 2000).

In describing lightness effects "contrast" refers to the fact that a white surround makes a gray center appear darker than a black surround. Following Barlow's (1953) and Kuffler's (1953) discovery of spatial opponent ganglion cells, it is generally believed that the white surround stimulates inhibition of the center, making that gray look darker. The black surround does not generate inhibition and that gray appears lighter. It is important to recall that these displays are usually much larger than the receptive fields of ganglion cells.

Assimilation is the name of the mechanism with the opposite effect (Gilchrist 1994). Grays with adjacent white no longer look darker than the same gray with adjacent black. Examples are Benary's Cross, White's Effect, Checkerboard and Dungeon Illusions. These effects have been used to suggest a top-down analysis of the scene, implying mechanisms based on the recognition of illumination, objects or junctions.

Recent experiments demonstrate that contrast is much more complex than predicted on the basis of inhibition by average luminance in the surround. Displays with a square gray central element and 8 square surround elements demonstrate significant sensitivity to the placement of white and black surround elements. Equal-average surrounds do not give equal gray appearances.

Other experiments show that periodic assimilation effects are sensitive to average luminance over very-large-receptive fields (McCann 2000a). All of the above assimilation effects have gray center lightnesses that correlate with large-receptive-field averages. One cannot assume that these experiments are evidence for unconscious inference. Contrast is the result of complex spatial interactions, while assimilation can be understood as large receptive field averages (McCann 2000b).

Segmented surrounds

This paper reports experiments using segmented black and white surrounds. Figure 24.1 illustrates a 1346 test target. The square gray center element subtends 1.25° with 8 surrounding elements (4 adjacent–4 diagonal). There are 256 combinations of white and black elements in 8 locations. A single black segment at position the top center (target 1) is assumed to be the same as all the other single adjacent black squares (targets 3 (east side), 5 (bottom), and 7 (west side)). Target 1 was tested and the stereoisomers, targets 2, 3, and 4 were not. Removing all the stereoisomers leaves 56 unique spatial surround tests.

The 3 × 3-segment test target and the same size white-surround matching display were both on an 18.75° × 11.25° gray background (Fig. 24.2). With 8-white-surround elements, grays matched 17.5 per cent maximum luminance [17.9 ± 2.5% MAM/17.3 ± 0.4% JMC]; with 8-black-surround, 68.2 per cent maximum luminance [67.9 ± 6.52% MAM/68.5 ± 6.52% JMC]. The results are analyzed using log luminance axes with 100 per cent scaled to 1.0. The matching value on this scale for the white surround is 0.23, and for the black surround is 0.85.

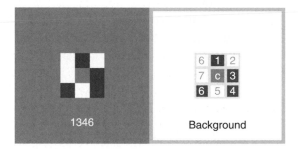

Figure 24.1 This figure shows a "1346" segmented test target (left) and a diagram of the nomenclature (right). The center [c] and the background were both constant and fixed at 17 per cent maximum luminance. The surround was segmented into 8 elements, numbered clockwise starting at the top center. Independently, the luminance of each surround segment could be set to 100 per cent or 3 per cent. This display has 3 per cent luminance in the 1, 3, 4, and 6 segments, hence its name.

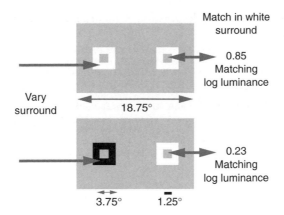

Figure 24.2 This figure diagrams the segmented surround experiment. In a dimly lit room, observers viewed an 18.75° by 11.25° background. On the left observers saw a variable 3.75° test surround and a constant 1.25° test center. On the right observers saw a constant 3.75° maximum luminance surround and an observer-controlled, variable intensity, 1.25°-matching center. The experimenter controlled the pattern of the segmented surround on the left. The observer varied the intensity of the right matching gray center in a constant maximum luminance surround. With all 100 per cent surround elements the observer average was 17.5 per cent (0.23 log luminance); with all 3 per cent surround elements the observer average was 68.2 per cent maximum luminance (0.85 log luminance).

The result from all 56 targets, for 8 trials each target, for two observers is shown in Fig. 24.3. The vertical axis is the average log matching luminance (LML). The horizontal axis identifies the segmented surround. The data have been sorted so that the number of black elements increases from left to right. The matches showed little correlation with the number of black segments, or the spatial average. If the number of black elements, or a surround average, were controlling contrast, then we might expect a series of flat steps with vertical risers at the change in number of black segments. Instead we found a marked dependence on the surround's spatial pattern. Target 2 (LML = 0.24) with one diagonal black segment is the same as target 0 (LML = 0.23) with an all white surround. However, target 1 with one adjacent black segment is lighter (LML = 0.32). Among the 6 targets with two black sectors, the average log matching luminances vary from 0.22 to 0.53. Among the 12 targets with three black sectors, the average log matching luminances vary from 0.26 to 0.56. Among the 14 targets with four black sectors, the average log matching luminances vary from 0.26 to 0.67. Among the 12 targets with five black sectors, the average log matching luminances vary from 0.29 to 0.74. Among the 6 targets with six black sectors, the average log matching luminances vary from 0.31 to 0.75. In the 2 targets with two black sectors, the average log matching luminances vary from 0.22 to 0.53. Target 2345678 (LML = 0.83) with one diagonal white segment is the same as the all black target 12345678 (LML = 0.85). However, target 2345678 with one adjacent white segment is darker (LML = 0.59). Instead of flat steps correlating with number of black sectors, we find that there is a very wide range of matches for each

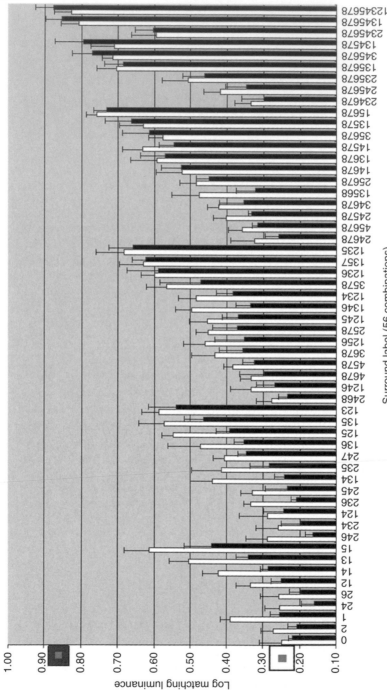

Figure 24.3 This figure shows matching data for all 56-surround arrays. The vertical axis plots the relative log luminance of observer's matches. The icon for the all white surround is placed at 0.23, and the icon for the black surround match is placed at 0.85 on the axis to illustrate the range of possible matches. The horizontal axis identifies the segmented surround. The data have been sorted so that the number of black elements increases from left to right. In each group the data are ordered by average log matching luminance.

set of constant number of black sectors. The matching data are inconsistent with the hypothesis that appearance is controlled by the average luminance of the surround.

Figure 24.4 is a plot of Segment Pattern versus Log Matching Luminance for all 14 patterns with 4 white and 4 black elements in the surround. They are sorted from left to right in order of increasing average log matching luminance. The two lowest LML values have 0 adjacent blacks. The next two patterns have one adjacent black. The next seven LML values have two adjacent blacks. The remaining five LML values increase with the number of adjacent blacks, but with more variability than previous patterns. The adjacent segment has more influence than the diagonal on matching luminance. The data from the 14 test targets with 4 white and 4 black elements are more consistent with the number of gray-black edges/gray-white edges than with the average luminance of the surround.

Figure 24.5 is the plot of number of gray-black edges versus log matching luminance for all 56 targets. The graph shows good correlation in that the data are clustered around the solid-line plot of average log luminance values for 0, 1, 2, 3, and 4 black segments. Nevertheless, the range of data around the average suggests that number of black segments is not a sufficient explanation of the data. A more complex spatial analysis is required.

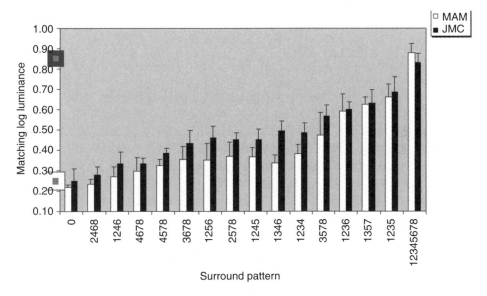

Figure 24.4 This figure shows matching data for all the 4-white/4-black surround targets. All 14 targets have the same number of surround elements. The vertical axis plots the relative log luminance of observer's matches. The icon for the all white surround is placed at 0.23, and the icon for the black surround match is placed at 0.85 on the axis to illustrate the range of possible matches. The horizontal axis identifies the segmented surround (illustrations above the bars). Matches vary from 0.26 to 0.67 LML depending on the placement of the white and black surround elements.

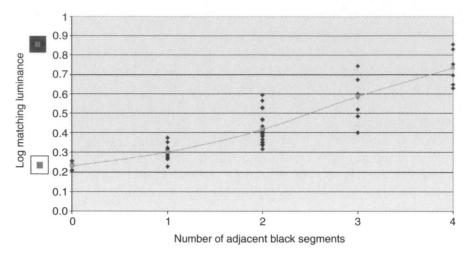

Figure 24.5 This figure shows the analysis of the number of black versus white edges for all 56 displays. The vertical axis is log matching luminance. The horizontal axis is a count of the number of black edges adjacent to the central gray segment. As shown in Fig. 24.4, the there is a degree of correlation between the log matching luminance and the number of adjacent edges for 4 white/4 black displays. Here we plot the data for all 56 displays. The solid line connects the matches for white (0) and black (4) along with the average matches for all displays having one black edge (1), two black edges (2), three black edges (3). The number of adjacent blank squares is a first order predictor of matching luminance, but a more sophisticated spatial model is required to fully account for the data.

It is important to note that although the data are reported in terms of number of gray–black segments, it is equally accurate to describe it as the number of gray–white edges. The essential result here is that the spatial pattern, and not the average of the spatial pattern, correlates with matching luminance. The mechanism controlling the appearance of the grays is not identified further by these experiments. Other experiments studying assimilation make that point very well.

The analysis of data from all 56 test targets shows that adjacent elements have much more influence than diagonal elements, although adjacent elements alone cannot account for the matching data. The appearance of grays with segmented surrounds having constant average luminance shows dependence on spatial pattern. Contrast effects with segmented surrounds are much more complex than predictions of models in which the radiance of a central area is compared with a spatial average of a concentric surround.

Assimilation

Although often associated with top-down cognitive interpretations, Benary's Cross, White's Effect, the Checkerboard and Dungeon Illusions can be explained by the spatial components of the stimulus. All four of these experiments demonstrate appearance shifts opposite to those found in simultaneous contrast. Here, grays with adjacent white no longer look darker than those surrounded by black. Unlike the above segmented contrast effects, these experiments show a correlation of appearance with spatial averages (McCann 2001*b*).

Top-down cognitive mechanisms, as well as T-junction segmentation algorithms (Ross and Pessoa 2000), are not necessary to account for observed lightness shifts in assimilation experiments. Large receptive fields can account for the observations. There is ample evidence that large receptive field pools are present in the visual system. Hecht *et al.*'s (1935) threshold sensitivity, Hubel and Wiesel's (1968) cortical measurements, and Blakemore and Campbell's (1969) adaptation experiments all demonstrate receptor pooling. The grays in the assimilation experiments in correlate with sampled averages using very large pools.

Contrast—assimilation antagonism

In contrast, white edges make grays look darker; in assimilation, white edges make grays lighter. The antagonism is apparent when you compare the assimilation found in the checkerboard illusion and contrast found in the very similar 1357 and 2468 segment pair (Fig. 24.6). The only difference the contrast displays on the left and the assimilation display on the right is the outer ring of black and white segments. It is as if this ring shuts off contrast and lets assimilation be apparent. One important feature is the outer ring be a periodic addition to the 9-segment inner area. If the outer ring is replaced with equal areas of white and black in an aperiodic pattern, then contrast remains and assimilation is not apparent (McCann 2001*c*).

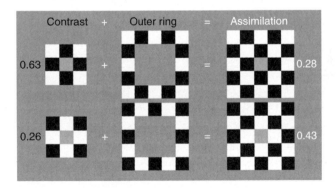

Figure 24.6 This figure shows the change in appearance for the central gray squares with the addition of more checkerboard squares. On the left observers reported "contrast" as shown above. The gray with 4 adjacent black squares had a matching log luminance of 0.63, while the one with 4 adjacent white squares had a matching log luminance of 0.26. The center shows the checkerboard ring of 16 square rings added to the "contrast" display to make the "assimilation" display. Observer matches for the gray squares in the center of displays on the right were 0.28 for 4 adjacent black squares and 0.43 for 4 adjacent white squares.

Summary

Contrast is a complex spatial mechanism that is evident with simple center-surround displays. It can be shut off, and reintroduced by the spatial pattern of outer-surround elements.

Assimilation in periodic displays is a simple mechanism found in the absence of contrast. It depends on the average value of very large-receptive fields.

References

Barlow, H. (1953). Summation and inhibition in the frog's retina. *Journal of Physiology, 119*, 69–88.

Barnes, C. S., Wei, J., & Shevell, S. K. (1999). Chromatic induction with remote chromatic contrast varied in magnitude, spatial frequency and chromaticity. *Vision Research, 39*, 3561–74.

Blakemore, C. & Campbell, F. W. (1969). On the existence of neurons in the human visual system selectively sensitive to the orientation and size of retinal images. *Journal of Physiology (Lond.) 203*, 237–60.

Gilchrist, A. (1994). *Lightness, Brightness and Transparency* (p. 136). Hillsdale: Lawrence Erlbaum Associates.

Hecht, S., Haig, C., & Wald, G. (1935). The dark adaptation of retinal fields of different size and location. *Journal of General Physiology 19*, 321–7.

Hubel, D. & Wiesel, V. (1968). Receptive fields and functional architecture of monkey striate cortex. *Journal of Physiology 195*, 215–43.

Kuffler, S. (1953). Discharge patterns and functional organization of mammalian retina. *Journal of Neurophysiology 16*, 37–68.

McCann, J. (1999). Lessons learned from Mondrians applied to real images and color gamuts. In: Proc. IS&T/SID Seventh Color Imaging Conference, (pp. 1–8). Scottsdale: IS&T.

McCann, J. (2001a). Calculating the Lightness of Areas in a Single Plane. *Journal of Electronic Imaging, 10*, 110–22.

McCann, J. (2001b). Image Processing Analysis of Traditional Gestalt Vision Experiments. In: Proc. AIC Conference (pp. 375–8) Rochester, NY.

McCann, J. (2001c). Assimilation and Contrast. In: Proc. IS&T/SID Ninth Color Imaging Conference, (pp. 91–6). Scottsdale: IS&T.

Ross, W. & Pessoa, L. (2000). Lightness from contrast: A selective integration model. *Perception and Psychophysics*, 1160–81.

Shevell, S. K. & Wei, J. (1998). Chromatic induction: Border contrast or adaptation to Surrounding light? *Vision Research, 38*, 1561–66.

Shevell, S. K. (2000). Chromatic Variation: A Fundamental Property of images. In: Proc. IS&T/SID Eighth Color Imaging Conference, (pp. 8–12). Scottsdale: IS&T.

CHAPTER 25

THE EFFECT OF GLOBAL CONTRAST DISTRIBUTION ON COLOUR APPEARANCE

K. WOLF AND A.C. HURLBERT

Introduction

Surface colours depend on their local context. The classic example of this dependence is simultaneous chromatic contrast, in which a contiguous or surrounding surface induces its complementary colour in the target surface: for example, a grey square against a green background appears pinkish (Chevreul 1868; Jameson and Hurvich 1961; Valberg 1974; Walraven 1976; Ware and Cowan 1982). In simple configurations, colour appearance is largely determined by the ratio of cone excitations (within cone types) between the surface and its immediate background (or by nonlinear functions thereof; see Lucassen and Walraven 1993), for matches made in asymmetric or fused haploscopic displays (Shepherd 1997; Chichilnisky and Wandell 1995; Hurlbert *et al.* 1998).

The chromatic content of distant surfaces may also influence the colour appearance of a target surface. For example, a remote red/green checkerboard attenuates the chromatic induction of a local, uniform red background on a central yellow patch (Shevell and Wei 1998). Although some studies suggest that remote influences are small (Valberg and Lange-Malecki 1990), or even sometimes explained by changes in local contrast (Brenner and Cornelissen 1998), at least some remote chromatic induction effects cannot be explained by linear spatial summation of contrasts (Schirillo and Shevell 2000; Zaidi *et al.* 1992). Remote induction effects depend on the distance and spatial frequency of the inducing surfaces (Brenner and Cornelissen 1991; Barnes *et al.* 1999; Smith *et al.* 2001), as well as on the mean and variance of their chromaticities (Shevell and Wei 1998). Local induction effects also depend on the variance of contrasts at the border between a surface and its background (Brown and MacLeod 1997) as well as on their spatial configuration (Brou *et al.* 1986).

The influence of local and remote context on surface colour may be directly linked to colour constancy. Under changes in natural illumination (such as daylight) the cone excitation ratios (within-type cone contrasts) between natural surfaces tend to be preserved (Foster and Nascimento 1994). Thus, the encoding of colour appearance by cone ratios between surfaces may enable the preservation of colour appearance under natural illumination changes. Computational theories of colour constancy further suggest that the accuracy of estimating the illumination colour improves with the number of distinct surfaces (e.g. Brainard and Wandell 1991). The influence of local and remote chromaticity variance on colour appearance may therefore also be a consequence of mechanisms for colour constancy.

This notion is supported by recent results showing that under temporal changes in the uniform background colour, its chromatic induction on a target surface is enhanced by consistent colour changes in remote surfaces (Wachtler *et al.* 2001). This "contrast enhancement" effect may be interpreted as a reinforcement of the illuminant colour estimate.

Here we test the hypothesis that increasing the number of distinct surfaces that change consistently with the local background causes stronger reinforcement of the illuminant colour signalled by the background change, using the temporal-change paradigm introduced by Wachtler *et al.* (2001). We also test whether segmenting the remote surfaces from the local background by increasing their luminance contrast against it, and thereby weakening the evidence that they belong to the same illuminant, attenuates the contrast enhancement effect. Whereas local chromatic induction appears to be largely monocular in origin (Shepherd 1997) and probably retinal (Chichilnisky and Wandell 1995), there is some evidence that remote induction effects occur beyond the retina at a binocular locus (Shevell and Wei 2000) and that spatial cone excitation ratios may be computed binocularly (Nascimento and Foster 2001). Long-range mechanisms that contribute to colour constancy most likely occur in higher visual cortical areas, as natural lesion studies suggest (Hurlbert *et al.* 1998; Ruettiger *et al.* 1999), although local contextual effects on colour and lightness responses have been demonstrated as early as primary visual cortex (Wachtler *et al.* 1999; MacEvoy and Paradiso 2001). In our final experiment, we probe for the locus of the "contrast enhancement" effect by presenting the remote inducers and the target surface to different eyes, using haploscopic viewing.

Methods

The task and stimuli

Observers performed a two-interval, forced-choice colour discrimination task, based on the paradigm of Wachtler *et al.* (2001), in which they compared the colour appearance of two central squares, presented in temporal succession against variable backgrounds.

Each trial consisted of the following sequence: prototypic stimulus (500 ms); mask pattern (500 ms); test stimulus (500 ms); neutral background (1000 ms). The prototypic stimulus consisted of a central square (size 2°; CIE coordinates $x = 0.321, y = 0.337$) surrounded by two concentric rings of remote squares (size 2°) 2°, 6°, and 8° distant, all against a 32° by 24° uniform, neutral background (CIE coordinates $Y = 18.7 \text{ cd/m}^2$, $x = 0.321, y = 0.337$). Eight of the remote squares had S-cone contrasts of $+0.5$, and the remaining eight -0.5, relative to the background chromaticity. In Experiment 1, we tested two conditions: the low luminance contrast condition, in which the central square was 7.5 per cent lower in luminance than the background, and the remote squares

3.5 per cent more luminant. In the high luminance contrast condition, these values were respectively -20 per cent and $+12$ per cent. Four black 1' points were arranged in a $1°$ square in the central square to promote fixation.

The full-screen mask was filled by $0.25°$ squares, whose colours were chosen uniformly at random from a set of 9 made by combining three luminances (the background luminance ±3.5 per cent) with three chromaticities (the chromaticity of the background in the subsequent test stimulus and ±0.5 S-cone contrast with respect to it). [The S-cone contrast, dS, is defined as $(s_p - s_b)/s_b$ where s_p is the modified MacLeod–Boynton coordinate of the square, $s_p = S_p/(L_p + M_p)$, and s_b is that of the background, with equivalent definitions for $l = L/(L + M)$, $m = M/(L + M)$, and L- and M-cone contrasts, e.g. $dL = (l_p - l_b)/l_b$. L, M, and S are the cone excitations calculated using the Smith-Pokorny cone fundamentals.]

The spatial configuration of the test stimulus was identical to that of the prototypic stimulus, but the chromaticities of the background and/or the remote squares could be shifted isoluminantly in the direction of increasing L-cone excitation relative to their prototypic colours. The shift in background chromaticity was fixed at an L-cone contrast of 0.05 relative to the neutral background. Hence four conditions were possible:

1. No shift for either background or remote squares.
2. Shift in remote squares only ("remote" change).
3. Shift in background only ("local" change).
4. Shift of both background and remote squares ("global" change).

The L-cone contrast of the central square in the test stimulus was varied between trials, the observer's task being to indicate by a button-press whether each value appeared "redder" or "greener" than in the first presentation. Responses were collected during the 1000 ms period of top-up adaptation between trials.

To enforce pre-adaptation, no responses were collected for the first two minutes of each experimental session. All four conditions were randomly interleaved in each session, except for Experiment 2.

Observer details

Six observers (2 males; age range 18–42) participated in Experiment 2; a subset of 4 participated in Experiment 1 and a subset of 5 participated in Experiment 3. A typical observing session consisted of four 15-min sessions of approximately 350 trials each.

Apparatus and calibration

Stimuli were generated using a Silicon Graphics O$_2$ workstation and displayed on a 20-inch SGI monitor, calibrated and checked for spatial chromatic homogeneity with a Minolta CS-100 chromameter. Halftoning doubled the colour resolution to 512 levels per phosphor.

Observers viewed the stimuli in complete darkness from a distance of 62 cm, using a chinrest to limit head movement. To provide a wide adaptational field, we lined the interior of a viewing box with white card, whose flat spectral reflectance we verified spectrophotometrically.

In Experiment 3, observers viewed the stimuli through a modified Wheatstone mirror haploscope individually adjusted for binocular fusion. A removable, white, septum divided both the viewing box and screen vertically into two light-tight halves.

Results and discussion

Experiment 1

We replicated the contrast enhancement effect described by Wachtler *et al.* (2001). Figure 25.1(a) illustrates that the L-cone contrast coordinates of the perceptually neutral point shift further towards "red" under the global background change, compared with the local change. Although the shifts in the perceptually neutral point are small, they are at or above successive discrimination thresholds measured against a fixed neutral background, and in agreement with the results of Wachtler *et al.* (2001). When only the remote squares change, there is no shift in the perceptually neutral point.

For all but one observer, increasing the luminance contrast between the different stimulus elements decreases the magnitude of the effect (Fig. 25.1(b)). Small changes in perceptual grouping may appreciably affect lightness perception (Adelson 1993) and colour appearance (Schirillo and Shevell 2000). Here, ungrouping the stimulus elements may reduce the importance that global coherence plays in determining whether a colour change is due to a change in illumination or surface material.

Experiment 2

We compared the effects of two different remote colour distributions, using the high contrast luminances described above. In the 2 colour distribution, the remote square S-cone contrasts were ±0.5 (8 squares of each), and in the 8 colour distribution, ±0.5, ±0.375, ±0.25, and ±0.125 (2 squares each), relative to the relevant background (Fig. 25.2).

Contrary to our expectations, the 2- and 8-colour conditions were equivalent for all but two (out of six) observers, for whom the 8-colour condition significantly increased the contrast enhancement caused by a global change. This result suggests that the mechanism responsible for contrast enhancement on the L-cone axis may be insensitive to variation solely along the S-cone axis. In other experiments (results not shown) we varied the remote chromaticities along the L-cone axis, and shifted only the S-cone contrast of the background. There we found no global contrast enhancement effect in all four observers tested (contrary to Wachtler *et al.* 2001), again suggesting that long-range chromatic interactions differ qualitatively across the cardinal axes (Brenner and Cornelissen 1991; Barnes *et al.* 1999).

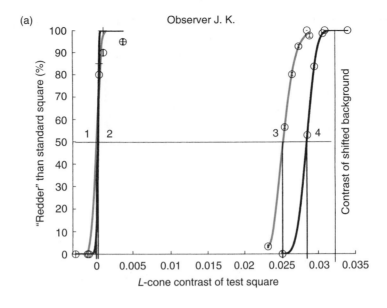

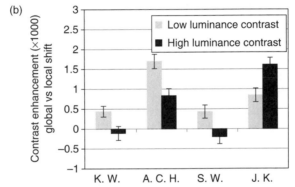

Figure 25.1 (a) The percentage of responses in which the test square is judged "redder" than the prototypic square are plotted against the L-cone contrasts (modified MacLeod–Boynton coordinates) of the test, relative to the neutral background, for observer J. K. Smooth curves are best-fitting Weibull functions. Numbers 1–4 label the curves corresponding to the 4 conditions described in the text. Each data point is the average of at least 45 trials. (b) Filled bars show the difference in L-cone contrasts ($\times 1000$) of the perceptually neutral square (50 per cent point on the fitted Weibull function) for the global change versus local change conditions ("contrast enhancement"). Gray bars: low luminance contrast condition. Black bars: high luminance contrast condition. Error bars are SDs of the difference.

Experiment 3

For the haploscopic experiments, we used a smaller stimulus (16° by 24°, in each eye) with only four remote inducers (of 2 colours, ±0.5 S-cone contrast; low luminance contrast condition) 4° distant from the center. The fixation dots were presented to both eyes to stabilize convergence. With the exception of one observer, who did not perform

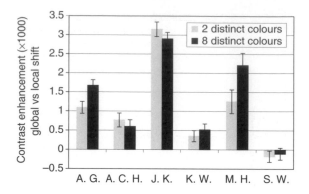

Figure 25.2 The magnitude of the contrast enhancement effect for each observer, plotted as in Fig. 25.1(b). Filled bars show the difference in L-cone contrast ($\times 1000$) of the perceptually neutral square (50 per cent point on the fitted Weibull function) for the global change versus local change conditions ("contrast enhancement"). Gray bars: 2 distinct colour condition. Black bars: 8 distinct colour condition. Error bars are standard deviations of the difference.

the experiment, all reported fusion of the combined stimulus to be straightforward and stable.

In each session, the central square was presented to one eye only, but the uniform background (either neutral or L-shifted) was presented to both. Results of right-eye and left-eye sessions were then pooled for analysis. Three separate conditions were interleaved in each session:

1. Remote squares presented only to same eye as central square ("same eye" condition).

2. Remote squares presented only to the opposite eye ("different eye" condition).

3. Remote squares absent on second stimulus presentation.

Figure 25.3 shows that the contrast enhancement effect disappears or is greatly reduced for all observers under haploscopic viewing. Whether the surrounding squares are presented to the same or the opposite eyes, the differences between the neutral thresholds for the global and local shift conditions are minimal.

Binocular interactions are unlikely to alter the chromatic appearance of the remote squares themselves, as such effects are small when there are no aligned borders in the two eyes (Whittle and Challands 1969; Shepherd 1997). Hence, it seems likely that the uniform background presented to the opposite eye overrides induction by the remote squares. As either explanation requires interaction at a binocular level, the remote contrast enhancement effect is unlikely to be monocular.

Wachtler *et al.* (2001) found that the magnitude of the effect was invariant to the number and radial distance of remote squares. A parsimonious explanation for these results is that observers briefly make an eye movement to the remote squares before judging the colour of the central square, allowing retinal adaptation during this period to

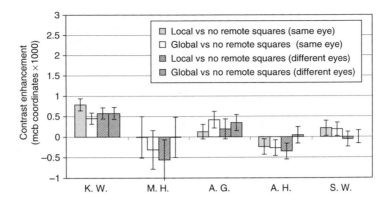

Figure 25.3 Contrast enhancement effects for Experiment 3 measured as the changes in the perceptually neutral *L*-cone contrast (×1000) caused by local or global shifts plotted relative to the reference threshold for the no-remote-squares background shift. Solid bars: same eye. Hatched bars: different eye.

cause the effect. In the light of our results and the finding that the contrast enhancement effect occurs for stimulus durations of 125 ms (Wachtler, pers. comm.), this monocular explanation appears unlikely.

Conclusion

Our results provide inconclusive support for the notion that contrast enhancement by remote inducers is linked to estimation of the illuminant colour in a constancy mechanism. Although perceptual grouping may influence the effect, the number of distinct *S*-cone contrasts does not. Given that the daylight locus moves roughly along the tritan line, it is also surprising that we failed to obtain a significant effect when *S*-shifting the background and remote squares. The hallmark of our results is the high degree of inter-individual variation in the magnitude of the contrast enhancement effect.

References

Adelson, E. H. (1993). Perceptual organization and the judgment of brightness. *Science 262:* 2042–44.

Barnes, C. S., Wei, J., & Shevell, S. K. (1999). Chromatic induction with remote chromatic contrast varied in magnitude, spatial frequency and chromaticity. *Vision Research 39:* 3561–74.

Brainard, D. H. & Wandell, B. A. (1991). A bilinear model of the illuminant's effect on color appearance. In *Computational Models of Visual Processing*, Eds: M. S. Landy & J. A. Movshon, MIT Press, Cambridge, MA.

Brenner, E. & Cornelissen, F. W. (1991). Spatial interactions in color vision depend on distances between boundaries. *Naturwissenschaften 78:* 70–3.

Brenner, E. & Cornelissen, F. W. (1998). When is a background equivalent? Sparse chromatic context revisited. *Vision Research 38:* 1789–93.

Brown, R. O. & MacLeod, D. I. A. (1997). Color appearance depends on the variance of surround colors. *Current Biology 7:* 844–9.

Brou, P., Sciascia, T. R., Linden, L., & Lettvin, J. Y. (1986). The colors of things. *Scientific American 246:* 84–91.

Chichilnisky, E. J. & Wandell, B. A. (1995). Photoreceptor sensitivity changes explain color appearance shifts induced by large uniform backgrounds in dichoptic matching. *Vision Research 35:* 239–54.

Chevreul, M. E. (1868). *The Laws of Contrast of Colour.* London, George Routledge & Sons.

Foster D. H. & Nascimento, S. M. C. (1994). Relational color constancy from invariant cone-excitation ratios. *Proceedings of the Royal Society B 257:* 115–21.

Hurlbert, A. C., Bramwell, D. I., Heywood, C., & Cowey, A. (1998). Discrimination of cone contrast changes as evidence for colour constancy in cerebral achromatopsia. *Experimental Brain Research 123:* 136–44.

Jameson, D. & Hurvich, L. M. (1961). Opponent chromatic induction: experimental evaluation and theoretical account. *Journal of the Optical Society of America A 51:* 46–53.

Lucassen, M. P. & Walraven, J. (1993). Quantifying color constancy–evidence for nonlinear processing of cone-specific contrast. *Vision Research 33:* 739–57.

MacEvoy, S. P. & Paradiso, M. A. (2001). Lightness constancy in primary visual cortex. *Proceedings of the National Academy of Sciences, USA 98:* 8827–31.

Nascimento, S. M. C. & Foster, D. H. (2001). Detecting changes of spatial cone-excitation ratios in dichoptic viewing. *Vision Research 41:* 2601–06.

Ruettiger, L., Braun, D. I., Gegenfurtner, K. R., Petersen, D., Schoenle, P., & Sharpe, L. T. (1999). Selective color constancy deficits after circumscribed unilateral brain lesions. *Journal of Neuroscience 19:* 3094–106.

Schirillo, J. A. & Shevell, S. K. (2000). Role of perceptual organization in chromatic induction. *Journal of the Optical Society of America A 17:* 244–54.

Shepherd, A. J. (1997). A vector model of colour contrast in a cone-excitation colour space. *Perception 26:* 455–70.

Shevell, S. K. & Wei, J. (1998). Chromatic induction: border contrast or adaptation to surrounding light? *Vision Research 38:* 1561–6.

Shevell, S. K. & Wei, J. (2000). A central mechanism of chromatic contrast. *Vision Research 40:* 3173–80.

Smith, S. C., Jin, P. Q., & Pokorny, J. (2001). The role of spatial frequency in color induction. *Vision Research 41:* 1007–20.

Valberg, A. (1974). Color induction: Dependence on luminance, purity, and dominant or complementary wavelength of inducing stimuli. *Journal of the Optical Society of America 64:* 1531–40.

Valberg, A. & Lange-Malecki, B. (1990). Color constancy in mondrian patterns—a partial cancellation of physical chromaticity shifts by simultaneous contrast. *Vision Research 30:* 371–80.

Wachtler, T., Sejnowski, T. J., & Albright, T. D. (1999). Responses of cells in macaque V1 to chromatic stimuli are compatible with human color constancy. *Society for Neuroscience* 25: 4(7.8).

Wachtler, T., Albright, T. D., & Sejnowski, T. J. (2001). Nonlocal interactions in color perception: nonlinear processing of chromatic signals from remote inducers. *Vision Research 41:* 1535–46.

Walraven, J. (1976). Discounting the background—the missing link in the explanation of chromatic induction. *Vision Research 16:* 289–95.

Ware, C. & Cowan, W. B. (1982). Changes in perceived color due to chromatic interactions. *Vision Research 22:* 1353–62.

Whittle, P. & Challands, P. D. C. (1969). The effect of background luminance on the brightness of flashes. *Vision Research 9:* 1095–110.

Zaidi, Q., Yoshimi, B., Flanigan, N., & Canova, A. (1992). Lateral interactions within color mechanisms in simultaneous induced contrast. *Vision Research 32:* 1695–707.

COLOUR SPACES AND THEIR VARIATION

SCHOPENHAUER'S "PARTS OF DAYLIGHT" IN THE LIGHT OF MODERN COLORIMETRY

JAN J. KOENDERINK

Schopenhauer's "parts of daylight"

Arthur Schopenhauer is the author of a little known booklet "*On Vision and Colours*" ("*Über das Sehn und die Farben*", conceived 1814, first edition 1815, second 1854, see Schopenhauer 1877). The philosopher was personally introduced to Goethe's (1984) "*Theory of Colours*" ("*Zur Farbenlehre*", orig. 1810) by the master, who apparently regarded the young man as a potential advocate of his idiosyncratic ideas. Master and pupil eventually came to bad terms though and Goethe even went as far as to "disinherit" the philosopher. Nevertheless Schopenhauer always continued to speak of Goethe with the highest respect. The story is told by Ostwald (1918*a*), with excerpts from an exchange of letters between the philosopher and the poet.

Schopenhauer considered his contribution as a major scientific achievement. He even translated his book into Latin in order to make it accessible to the world at large and expected science to eventually catch up. In that he was mistaken as history has—by now—amply shown. There are various reasons for this, among them being the fact that some of Schopenhauer's great expectations were misplaced because of weaknesses or errors in his arguments. This is not to say that the theory is worthless though. There is much in it that is valuable although it has been ignored by established colour science (in this Chapter I really mean "colorimetry" when I write "colour science").

I cannot even start to attempt to analyse Schopenhauer's theory from every angle here. For instance, I will not enter into discussion concerning the physical, physiological, and/or psychological origins of colour, nor of colours as *qualia*. Instead, I will confront Schopenhauer's ideas with a colorimetric framework that stands somewhat removed from these questions. In reading the original one often needs to be careful, for when Schopenhauer talks about the "activity of the retina" this can often be interpreted colorimetrically (the "full activity" is also called "white" or "(day-)light") rather than physiologically. I do not think one should take the philosopher too literally here, since he was obviously trying hard to appear scientific by any means.

Like Goethe, Schopenhauer considered colour to be "shadowlike" (a notion derived from the ancient Greeks), that is to say, as strictly less than daylight. Thus he writes: "*Inactivity of the retina is darkness. Thus a colour is at least partly darkness. . . . The qualitative partition entails the wedding of light and darkness, whose appearance is colour.*" The "activity of the retina" also appears as "white" or "(day-)light". Here "daylight" may be understood as the colour of a perfectly white object under "average" conditions. In itself, daylight is assumed to be a simple (perhaps the simplest) entity. Thus Newton's understanding of daylight as a "confused mixture" (of "homogeneous light") appeared abhorrent to Goethe. Goethe also thought the facts to speak clearly against Newton's notion. When he put a prism in front of his eye and looked at a featureless whitewashed wall, he saw no colours at all, and immediately realized that Newton had to be wrong.

Goethe saw colours only when he looked (through the prism) at edges or white stripes on black or black stripes on white. These "boundary colours" ("*Kantenfarben*") came in two varieties, one series running from dark red over yellow to white, the other from light green over cyan to black. Which variety he obtained depended upon the orientation of the boundary with respect to the refracting edge of the prism. When looking at white stripes on black he saw the colours of the Newtonian spectrum, an inverted spectrum (which lacks the magentas) and when looking at black stripes on white he saw another spectrum that contained the magentas but lacked the greens. In modern terms we would say that the boundary colours (see Figs 26.1 and 26.2) form a basis for the brightest surface colours (Schrödinger's "optimal colours", see below), just like Newton's "homogeneous lights", where both are considered as aperture colours. Whereas monochromatic beams occur only as aperture colours, the boundary colours can be realized both as aperture and as surface colours. The boundary colours are actually realizable though, whereas

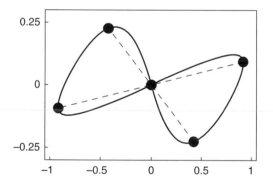
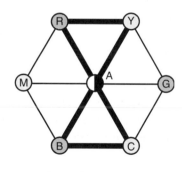

Figure 26.1 When you cut the daylight spectrum at some wavelength you obtain two parts. On the left I consider these parts in CIE 1964 XYZ-space. I have projected the colours of these parts parallel to the achromatic direction on the XZ-plane. When the cut locus is varied the projections trace out a figure eight shaped loop (which has historically played an important role in the theory of the colour solid). The colours of the parts for the optimum Schopenhauer cuts are indicated (see Figs 26.4–26.6). Of course the colours of a pair are necessarily complementary. On the right I show the same construction for the RGB-cube. Here the loop is made up of two equilateral triangles (vertices achromatic (A), red (R), yellow (Y) and achromatic, blue (B), cyan (C); the "achromatic" (A) doubles for white and black). Notice the similarity of the real thing to the simple relations in the RGB-cube.

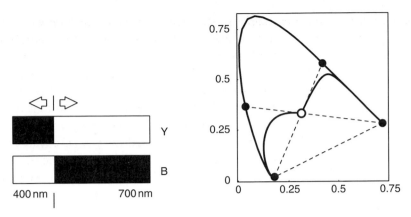

Figure 26.2 On the left the spectrum is divided into two supplementary (and thus complementary) parts, here (roughly) yellow and blue. As you shift the cut locus the colours progress through the series of Goethe's "*Kantenfarben*". On the right the spectrum locus in the CIE xy-diagram. The open dot is the achromatic point for natural daylight (CIE illuminant D65). The loci of boundary colours are smooth curves that connect the spectrum limits with the achromatic point. The closed dots indicate the short and long wavelength spectrum limits and their complementaries. These divide the spectrum locus into three stretches. Alternatively, the lines connecting a spectrum limit with its complementary define "cuts" that divide the daylight spectrum into two parts.

the homogeneous lights are not (monochromatic beams are ideal entities that cannot be physically realized, only approximated). The boundary colours are also preferable from a mathematical point of view, but these are subtleties that were beyond Newton's and Goethe's horizons (and Goethe despised mathematics anyway). The point of whether daylight is a confused mixture or not is a moot one. Personally I hold that a loaf of bread is not composed of slices before the actual act of slicing has taken place. If you agree with me, then daylight can indeed be said to be decomposable into homogeneous lights, but cannot be said to be composed of them.

Since—according to Goethe's Colour Science—colours are "shadowlike", they originate when one takes something away from the white. The idea to partition daylight into parts, some of which are missing in obviously coloured objects, is then a natural one. In Schopenhauer's view the very essence of colour is the bi- or tri-partition of daylight. One can split daylight into complementary pairs in infinitely many ways. "Supplementary" is perhaps a better term than "complementary", because the members of a pair necessarily combine to white ("daylight"). This was a major source of disagreement with Goethe who flatly denied that combination of any two colours could ever yield white. Goethe based this notion on the study of colour tops. Indeed, in this case of partitive mixture one may produce at best greys, but never white. Schopenhauer combined spectra additively (by superposition of mutually incoherent beams) and saw white when red overlapped with cyan or yellow with blue. This reminds one of the later work by Helmholtz (1855) which triggered Graßmann's (1853) fundamental paper since it conflicted with Newton's (1952) predictions.

The bi-partitions may yield pairs of very different vividness in the sense that the two colours may vary widely in brightness and saturation (or "colour", "black", and "white content" in the sense of Ostwald). For instance, a bipartition into black and white has two achromatic components. There exist "optimal" ways to split daylight in the sense that both components are maximally vivid hues. This happens when one cuts the visual region at two complementary photon energies or at a single location for which no complementary exists. The parts then are Ostwald (1917) "semichromes" ("*Farbenhalb*") (see Fig. 26.3). In the case of a single cut the pairs are red–cyan and blue–yellow (Figs 26.4 through 26.6), and thus the idea may be seen as a precursor of Hering's (1920) opponent colours. It is indeed intuitively obvious that when one slightly

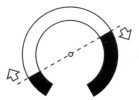

Figure 26.3 The idea behind Ostwald's "semichromes". The Newtonian spectrum is bent into a "colour circle", but (unlike Newton) Ostwald is aware of the "purples gap". Complementary monochromatic pairs are plotted as antipodes of the colour circle, otherwise the metric is arbitrary. When you select a "*Farbenhalb*" (half-colourcircle) by removing all spectral power in the black areas you obtain a "semichrome". When you rotate the cut locus as indicated you generate a periodic sequence of semichromes, thus you have generated the colour circle from the spectrum (which is a linear, open segment and thus has a different topology). It is possible to prove that the semichromes are the "best" object colours for a given hue, thus Ostwald also refers to them as "*Vollfarben*" (full colours). (The full colours have maximum monochromatic content as was proven by Schrödinger.) The procedure yields all possible full colours, also those of "non-spectral" hue (the purples).

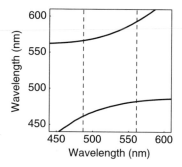

Figure 26.4 When you cut the daylight spectrum into two parts, at a wavelength indicated on the abscissa, the dominant wavelengths of the parts (on the ordinate) run from one spectrum limit to the complementary of the other spectrum limit. One branch runs from (dark) blue to (pale) cyan, the other from (pale) yellow to (dark) red. These branches are Goethe's "boundary colours". The dotted lines indicate the best Schopenhauer cuts for a binary section of daylight (see also Figs 26.5 and 26.6).

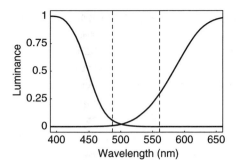

Figure 26.5 When you cut the daylight spectrum into two parts, at a wavelength indicated on the abscissa (see also Figs 26.4 and 26.6), the luminance of the achromatic component of the parts (on the ordinate) runs between total darkness and the full daylight spectrum. The dotted lines indicate the best Schopenhauer cuts for a binary section of daylight. Evidently the achromatic component of the parts is quite small.

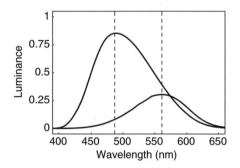

Figure 26.6 When you cut the daylight spectrum into two parts, at a wavelength indicated on the abscissa (see also Figs 26.4 and 26.5), the luminance of the monochromatic component of the parts (on the ordinate) assumes a (global) maximum at one of the best Schopenhauer cuts (this is indeed my definition of these cut loci). The dotted lines indicate the best Schopenhauer cuts for a binary section of daylight. The maximum luminances of the monochromatic components are appreciable as compared with full daylight spectrum. Evidently the monochromatic components of the parts are very significant. Schopenhauer's notion of daylight consisting of red and cyan or of yellow and blue makes sense. There really are just two optimum ways to cut the daylight spectrum into two parts.

perturbs a semichrome partition one member will become darker (hence less coloured) and the other brighter and less saturated (thus also less coloured). A formal proof involves the Helmholtz decomposition into achromatic and monochromatic components. (One (formally) writes a colour as the weighted sum of the achromatic beam and a monochromatic beam of unit power and the suitable wavelength. This is always possible: the description was introduced by Graßmann (1853) and Helmholtz (1896).) Both parts are "full colours" ("*Vollfarben*") in Ostwald's terminology, for which the monochromatic content is the maximum possible for the given chromaticity.

Although there exist infinitely many pairs of (supplementary) semichromes, some are apparently more "natural" than others in the sense that "people of various cultures" agree on their names. (Schopenhauer makes such remarks, nowadays one would quote Berlin and Kay (1969) on the topic.) Examples are red–cyan, yellow–blue, and green–magenta. These are related though because cyan is a combination of green and blue, yellow of red and green, and magenta of blue and red. Schopenhauer does not venture a further explanation (except from the numerically "simple ratios" of the special bipartitions—see below), but one might speculate that the spectrum limits might be involved (see Figs 26.4–26.6), since these give rise to a "natural" division of semichrome pairs into pairs of "boundary colours" (Goethe's "*Kantenfarben*") and pairs of Newtonian or non-Newtonian "optimal colours" (see below).

Schopenhauer thus considered daylight to be composed of red, green, and blue parts. Various combinations of the parts then yield cyan, magenta, and yellow (when one part is missing) or even white (when no part is missing). So far, so good. As I will argue below, these ideas can be given a quite respectable foundation in the established framework of colorimetry.

Schopenhauer went on to speculate that the parts stand in certain relations to each other, more specifically he speculated that the "sizes" of the parts stand in simple ratios to each other. (*He writes*: "... *black and white, while not ratios, thus not partitions, are not proper colours, only limits. Colour theory proper deals with bipartitions, and the purity of a colour depends on the simplicity of the ratio.*") In this way he saw the possibility of arriving at a principled theory of colour harmony, emulating the theory of harmony of musical sounds. (Schopenhauer writes: "*Why the special importance of these six (colours)? Because in these cases the bipartition gives rise to simple ratios. Just as the musical scale contains only seven cardinal pitches on the continuous sequence.*") The problem is that it is quite unclear what Schopenhauer might have meant by the "sizes" of the parts, even more unclear how one might ever arrive at a rational colorimetric basis of such. In my opinion these speculations are void (but see below for a possible interpretation).

Is there a "natural" definition of "parts of daylight" in the framework of colorimetry?

"Colorimetry" is a discipline that was developed in the nineteenth century as a tool to "measure colour". Major contributors were James Clerk Maxwell (1860), Hermann von Helmholtz (1855) and Hermann Graßmann (1853). It is important to understand that colorimetry works because of severe response reduction. A human observer is required to discriminate between two beams of radiation (these appear as patches of light in the visual field), the only acceptable response being same or different. This is the crux of the matter, though practical considerations lead to an additional and often severe stimulus reduction, and so forth. Here I consider only beams of radiation that are sufficiently characterized through spectral photon number density as a function of photon energy. Thus I ignore coherence and polarization properties. Moreover, I assume that spatiotemporal structures and (psychophysical) methodological variables are kept fixed. Then, the space of beams of radiation is an infinite dimensional Hilbert space of spectra. This Hilbert space becomes foliated into equivalence classes by the colorimetric paradigm and each equivalence class of beams is denoted a "colour". Notice that in this fairly abstract procedure the observer is never permitted to venture an opinion concerning the colour experience of any beam though! The problem of *qualia* thus does not arise in colorimetry by construction.

One finds empirically that the set of colours is highly structured. For most observers it is a convex, pointed (i.e. confined to a half-space) cone (the apex corresponding to the empty beam) in a three-dimensional linear space. For some observers the space is only two-, or even one-dimensional (zero dimensional if one includes blind people). In an abstract geometrical sense the "colour space" is a three-dimensional projection of the positive part of the infinite dimensional space of beams ("positive part" meaning beams whose spectral density is non-negative throughout the spectrum). This makes "colour space" a subspace of the space of beams, nowadays often called "fundamental (visual) space" (Cohen and Kappauf 1982). The nineteenth century "colour space" is a representation (isomorphic image) of this subspace as a three-dimensional linear space. A point in colour space thus represents an infinitely dimensional (dimension three less than the infinite dimension of the space of beams) subspace of the space of beams defined by the corresponding point (a spectrum) in fundamental space, augmented with the "black space". The black space contains all (necessarily virtual) beams that cannot be discriminated from the empty beam. The black space is the invariant description of colour vision as determined by colorimetry. Creatures that share the black space are colorimetrically identical. The black space is the complete and most concise summary of all possible judgements of perceptual equality of beams. Moreover, it is fully independent of the (conceptually arbitrary) choice of primaries. It is in a way all colorimetry in the strict sense has to offer.

It is often convenient to denote a certain beam as a "fiducial", often called the "achromatic beam". From the perspective of colorimetry this is an essentially arbitrary act. Notice that it matters whether one assigns a fiducial colour or a fiducial beam. Here I will assume that a certain beam is selected and denoted "average daylight". I will assume that the spectral density is strictly positive throughout the spectrum. I can describe the fiducial beam as the linear superposition (a Lebesgue integral) of an infinite number of "monochromatic beams". In practice one divides the spectrum into bins and regards spectra as finite sums over the bins within the "visual region" of the spectrum. This avoids technical problems with arbitrarily fine spectral structure. I will refer to a single bin of the fiducial beam as a "monochromatic" component without much need for confusion. The colours of the monochromatic components describe the "spectrum locus" of average daylight in colour space.

When one considers a colour modulo its intensity (where any measure of "intensity" will do, for example, luminance) one obtains half-lines with apex at the origin as equivalence classes. These are conventionally known as "chromaticities". "Chromaticity space" is the space of lines through the origin of colour space, thus—in formal mathematical language—a "projective plane". (Since the lines through a point can be placed in a one-to-one relation with the points of a plane, the line bundle is formally isomorphic with a plane though it may "look" like a three-dimensional entity.) The chromaticities of the monochromatic components describe a (semi-)conical surface, the "spectrum cone". The spectrum locus runs over this surface of course. The convex hull of the spectrum cone is a conical volume with apex at the origin, confined to a half-space ("pointed"). The monochromatic chromaticities lie fully on the boundary of this volume (indeed, necessarily, because the spectrum cone mantle is convex), but don't exhaust it. They fill a sector of the boundary limited by the two "spectrum limits". The remaining part of the boundary is the (necessarily planar) "sector of purples". The spectrum part of the boundary is smoothly curved, although not all that different from a dihedral with crease at some place in the middle of the spectrum ("green") as Maxwell (1860) discovered.

The chromaticity of the fiducial beam lies necessarily in the interior of the spectrum cone and thus defines two special planes with the chromaticities of the spectrum limits, which divide the volume of the interior into four parts. Two parts correspond to the high and low photon energy regions of the spectrum ("blues" and "reds"), one part to the medium photon energy region ("greens") and a final part to mixtures of high and low photon energy regions ("purples" or "magentas"). This subdivision of the spectrum region into three parts ("reds", "greens", and "blues") is an immediate consequence of the choice of a fiducial chromaticity. It is one obvious candidate when one looks for a colorimetric definition of Schopenhauer's parts of daylight (see Figs 26.4–26.6). In this division of colour space reds and blues can be paired off into "complementary pairs" (meaning that the colours of such a pair can be mixed such as to yield the fiducial colour) whereas all "greens" lack such a complementary (a state of affairs discovered empirically by Helmholtz (1855) in marked opposition to Newton's (1952) predictions).

Perhaps a better way to find "parts of daylight" in colorimetry is to try to find the "optimal cuts" in a (tri-)partition of the fiducial spectrum (see Figs 26.7 and 26.8). That means the assignment of two photon energies that divide the visual region into low,

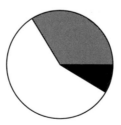

Figure 26.7 The "parts of daylight" for the optimum trisection. The ratios are very close to R : G : B = 3 : 6 : 1 in any reasonable definition, for example, the luminance of the components (32 : 59 : 9) or the luminance of the monochromatic contents of the components (34 : 58 : 8). It is quite unclear which definition Schopenhauer intended. In any case, Schopenhauer's notion that the ratios would necessarily be "simple" has no basis in fact.

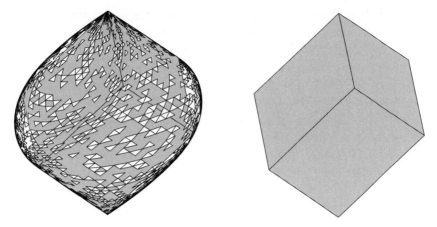

Figure 26.8 On the left the "Schopenhauer RGB-crate" inside Schrödinger's optimal colour solid (I have only plotted 30 per cent of the faces of a triangulation of its surface in order to render it "transparent"), on the right the crate alone. The crate is in most respects similar to the RGB-cube of computer graphics. It is the unique crate that exhausts a maximum volume (65 per cent) of the colour solid. Thus the probability of any object colour to have positive (or non-negative) RGB contents is highest. In practice the overwhelming majority of object colours are inside the crate, since near optimal colours are quite rare (their spectral albedo has to be all or none with at most two transitions in the visual region). Thus the crate is indeed quite special and allows a very convenient representation of object colours.

medium and high photon energy stretches. One way to define "optimal" would be to maximize the volume of the tetrahedron spanned by the "red" (low photon energy part), "green" (medium photon energy part), "blue" (high photon energy part) and "black" (zero beam, origin) colours. This is a simple extremal problem, whose solution is that the cut between the low and medium photon energy regions should be at a photon energy complementary to the colour of the high photon energy region, whereas the cut between the high and medium photon energy regions should be at a photon energy complementary to the colour of the low photon energy region. The result one obtains is (numerically) not too different from that of the former method in the case of average daylight (say the CIE D65 spectrum).

The relation to object colours

"Object colours" in a very restricted definition (but one that is especially adapted to colorimetric considerations) are the colours of Lambertian surfaces described fully through a spectral albedo between zero and one throughout the spectrum, irradiated with a fiducial beam. Then one simply weighs the spectrum of the irradiance with the spectral albedo and determines the colour of that beam. All object colours—in this extremely simplified framework—are copies of the fiducial beam with the monochromatic components selectively darkened (because of the albedo). Object colours are thus a variety of "darkened daylight", very much in Goethe's spirit of colours as "shadow-like entities". The Lambertian assumption is necessary in order to avoid the influence of viewing direction on the retinal irradiation.

In the case of object colours the "fiducial beam" is a much more natural entity than in the colorimetry of beams. There simply are no object colours without the assignment of the fiducial beam!

Colours (in the colorimetric sense, that is, points in colour space) can occur at arbitrarily large distances from the origin because beams can be arbitrarily powerful. Thus colour space extends to infinity. This is different in the case of object colours. White is the most one gets, namely the colour of the fiducial beam itself. All other object colours are darker than white in the sense that something has to be added to them in order to reach white. Colour space becomes a finite volume, the so-called colour solid (see Fig. 26.8). This was grasped early in the history of colour science (e.g. by the painter Runge 1810; a letter by Runge is printed as an appendix in Goethe's "*Zur Farbenlehre*"), though the first (correct) formal treatment is by Schrödinger (1920).

When one partitions the visual region into three parts one immediately obtains a number of colours. Without doing anything one has black. The parts are red, green, and blue. Binary addition yields cyan, magenta, and yellow. When one adds the three parts one obtains white of course. The eight colours yellow, green, cyan, blue, magenta, red, and black and white lie on the vertices of a parallelepiped inscribed in the colour solid. A natural definition of the cuts (the "parts of daylight") would be via an optimalization of the volume of this parallelepiped. When one does the exercise one finds the same result as before (Neugebauer 1937). The sequence yellow, green, cyan, blue, magenta, red (and yellow again) is the "equator" of the parallelepiped, when one regards white and black as the "poles". It has the topology of the colour circle.

When one takes the three Schopenhauer parts R (red), G (green), and B (blue) as primaries, one can write almost any object colour (namely all those within the parallelepiped) as $rR + gG + bB$, with $0 <= r, g, b <= 1$. It is the best possible RGB-approximation to the actual colour solid (see Fig. 26.8).

Since white (W) is composed of red, green, and blue parts, any "luminance function" will produce numbers that might be interpreted as Schopenhauer's "divided activity of the retina". Let the luminance function be the linear functional L, then clearly $L(W) = L(R) + L(G) + L(B)$, thus the fractions fR, fG, fB with $fR = L(R)/L(W)$, etc., add to 100 per cent and can be interpreted as "Schopenhauer fractions". We find (approximately) $R:G:B = 3:6:1$. Alternatively, we may use the luminances of the monochromatic components in a Helmholtz decomposition. Again we find (again, approximately, the precise values differ slightly from the former case) $R:G:B = 3:6:1$. It is not clear what Schopenhauer had in mind (of course he had to reason without any knowledge of colorimetry). Schopenhauer suggests that his ratios are not additive (e.g. $R:G:B = 3:6:1$ would not imply $Y:B = 9:1$ because $Y = R + G$), thus he did not think in terms of something similar to luminance. The second method mentioned above is not additive, because addition of beams generally converts monochromatic content into achromatic content. (Think of the addition of yellow (R+G) and blue, the result is purely achromatic (R + G + B equals daylight), whereas the components are chromatic.)

The colour sequences black, blue, cyan, white and white, yellow, red, black are samples from the so called Goethe "boundary colours", the colours one sees through a prism when one looks at a white-black boundary (Bouma 1947). There is a symmetry between the two series in that the pairs (black, white), (blue, yellow), (cyan, red) and (white, black) all add to white, hence are "supplementary" (and consequently complementary) colours. The boundary colour loci describe spirals of opposite chirality on the boundary of the colour solid and divide this boundary into two parts (see Fig. 26.9). One part consists of "Newtonian colours" in the sense that they correspond to spectral selection via a slit of variable position and width. The other part contains "non-Newtonian" colours in the sense that they cannot so be obtained and thus are not "spectral" in any obvious sense. In order to obtain these colours one must block a part (of variable position and width) of the spectrum, passing both spectral ends.

The colours on the boundary of the colour solid are the so-called Schrödinger (1920) "optimal colours". They are the most luminous object colours for a given chromaticity. Their spectral albedos are either one or zero with not more than two transitions. When there is only a single transition (which is non-generic, that is, a random optimal colour has two transitions with probability one) one has a boundary colour, otherwise a generic optimal colour.

The Schopenhauer parts of daylight as defined here are obviously optimal colours. Red, blue, cyan, and yellow are boundary colours, green is a Newtonian optimal colour and magenta a non-Newtonian one.

Not all optimal colours are very vivid, for obviously many will be close to white or black. The most vivid colours are the ones farthest from the grey axis (the "equator" of the colour solid) and these can be shown to be precisely the Ostwald "semichromes", for

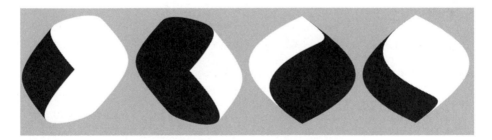

Figure 26.9 The "Newtonian" (black) and the "non-Newtonian" (white) optimal colours subtend equal and congruent areas of the surface of the colour solid. They correspond pair-wise via the central symmetry, thus there exist equally many of each. The boundary between the families is made up of two spirals of opposite chirality that connect the white point to the black point. These are the Goethe "*Kantenfarben*" which also appear (in different guise) in the Fig. 26.1 (the figure eight loop), Fig. 26.2 (the curves connecting the spectrum limits to the achromatic point) and Figs 26.4–26.6.

which the transitions are at complementary photon energies. Some of the "semichromes" have one transition at a spectrum limit, only one within the spectrum, and thus are also Goethe boundary colours. Examples are red and blue. "Pure" red is the low photon energy spectrum from the spectrum limit up to the complementary of the high photon energy spectrum limit. Slight perturbations either make the red purplish, because the semichrome includes part of the high photon energy region of the spectrum, or yellowish, because more of the medium photon energy region is added in. A similar reasoning applies to "pure" blue.

This tripartition into a red, green, and blue depends on the spectrum, not just the colour of the irradiance. This may or may not be considered a drawback. There are ways to deal with this, but in order to keep in the spirit of Schopenhauer's "parts" I will stick to the definition of "white" as a fiducial beam, not a fiducial colour.

Relation to Ostwald's "Principle of Internal Symmetry"

Wilhelm Ostwald (1918b) framed an interesting "Principle of Internal Symmetry" which he used to mensurate the colour circle. The idea is simple (see Fig. 26.10). Let the sequence $c(0), \ldots, c(2n - 1)$ denote "cardinal colours", that is, be the steps of a discrete, $2n$-step colour circle (thus $c(2n)$ equals $c(0)$ again). Then $c(i)$ and $c(i + n)$ are antipodes and thus should be taken as complementary. One needs only to space $c(0), \ldots, c(n - 1)$ in

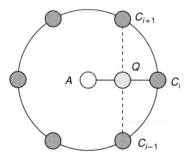

Figure 26.10 The "Principle of Internal Symmetry" (PIS) according to Ostwald. Start by distributing an even number of cardinal colours on the colour circle (a multiple of six makes most sense). Make sure that they come in complementary pairs (hence the need for an even number). Then the aim is to distribute the colours (when you shift one the complementary shifts with it, Ostwald says the colours are "like beads on a string") evenly. According to the PIS this means that the even mixture of the two neighbours of a colour has the same hue as that colour. (Q the same colour as $(C_{i+1} + C_{i-1})/2$, that is, A, Q, and C_i are collinear.) The principle can easily be formalized mathematically and leads to a simple and stable algorithm to mensurate curves in colour space according to "arc length" (as defined by the principle). One shows that this arc length is an affine invariant, that is, the (arbitrary) choice of primaries does not matter. Thus Ostwald's principle makes solid colorimetric sense. Sadly, most authors (I know of only a few exceptions, mostly from the pre Second World War period) have chosen to misunderstand and/or ridicule the principle.

some way, then the others automatically fall into place (as Ostwald says: "The colours are like beads on a string"). In order to arrive at the desired even spacing Ostwald stipulates that the mixture $c(i-1) + c(i+1)$ should have the same hue (dominant wavelength in colorimetry) as that of $c(i)$. This the "Principle of Internal Symmetry" (see Richter 1930 and Bouma 1946). It was foreshadowed in a letter by Graßmann (Graßmann 1879, Ostwald does not quote Graßmann's letter, though I do not exclude (nor do I know for certain) that he knew it) and in Gustav Fechner's (1876–97) book on aesthetics (Ostwald knew Fechner personally and held him in high regard but does not mention this). It is a surprising fact that Ostwald's mensuration yields results that are in excellent agreement with those of pure eye measure. This is apparent from Ostwald's colour atlas. Numerical calculation reveals that the Principle of Internal Symmetry reproduces Munsell's eye measure results to within about one step on a 24-step scale. This is about as good as might be expected since the (few) eye measure results that have been published differ by similar amounts among each other. It is indeed surprising because colorimetry doesn't involve any eye measure at all, but only judgements of equality.

The colour circle that results from the Schopenhauer partition of daylight is the sequence yellow, green, cyan, blue, magenta, red, and back to yellow. Because cyan is green plus blue, magenta blue plus red, and yellow, red plus green, this colour circle is automatically mensurated according to the Principle of Internal Symmetry. Thus Schopenhauer's parts automatically lead to a "well tempered" colour circle (see Fig. 26.11).

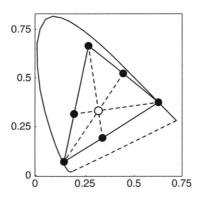

Figure 26.11 When you look for the optimum trisections of daylight (such that additive mixtures of the parts claim the largest possible volume of the colour solid) you find that there exists a unique solution. The three parts may be denoted "red", "green", and "blue", and together they reproduce daylight, added in pairs they yield "cyan", "magenta", and "yellow". Here I have plotted the Schopenhauer YGCBMR colour circle in the CIE xy chromaticity diagram. The colours lie on a triangle that closely approximates the locus of the Ostwald full colours, thus the colours by reflection (of daylight) with the highest possible monochromatic content (remember that the spectrum locus is a locus of black colours by reflection!).

Reappraisal of Schopenhauer's notion

Although Schopenhauer's high hopes of arriving at a principled basis of colour harmony seem futile, the concept of colours as "parts of daylight" is a valuable one. As I have shown the tripartition is very natural, namely the unique solution to the problem of inscribing a "best fitting crate" (a parallelepiped) into the colour solid that exhausts the greatest fraction of its volume.

The best fitting crate can be used to approximate the colour solid very effectively and allows one to describe all object colours that fit into the best fitting crate in terms of their red, green, and blue (RGB) content, these contents being numbers (fractions) in the range $[0, 1]$. This is analogous to the conventional RGB colours of the CRT screens with R, G, and B in the range $0 \ldots 255$ (byte values). When one converts colorimetric values to RGB colours that way one indeed obtains a convenient method to render (or rather "suggest", because colorimetrically the notion is void of course!) colorimetric values on the CRT screen.

To approximate the actual colour solid with a simple RGB crate is attractive, because it leads to a very convenient and intuitive description of surface colours. It is an exact description that fits seamlessly into the formalism of colorimetry, in which surface colours are denoted by their rgb-values. For colours inside the crate these values lie between zero and one. Clearly, it would seriously detract from the attractiveness if it were the case that many colours existed for which rgb-values turn out to be negative or in excess of unity. The crate approximation is only of interest when almost all object colours fall within the interior of the crate. A question that naturally arises is how good such a crate approximation actually is. The answer cannot be a simple one. It is indeed simple enough to find the fraction of the volume of the colour solid that is exhausted by the best fitting crate. (It is 65 per cent for natural daylight.) But the volume that falls outside of the best-fitting crate (35 per cent of the volume) contains object colours that are extremely rare, thus the fraction is not that informative. If one generates random object colours from a uniform distribution of spectral albedo at each wavelength, they are median (50 per cent) greys with overwhelming probability. In order to obtain some vivid colours one has to put severe constraints upon the random generator. You should strongly bias the distribution against violent spectral variations in order to obtain vivid colours with some probability. Such constraints capture one's prior information concerning the frequency of occurrence of particular spectral albedos. The knowledge of the human biotope (over evolutionary significant periods) is too scant to be able to venture a guess. However, it is quite clear that the best fitting crate will contain the overwhelming majority of object colours that one is likely to encounter in daily life.

The precise cut loci for the Schopenhauer parts depend upon the spectrum of the irradiance. Even if the colour of the source is the same, the partitions may vary, because the spectrum is not determined by the colour. If one switches from daylight to tungsten light (say) one has to cut the visual region at different locations in order to obtain a best-fitting crate. It is a priori likely that colours of the parts will be very similar though and that they will mainly differ in luminance. This is indeed corroborated by straightforward numerical calculation. This suggests that one may use the mapping between crates as a "constancy" mechanism, and that this mechanism is likely to be very close indeed to a von Kries (1904) scheme.

One can indeed use the idea of parts to estimate the spectral albedo of the material and use this estimate to predict the colour change under variation of the irradiance (Ostwald 1919). This is of course related to the "colour constancy problem". The spectral albedos in the "parts" description correspond in a one-to-one fashion to the colours because they form a three-parameter family. This is similar to the simplified spectrometry proposed by Ostwald. It is only an approximation (of course), but it is surprisingly effective, quite probably "good enough" to let biological implementations "get by".

Such considerations show that Schopenhauer's long forgotten notion of (object) colours as "parts of daylight" is a viable one by today's standards and can easily be given practical applications.

References

Berlin, B. & Kay, P. (1969). *Basic Colour Terms, Their Universality and Evolution*. Berkeley: University of California Press.

Bouma, P. J. (1946). Zur Einteilung des Ostwaldschen Farbtonkreises. *Experientia, 2*, 99–103.

Bouma, P. J. (1947). *Physical Aspects of Colour*. Eindhoven: N.V. Philips Gloeilampenfabrieken.

Cohen, J. B. & Kappauf, W. E. (1982). Metameric Colour Stimuli, Fundamental Metamers, and Wyszecki's Metameric Blacks. *Am. J. Psychol., 95*, 537–64.

Fechner, G. T. (1876–97). *Vorschule der Ästhetik*. Leipzig: Breitkopf.

Goethe, J. W. von (1984). *Farbenlehre, mit Einleitungen und Kommentaren von Rudolf Steiner*. Stuttgart: Verlag Freies Geistesleben.

Graßmann, H. (1853). Zur Theorie der Farbenmischung. *Ann. Phys., 89*, 69–84.

Graßmann, H. (1879). Bemerkungen zur Theorie der Farbenempfindungen. *Va.Selbstanzeige von V.Königsb.Rep., II*, 213–21.

Helmholtz, H. von (1855). Über die Zusammensetzung von Spektralfarben. *Poggendorfer Ann., 94*, 1–28.

Helmholtz, H. von (1896). *Handbuch der Physiologischen Optik*. Hamburg: Voss.

Hering, E. (1920). *Grundzüge der Lehre vom Lichtsinn*. Berlin: Julius Springer.

Kries, J. von (1904). Die Gesichtsempfindungen. In: Nagel's *Hndb. d. Physiol. d. Menschen, 3* (p. 211).

Maxwell, J. C. (1860). On the Theory of Compound Colours, and the Relations of the Colours of the Spectrum. *Phil. Trans. Roy. Soc.*, 57–84.

Newton, I. (1952). *Opticks*. New York: Dover Publications.

Neugebauer, H. E. J. (1937). Ueber den Körper der optimalen Pigmente. *Z. f. wiss. Phot., 36*, 18–24.

Ostwald, W. (1917). Das absolute System der Farben. *Z. f. Phys. Chem., 92*, 222–6.

Ostwald, W. (1918*a*). *Goethe, Schopenhauer und die Farbenlehre.* Leipzig: Unesma.

Ostwald, W. (1918*b*). *Die Farbenlehre: Mathetische Farbenlehre.* Leipzig: Unesma.

Ostwald, W. (1919). *Die Farbenlehre: Physikalische Farbenlehere.* Leipzig: Unesma.

Richter, M. (1930). Zur Einteilung des Ostwaldschen Farbtonkreises. *Licht*, 12–15.

Runge, Ph., O. (1810). *Farben-Kugel oder Construction des Verhältnisses aller Mischungen der Farben zu einander, und ihrer vollständigen Affinität, mit angehängtem Versuch einer Ableitung der Harmonie in den Zusammenstellungen der Farben.* Hamburg: Friedrich Perthes.

Schopenhauer, A. (1877). Über das Sehen und die Farben (Theoria colorum physiologica). In Julius Frauenstädt (Ed.), *Arthur Schopenhauer's sämmtliche Werke: Schriften zur Erkenntnislehre, II-1* (pp. 1–93), *III-1* (pp. 1–58). Leipzig: F. U. Brodhaus.

Schrödinger, E. (1920). Theorie der Pigmente von grösster Leuchtkraft. *Ann. Phys., 62*, 603–22.

CHAPTER 27

REPRESENTING AN OBSERVER'S MATCHES IN AN ALIEN COLOUR SPACE

KENNETH KNOBLAUCH

L, M, and *S* spectral sensitivities and cone excitation space

In normal human colour vision, light is initially encoded in the quantum catch rates in three classes of photoreceptor, L, M, and S cones. The spectral sensitivities of these three systems are treated as linear, single-valued functions on the space of lights. The values of these three functions on lights are represented in *LMS*-cone excitation space.

We take as our point of departure the parameterized space curve $\tau : \Lambda \to \Re^3$, where Λ is the interval $(400, 700 \text{ nm})$ in $\Re$ and $\tau(\lambda) = (L(\lambda), M(\lambda), S(\lambda))$. This trajectory defines the triple of *LMS* values as a light changes wavelength at unit energy and is called the spectrum locus (Fig. 27.1(a)). We note that the spectrum locus is non-planar, that is, it is a space curve with non-zero torsion. If instead of unit energy, the lights are equated for one of the cone spectral sensitivities, the locus becomes planar. For example, equating the lights for an excitation level k of the L cones gives the trajectory

$$\tau_L(\lambda; k) = \frac{k}{L(\lambda)}(L(\lambda), M(\lambda), S(\lambda)) = k\left(1, \frac{M(\lambda)}{L(\lambda)}, \frac{S(\lambda)}{L(\lambda)}\right) \tag{1}$$

which lies in the plane $L = k$ (Fig. 27.1(b)). Note that all convex linear combinations of the points on this curve are coplanar, as well. It is trivial to show that a trajectory and its convex linear combinations are also coplanar if and only if the energy is equated for any linear combination of the three spectral sensitivities. A well-known example is the MacLeod–Boynton chromaticity diagram in which the spectrum locus is confined to the plane $L + M = 1$ (MacLeod and Boynton 1979).

Rod excitation in cone space

Consider now the spectrum locus generated for lights equated for the rod photoreceptors (Fig. 27.1(c)). The rod spectral sensitivity is taken here to be the $V'(\lambda)$ curve, which defines scotopic spectral efficiency (Wyszecki and Stiles 1981). Similar to eqn (1) the rod-equated spectrum locus is defined as

$$\tau_{V'}(\lambda; k) = \frac{k}{V'(\lambda)}(L(\lambda), M(\lambda), S(\lambda)) \tag{2}$$

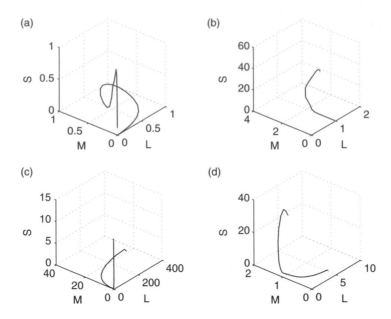

Figure 27.1 The solid curve in each graph indicates the spectrum locus plotted in *LMS*-cone excitation space for lights equated on the basis of (a) energy, (b) *L*-cone excitation, (c) rod excitation, and (d) protanomalous long-wavelength cone excitation. Cone spectral sensitivities are based on those of DeMarco *et al.* (1992). Rod spectral sensitivity is based on $V'(\lambda)$ (Wyszecki and Stiles 1981). Note that the axes have been rescaled as each figure required for display purposes.

where k is the level of rod excitation. The rod spectral sensitivity cannot be expressed as a linear combination of the cone spectral sensitivities. Thus, this space curve is non-planar. Each point on this curve indicates the coordinates of a monochromatic light at an energy that equates it in excitation for the rods. Convex combinations of points on the spectrum locus correspond to mixtures of wavelength that are also equated for rod excitation. For excitation level k, these points can all be described by

$$k\left(\int_{400}^{700} \alpha(\lambda)\frac{L(\lambda)}{V'(\lambda)}d\lambda, \int_{400}^{700} \alpha(\lambda)\frac{M(\lambda)}{V'(\lambda)}d\lambda, \int_{400}^{700} \alpha(\lambda)\frac{S(\lambda)}{V'(\lambda)}d\lambda \right) \qquad (3)$$

where $k\alpha(\lambda)/V'(\lambda)$ is the spectral radiance distribution,

$$\int_{400}^{700} \alpha(\lambda)d\lambda = 1 \qquad (4)$$

and $\alpha(\lambda) \geq 0$, for 400 nm $\leq \lambda \leq$ 700 nm. This is so because even though the rod spectral sensitivity cannot be expressed as a linear combination of the cone spectral sensitivities, it is itself linear. Since the curve is non-planar, the set of all such convex combinations defines a solid of constant rod excitation. Each point in this solid corresponds to a set of spectral distributions whose rod excitation equals that generated by the spectral distributions associated with every other point in the solid. This solid represents all such spectral distributions. We will call it a Constant Rod Excitation Solid or CRES.

There is an important difference, however, between a CRES and the Constant L-cone Excitation Plane, a CLEP (or any other linear combination of the cone spectral sensitivities, for that matter). Suppose a small change, ε, in the excitation level. In the case of a CLEP, a new plane will be generated parallel to the first which corresponds to an excitation level of $k + \varepsilon$. The mapping of LMS to excitation level is many to one, so that the two CLEPs will not share any points in common. In the case of a CRES, however, a new CRES with increment of excitation ε sufficiently small will overlap with the previous CRES. Thus, a given value of LMS does not correspond to a unique level of rod excitation. While a given coordinate can be in many CRES's, that is, represent many different levels of rod excitation, each excitation level will correspond to a different family of spectral distributions, that is, convex combinations of points of the spectrum locus necessary to generate the point in the CRES. Thus, when we try to represent a light with respect to an alien spectral sensitivity, that is one from an observer whose characteristics are different from those of our color space, we are obliged to retain $\alpha(\lambda)$, which with the alien spectral sensitivity determines the spectral distribution of the light.

Anomalous trichromatic metamers in normal cone space

Consider now an anomalous trichromatic observer who shares two of the cone photopigments with a normal observer but for whom the third has a different spectral sensitivity. To use a specific example, we will consider a protanomalous observer who has normal S and M cones but whose long-wavelength sensitive cone has a different spectral sensitivity, $P(\lambda)$. We can treat this case similarly to that of the rods. The spectrum locus generated by lights equated for the $P(\lambda)$-cones is

$$\tau_P(\lambda; k) = \frac{k}{P(\lambda)}(L(\lambda), M(\lambda), S(\lambda)) \tag{5}$$

Because $P(\lambda)$ is not a linear combination of the cone sensitivities of a normal trichromat, the spectrum locus is non-planar (Fig. 27.1(d)). The convex sum of all points on this curve generates a solid that represents all the spectra that produce a constant P excitation. As for the rods, a given point in LMS space does not represent a unique excitation of P.

Consider now the lines on which S and M are constant, protanopic confusion lines. The intersection of these confusion lines with the constant P-solid will produce points or line segments that correspond to sets of metamers for a protanomalous observer. Thus, we have demonstrated that the metamers of an anomalous observer fall on dichromatic confusion lines in normal color space. As with the rods, the spectral radiance distribution that generated each point on these segments must be retained.

We could reverse the situation and consider the solid of constant L-cone excitation in the protanomalous cone excitation space. Families of metamers for the normal trichromat map into line segments that result from the intersection of the constant L-cone excitation solid and the lines along which S and M are constant. We would see then the range of protanomalous cone excitations generated by a *set of lights* producing a constant *LMS* response. In other words, what we represent by these line segments is the range of excitations produced in the color space of one observer by a set of lights that are metameric for another observer.

Human and camera observers

A typical color camera has three sensors each with a spectral responsivity curve, $R_1(\lambda), R_2(\lambda), R_3(\lambda)$. With actual cameras, these curves are not, in general, linear combinations of the human cone spectral sensitivities. Thus, the camera represents a different observer than the human observer, with different metamers. The preceding discussion suggests a method for visualizing the differences between these observers.

For a given light, $E(\lambda)$, calculate the excitation of each of the three sensors, k_i. Then, for each of the three excitations, generate a constant excitation solid in *LMS* space. The general expression for the coordinates of these solids is

$$k_i\left(\int_{400}^{700} \frac{\alpha_i(\lambda)}{R_i(\lambda)}L(\lambda)d\lambda, \int_{400}^{700} \frac{\alpha_i(\lambda)}{R_i(\lambda)}M(\lambda)d\lambda, \int_{400}^{700} \frac{\alpha_i(\lambda)}{R_i(\lambda)}S(\lambda)d\lambda\right), \quad i = 1-3 \quad (6)$$

The points of intersection of the three solids are those for which the coordinates generated by eqn (6) are the same for each i. The three solids must intersect in at least one point, the point corresponding to the light, $E(\lambda)$. The set of lights that are camera metamers correspond to a subset of the points of intersection of the three solids. The camera metamers are those points that have the same spectral radiance distribution for the three equal excitation solids, that is, the points of intersection for which

$$k_1\frac{\alpha_1(\lambda)}{R_1(\lambda)} = K_2\frac{\alpha_2(\lambda)}{R_2(\lambda)} = k_3\frac{\alpha_3(\lambda)}{R_3(\lambda)} \tag{7}$$

for 400 nm $\leq \lambda \leq$ 700 nm. Points in the three solids that satisfy eqn (7) are points of intersection. However, the converse is not necessarily true.

Convexity, eqn (4), places the following constraint on the choice of weights for one sensor

$$0 \leq \alpha_1(\lambda) \leq \min\left(\frac{k_2}{k_1}\frac{R_1(\lambda)}{R_2(\lambda)}, \frac{k_3}{k_1}\frac{R_1(\lambda)}{R_3(\lambda)}\right) \tag{8}$$

Given the value of α_1, the other two weighting functions are determined as

$$\alpha_2(\lambda) = \frac{k_1}{k_2}\frac{R_2(\lambda)}{R_1(\lambda)}\alpha_1(\lambda)$$

$$\alpha_3(\lambda) = \frac{k_1}{k_3}\frac{R_3(\lambda)}{R_1(\lambda)}\alpha_1(\lambda)$$

$$(9)$$

from eqn (7). In practice, the lights, spectral sensitivities, and weighting functions are defined discretely over wavelength. Even sampled every 10 nm, however, there is a large number of degrees of freedom in defining possible points of intersection.

Conclusions

This article describes a procedure for evaluating the range of excitations in one observer's color matching space generated by the set of metamers from a different observer's space. The approach outlined lends itself to visualizing the results geometrically, which is often helpful in generating intuitions about multi-dimensional problems. This kind of calculation should be useful in characterizing individual differences. For example, one could represent the range of metamers around a given point for the CIE 1931 observer in the chromaticity diagram of the Judd observer. Comparison with MacAdam's ellipses would permit an evaluation of the metameric lights for the1931observer that were most discriminable to the Judd observer. Ezquerro *et al.* (2001) have recently employed a related approach to analyze individual differences in colorimetric observers. They generated large sets of metameric spectral distributions for each of several observers using a Monte Carlo procedure and compared the clouds of points in a common chromaticity diagram with discrimination ellipses. The approach also might be relevant for practical applications, as in specifying the limits of gamut matching between different media.

There are other methods for exploring the differences between observers. For example, using the singular value decomposition, one can calculate an orthonormal basis for the null space for an observer's matches. The basis elements correspond to spectral distributions that, when added to a light, do not change its tristimulus values. Such theoretical lights are also called "metameric blacks" (Wyszecki and Stiles 1981).

By projecting one observer's spectral sensitivities on another observer's null space, one obtains a basis for a set of lights whose differences are visible to one observer but not the other. In general, however, the basis functions obtained are not all positive which renders it difficult to determine the mixtures that correspond to real (non-negative valued) lights. In the approach described here, convex combinations of the spectrum locus generate all metamers. In this way, all solutions are guaranteed to correspond to real lights.

Finally, a further step would be to restrict consideration to linear models of lights and surfaces. The differences under such restricted models might better correspond to the metameric differences between observers likely to be obtained in natural situations.

Acknowledgment

I am grateful for the helpful comments of Françoise Viénot and Robert Sève.

References

DeMarco, P., Pokorny, J., & Smith V. C. (1992). Full-spectrum cone sensitivity functions for X-chromosome-linked anomalous trichromats. *Journal of the Optical Society of America A*, 9, 1465–76.

Ezquerro, J. M., Carreño, F., Zoido, J. M., & Bernabeu, E. (2001). The use of metamers to compare the color vision of observers. *Color Research and Application*, 26, 262–9.

MacLeod, D. I. A. & Boynton, R. M. (1979). Chromaticity diagram showing cone excitation by stimuli of equal luminance. *Journal of the Optical Society of America*, 69, 1183–86.

Wyszecki, G. & Stiles, W. S. (1981). *Color Science: Concepts and Methods, Quantitative Data and Formulae*. New York: Wiley.

CHAPTER 28

MACULAR PIGMENT: NATURE'S NOTCH FILTER

J. D. MORELAND AND S. WESTLAND

Introduction

Macular pigment (MP) is a natural filter with "notch" transmission characteristics. The human population range of its peak absorbance extends over 1 log unit (Bone and Sparrock 1971) (see Fig. 28.1).

   The effect of MP variance has been reported by Wright (1947) for the White point and by von Schelling (1950) more generally. Rotation around the Illuminant point has been noted by Moreland and Dain (1995), Smith and Pokorny (1995) and Mollon and Regan (1999). None of these studies considered chromatic adaptation.

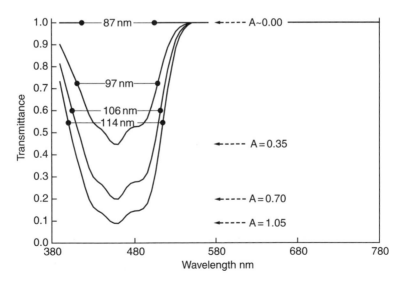

Figure 28.1 Macular pigment is a natural filter with "notch" transmission characteristics. The population range of the peak absorbance A extends over 1 log unit and the full-width half-depth block band increases with A.

Method

We assess the effect of MP on surface colours in Normal and Anomalous (X-linked) Trichromats for a database of 1782 reflectance spectra (513 natural and 1269 Munsell paper surfaces). Chromaticities are computed by convolving the reflectance spectra with CIE Illuminant C, the Normal and Anomalous cone fundamentals of De Marco *et al.* (1992) and a range (peak absorbances −0.35, 0, 0.35, and 0.7) of MP filters (Stockman *et al.* 1999). Chromaticities are presented in an analogue of the MacLeod–Boynton (1979) cone excitation diagram and the symbols "L" and "S", respectively are used as shorthand for the abscissa, $L/(L + M)$, and the ordinate, $S/(L + M)$, of that diagram. The von Kries adaptation correction is applied: adaptation being presumed to be complete, since changes in individual pigment concentration over time are usually very gradual (Hammond *et al.* 1997). Changes of variance in the "L" and "S" directions are computed globally for the 1782 spectra as well as locally for 25 non-overlapping rectangular colour cells. These cells are constructed by arranging 5 vertical bands, centred on Illuminant C, each containing some 356 spectra and then dividing each band into 5 cells each containing some 71 spectra. Additionally, the grid formed by the mean colours of the 25 cells is used to compute local changes in "L" and "S" geometric spacing for 20 nearest-neighbour pairs. All computations are performed using MatLab software.

Results and discussion

The results, presented here, are Enhancement Factors based on global standard deviations, means of the 25 local standard deviations and means of the 20 nearest-neighbour grid spacing. An Enhancement Factor is the ratio of a value, obtained at a particular level of MP, to that obtaining for −0.35 peak absorbance. The latter effectively removes the MP complement of an average 2° observer (Stockman *et al.* 1999).

The MacLeod–Boynton diagram is not uniform and this is a potential source of bias, particularly for results obtained with the global estimate. The other two measures, being local, are less affected by that bias. The division into equally populated cells was made to ensure statistical parity.

Table 28.1 lists the mean Enhancement Factors based on local standard deviations (SD) for Normals, Protanomals, and Deuteranomals. Trends for the "S" axis are similar for all three observers, showing an enhancement of some 7–8% close to the upper population limit for MP. Changes in the "L" direction are more variable between observers: those for Normals and Deuteranomals show continuous increases while that for Protanomals barely departs from unity. This variability is the subject of a further study.

The other two measures of enhancement, computed from grid spacing and from global variance, are compared with mean local SDs for Normals in Table 28.2. These two measures are not only considerably smaller for the "L" direction but, with values less than unity, show evidence of compression. In the "S" direction, enhancement factors based on

Table 28.1 Local enhancement factors for normals, protanomals, and deuteranomals

Added macular pigment. Peak absorbance	Enhancement factors based on local SDs					
	Parallel to the "L" axis			Parallel to the "S" axis		
	Normal	Protanomal	Deuteranomal	Normal	Protanomal	Deuteranomal
−0.35	1.00	1.00	1.00	1.00	1.00	1.00
0	1.00	0.97	1.07	1.04	1.03	1.04
0.35	1.05	0.98	1.12	1.06	1.06	1.07
0.70	1.09	1.00	1.16	1.08	1.07	1.08

Table 28.2 Comparison of three enhancement factors for normals

Added macular pigment. Peak absorbance	Enhancement factors					
	Parallel to the "L" axis			Parallel to the "S" axis		
	Local SDs	Grid spacing	Global SDs	Local SDs	Grid spacing	Global SDs
−0.35	1.00	1.00	1.00	1.00	1.00	1.00
0	1.00	0.99	1.00	1.04	0.97	1.08
0.35	1.05	0.97	0.99	1.06	1.00	1.13
0.70	1.09	0.96	0.99	1.08	1.00	1.15

global SDs are twice as large as those based on local SDs. This difference may reflect bias in the global measure produced by the gross non-uniformity of the MacLeod–Boynton Diagram. In contrast with local SDs, grid spacing in the "S" direction hardly changes. This disagreement is puzzling since both measures are local.

Increases in MP concentration produce a general clockwise rotation of chromaticity around the illuminant point (see Fig. 28.2) for Normals, in agreement with Moreland and Dain (1995), Smith and Pokorny (1995), Mollon and Regan (1999), as well as for Anomals. The chromaticity shifts, associated with rotation, increase with distance from the Illuminant point. There is additionally a shear component, with a similar centrifugal increase. Both rotation and shear strongly influence Factors based on grid spacing.

Factors based on local SDs depend on the choice of cell boundaries. Our decision to equate cell populations (for statistical parity) produces cells with quite disparate areas and shapes. Systematic changes in rotation and shear within some eccentric cells yields high local enhancement factors (see Fig. 28.3).

Such local factors may have practical relevance. Using cell demarcation in the biologically informed context of discriminating ripe fruit (a compact cell) against tropical forest foliage (a cell elongated in the "S" direction), Mollon and Regan (1999) have

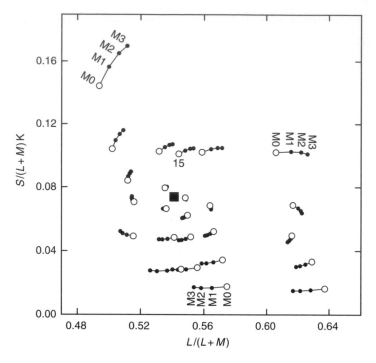

Figure 28.2 Changes in chromaticity with increasing macular pigment, after correcting for adaptation. Chromaticities are means for twenty-five cells, each containing some seventy-one separate colours. Square: Illuminant C. Peak absorbances, −0.35, 0, 0.35, and 0.70, are labelled M0–M3, respectively on selected loci. The constant K (4.93) applied to the ordinate improves the "uniformity" of the diagram in the region illustrated. Its effect is cosmetic; leaving the calculation of Enhancement Factors unchanged. The cell 15 locus is labelled: see Fig. 28.3.

demonstrated how MP in the primate retina may be related to the evolutionary fine-tuning of cone photopigment spectra.

It is relevant to consider here how the von Kries correction could affect our three Enhancement Factor measures. This correction addresses the issue of colour constancy, by stabilising the chromaticity of a changing illuminant but it introduces its own distortion of colour space around the Illuminant point. In particular, the negligible change of "S" grid spacing (Table 28.2) with MP conflicts with the experimental finding of "tritan" confusions, associated with the absorbance of filters simulating MP, in the Farnsworth 100-hue test (Moreland and Dain 1995). Of our three Enhancement Factor measures, only the one based on local variances is potentially capable of reducing the effects of such distortion. However, in order to achieve that potential, careful revision of cell partitioning would be required.

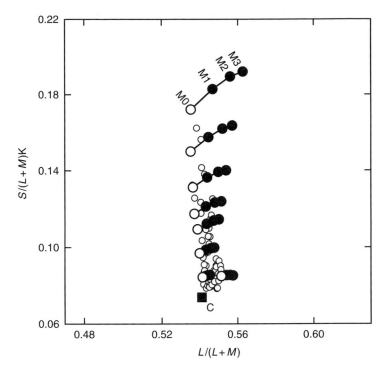

Figure 28.3 Chromaticity shifts within Cell 15 (see Fig. 28.2). Square: Illuminant C. Empty circles: chromaticities for −0.35 peak MP absorbance. Large circles: 8 selected colours showing shifts that increase systematically with distance from C. Absorbance labelling as in Fig. 28.2.

References

Bone, R. A. & **Sparrrock, J. M. B.** (1971). Comparison of macular pigment densities in human eyes. *Vision Research, 11,* 1057–64.

DeMarco, P., Pokorny, J., & **Smith, V. C.** (1992). Full-spectrum cone sensitivity functions for X-chromosome-linked anomalous trichromats. *Journal of the Optical Society of America A, 9,* 1465–76.

Hammond, B. R., Johnson, E. J., & **Russell, R. M.** (1997). Dietary modification of human macular pigment. *Investigative Ophthalmology & Visual Science, 38,* 1795–801.

MacLeod, D. I. A. & **Boynton, R. M.** (1979). Chromaticity diagram showing cone excitation by stimuli of equal luminance. *Journal of the Optical Society of America, 69,* 1183–6.

Moreland, J. D. & **Dain, S. L.** (1995). Macular pigment contributes to variance in 100 hue tests. *Documenta Ophthalmologica Proceedings Series, 57,* 517–22.

Mollon, J. D. & **Regan, B. C.** (1999). The spectral distribution of primate cones and of macular pigment: Matched to properties of the world? *Journal of Optical Technology, 66*(10), 847–52.

von Schelling, H. (1950). A method for calculating the effect of filters on color vision. *Journal of the Optical Society of America, 40,* 419–23.

Smith, V. C. & Pokorny, J. (1995). Chromatic-discrimination axes, CRT phosphor spectra, and individual variation in color vision. *Journal of the Optical Society of America A, 12,* 27–35.

Stockman, A., Sharpe, L. T., & Fach, C. (1999). The spectral sensitivity of the human short-wavelength sensitive cones derived from thresholds and color matches. *Vision Research, 39,* 2901–27.

Wright, W. D. (1947). *Characteristics of normal and defective colour vision.* London: Kimpton.

CHAPTER 29

HOW TO FIND A TRITAN LINE

H. E. SMITHSON, P. SUMNER, AND J. D. MOLLON

Introduction

Modern experiments on colour vision often seek to isolate one of the cardinal directions of colour space. These were identified psychophysically by Krauskopf *et al.* (1982), and correspond to two physiologically distinct channels in the retina and lateral geniculate nucleus (Derrington *et al.* 1984; Dacey 2000). One channel compares long-wave-sensitive (L) cone signals with middle-wave-sensitive (M) cone signals, and the other compares short-wave-sensitive (S) cone signals with some combination of L- and M-cone signals. The physical lights required to isolate one of the cardinal directions depend not only on the spectral sensitivity of the photoreceptors, but also on spectrally selective prereceptoral filtering. Spectral transmission properties of the lens vary with age (Pokorny *et al.* 1987) and there are large variations in the normal population in the amount and distribution of macular pigment (Moreland and Bhatt 1984; Hammond *et al.* 1997). Existing psychophysical procedures to determine an individual's tritan confusion line (i.e. the axis of colour space that modulates only the excitation of the short-wave cones) are the Webster method (Webster *et al.* 1990; Webster and Mollon 1994), and the minimally distinct border method (Tansley and Boynton 1976; Boynton and Kaiser 1978). We present here a new psychophysical method designed to locate—for an individual observer and for a specific position in the visual field—the tritan line.

We exploit the phenomenon of "transient tritanopia" (Mollon and Polden 1975). In the classical experimental arrangement, the threshold is measured for a violet probe stimulus first on a steady yellow field and then against a dark background shortly after the yellow field has been turned off. Paradoxically the threshold is higher against the dark field and may remain so for several seconds after the yellow field has been extinguished. To explain transient tritanopia, Pugh and Mollon (1979) have proposed that the S-opponent channel is optimally sensitive in the middle of its operating range, but has a compressive response function, so that it becomes less sensitive when driven to one or other extreme of its response range. After the offset of the yellow field, the S-opponent channel is polarized, perhaps because a restoring force that opposes the yellow field continues to act for a short time. In the present experiment we measure, not the absolute threshold for detection, but the threshold for detecting a chromatic difference along a particular direction in colour space, that is, the threshold for distinguishing between a neutral background and a coloured target defined by a particular hue angle (see Fig. 29.1). We

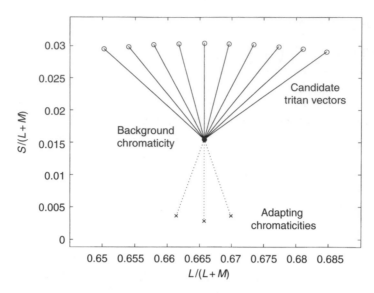

Figure 29.1 A plot showing the MacLeod–Boynton chromaticity co-ordinates of our stimuli. The filled circle represents the background chromaticity (approximately equal energy white). The array of ten vectors, plotted as solid lines, represent the ten candidate tritan directions. They were chosen to span a range including the tritan confusion line for the Judd (1951) 2° observer, that is, a vertical line in this plot. In our experiments, chromatic contrast between test and background was modified with a staircase until a threshold was found. Starting chromaticities are indicated with open circles. We suggest that the vector exhibiting the maximum transient tritanopia effect corresponds to an individual's tritan line. In Experiment 1, we compared the effects of three different adapting field chromaticities, shown on the plot as (×) symbols.

measure such thresholds shortly after extinction of a long-wave field and we repeat these measurements for different hue angles of the target. We predict that the threshold for detecting a chromatic change will be maximally elevated for the axis of colour space that offers no modulation of the L/M-opponent mechanism. For in this direction—the tritan line that we are seeking—detection must depend only on the S-opponent mechanism.

In an alternative tradition, one might expect that adaptation would produce maximal loss in sensitivity for test stimuli that were complementary to the adaptation, whatever axis was chosen for the chromaticity of the adapting field. This would be fatal for a method of finding a tritan line, since the result would depend on the choice of adapting field chromaticity and the method becomes circular. If, however, conditions of transient tritanopia tap the opponent stage of colour processing and selectively desensitise the S-opponent mechanism while leaving the L/M-opponent mechanism little changed, moderate changes in adapting chromaticity should not rotate the vector exhibiting maximal loss of sensitivity.

In Experiment 1 we test this prediction. In Experiment 2 we increase the viewing distance, thereby moving the stimulus to a retinal area with higher macular pigment density, and we test whether our method is able to reveal the associated change in tritan line.

Methods

Experiment 1

All stimuli were presented on a calibrated CRT. The chromaticities used in these experiments are conveniently described as vectors from the background chromaticity (equal energy white) and in each case we specify the clockwise angular rotation from the theoretical tritan axis $(+S/(L+M))$ in MacLeod–Boynton space. The aim is to identify the chromaticity vector that exhibits the largest loss of sensitivity under conditions of transient tritanopia. Ten test vectors were chosen spanning a range that covered both sides of the theoretical tritan axis, from 312° to 54° in MacLeod–Boynton space. Three different adaptation vectors were used: 160°, 180°, and 200°. The length of the adaptation vector was constrained by the available monitor gamut: a distance of 0.0126 units in MacLeod–Boynton space was the maximum possible with our arrangement (see Fig. 29.1).

Observers were first required to view a spatially uniform ($60 \, \text{cd/m}^2$) adapting field for two minutes, and then the trial sequence began. After each top-up adaptation period the display changed abruptly to equal energy white ($22.5 \, \text{cd/m}^2$), and after 400 ms a chromatic probe stimulus was presented. In order to maintain the subject's adaptive state, the duty cycle was fixed, with 7.25-s adaptation every 8 s. The sequence of events in a trial is depicted schematically in Fig. 29.2. Baseline thresholds were also measured for each of the probe stimuli. For the latter measurements, there was an initial two minute adaptation to equal energy white, but trial timings were under the subject's control.

The test stimuli resembled Ishihara plates in that spatial luminance noise ($\pm 7 \, \text{cd/m}^2$) was used to ensure that neither luminance differences nor edge artefacts could be used as a cue for discriminating the chromatic target against the field (Regan *et al.* 1994). The chromatic target formed a 90° segment of a ring. At the viewing distance of 1 m, the thickness of the chromatic arc was 1.55 degrees of visual angle and the separation between fixation and test loci was a minimum of 3 degrees. We chose this arrangement in order to use an area of retina that is relatively homogeneous for short-wave cones and for macular pigment. By presenting the chromatic test in one of four possible locations, chosen at random and at equal eccentricities, we discouraged the observer from moving fixation and forcing the stimuli to a retinal region where the macular pigment density, and thus the tritan line, were different.

A spatial 4AFC task was used: the observer was required to locate the position of the coloured patch, and the chromatic distance between this test patch and the background was modified with a staircase until a threshold was found. In each block of measurements a single candidate chromaticity vector was tested and two randomly interleaved staircases tracked the threshold for 75 per cent discrimination. Conditions were blocked in order that subjects could derive the optimal strategy for detecting each candidate chromaticity. Five blocks with the same adapting chromaticity were presented in a single experimental session. The order of blocks was counterbalanced for test chromaticity, and sessions were counterbalanced for adapting chromaticity, including the no-adaptation, baseline

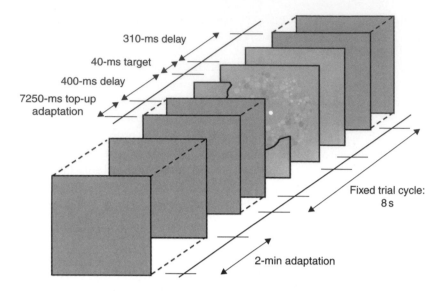

Figure 29.2 See also colour plate section. A schematic diagram showing the sequence of events in a trial. The initial two minute adaptation is followed by a repeated trial-cycle comprising a period of top-up adaptation followed, after 400 ms, by a 40-ms test array. The test arrays resemble Ishihara plates in that spatial luminance noise is used to mask luminance artefacts. The chromatic target formed a 90° arc that was presented in any one of 4 quadrants chosen at random. Ten different probe chromaticity vectors were tested as candidates for the tritan line. In Experiment 1 we compared three different adapting chromaticities. In Experiment 2 we increased the viewing distance, from 1 to 4 m, to determine whether the tritan axis rotated when the eccentricity of the target was reduced from 3 to 0.75 degrees of visual angle.

condition. To allow after-effects to dissipate there was a minimum interval of 30 minutes between sessions.

Experiment 2

We repeated the measurements for an adapting field with a hue angle of 180°, but increased the viewing distance from 1 to 4 m. The separation between the fixation point and the test loci was thus reduced from 3.00 degrees to 0.75 degrees of visual angle, and the width of the chromatic arc was reduced from 1.55 degrees to 0.39 degrees of visual angle.

Results

Observers R. E. S. and J. D. M. have normal colour vision, and are experienced psycho-physical observers. R. E. S. was naïve to the purposes of the study; J. D. M. is one of the authors. Baseline thresholds for both observers plot as ellipses in MacLeod–Boynton space, with the major axis oriented along the L/M-opponent direction. Since the scaling of the S-opponent axis of MacLeod–Boynton space is arbitrary, we describe the data in a scaled version of MacLeod–Boynton space $(S/(L+M) \times 4.0)$, chosen such that baseline thresholds plot as a circle, and baseline sensitivity, considered in the scaled space, is approximately equal across all vectors.

Data from Experiment 1 are plotted in Fig. 29.3. Values along the abscissa are probe chromaticities, defined as clockwise angular rotation from the theoretical tritan line in

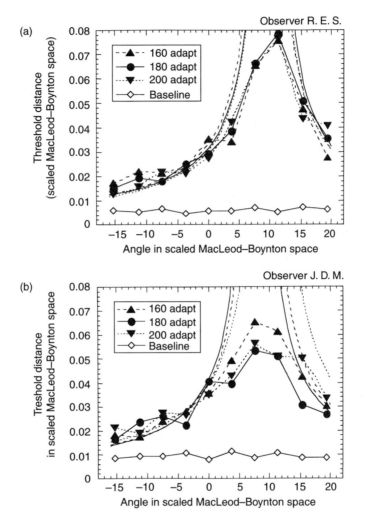

Figure 29.3 Data from Experiment 1, (a) for observer R. E. S., (b) for observer J. D. M.. Thresholds are expressed in a scaled version of MacLeod–Boynton space ($S/(L + M) \times 4.0$) such that baseline performance, considered in the scaled space, is approximately equal over all test angles. Values along the abscissa are probe chromaticities, defined as clockwise angular rotation from the theoretical tritan line in scaled MacLeod–Boynton space. Values on the ordinate are thresholds for the baseline condition (open diamonds), or following offset of the adapting field (solid up-triangles 160°, solid circles 180°, solid down-triangles 200°). Smooth curves describe theoretical performance determined only by the available L/M-opponent signal. Line-style for the three conditions matches that used for the data.

scaled MacLeod–Boynton space (expansion of the $S/(L + M)$ axis has transformed the range of test vectors from 102° to 34°). Thresholds for the baseline condition (open diamonds) plot as a horizontal line after scaling, and thresholds following offset of the adapting field (solid up-triangles, down-triangles, circles) show elevations from baseline, indicating a transient tritanopia effect. We suggest that the maximum elevation locates the tritan line.

In order formally to locate the position of the tritan line, we have developed the simple template represented by the smooth curves of Fig. 29.3. The template is intended to describe the thresholds that would be obtained if the S-opponent channel were completely desensitised and thresholds depended only on the L/M signal. For the Judd observer, whose fovea is represented by the standard MacLeod–Boynton chromaticity diagram, we can directly estimate the sensitivity of the L/M channel to each test vector, that is, we can estimate the length of the vector that is needed to give some specified threshold contrast in the L/M channel. The resulting threshold function must be symmetrical around the tritan line, asymptoting to infinity where contrast in the L/M channel falls to zero. We use a least-squares procedure to fit this template to the empirical data with just two free parameters, a vertical scaling factor to allow for individual differences in the sensitivity of the L/M channel and a horizontal scaling factor to accommodate the shifts in the tritan line that we are interested in. Since the phosphors of the monitor are fixed, the effect of variation in pre-receptoral filters such as macular pigment is to displace the set of test chromaticities by a nearly constant factor, and so our symmetrical template is a useful first approximation for locating the tritan line.

Despite the large differences in adapting field chromaticity, the three curves give comparable estimates for the tritan vector for each observer. For R. E. S. the curve for the 160° adapting field shows a peak at 33.7° in MacLeod–Boynton space (9.48° in the scaled space), and curves for 180° and 200° fields show a peak at 33.9° (9.53° in the scaled space). For J. D. M., critical vectors are 31°, 29°, and 35° (8.5°, 7.8°, 10.1° in the scaled space) for adapting fields of 160°, 180°, and 200° respectively. There is no evidence, from either observer, that the estimate of the tritan line is systematically biased by the L/M component of adaptation. The variation we observe in the estimate of the tritan line is small: a range of 6° in MacLeod–Boynton space for one observer, and a range of 0.2° for the other observer. The transient tritanopia method is robust to changes in adapting field chromaticity of ±20° rotation from the theoretical tritan axis in MacLeod–Boynton space, a range of 40°.

The data for Experiment 2 are plotted in Fig. 29.4. Again, smooth curves describe theoretical performance determined only by the available L/M-opponent signal. For observer R. E. S. the peak effect occurs for a vector of 8° in MacLeod–Boynton space (2.1° in the scaled space) and for J. D. M. the peak occurs at 12° in MacLeod–Boynton space (3.1° in the scaled space). Thus when the viewing distance was increased from 1 to 4 m, the tritan vector in MacLeod–Boynton space for our observers shifted from 34° to 8° (R. E. S.) and from 29° to 12° (J. D. M.).

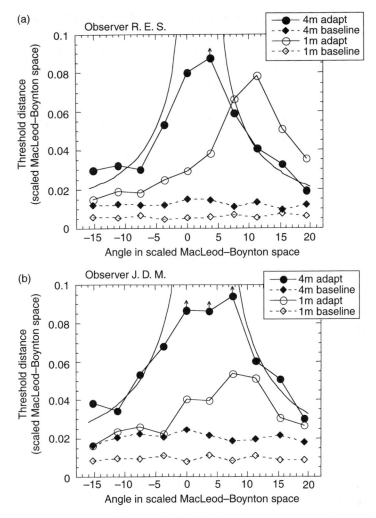

Figure 29.4 Data from Experiment 2, (a) for observer R. E. S., (b) for observer J. D. M.. The axes are the same as for Fig. 29.2. Filled symbols represent data obtained at a viewing distance of 4 m (circles adapt 180°, diamonds baseline). Upward pointing arrows, on the maximum point for R. E. S. and on the three central points for J. D. M., show conditions in which an out-of-range stimulus was requested, at least once, during the progression of the staircase. When this occurred the closest possible chromaticity was presented and the trials continued—the points are however an underestimate of the 75 per cent detection threshold. Smooth curves describe theoretical performance determined only by the available L/M-opponent signal. Open symbols represent data obtained in Experiment 1 with a 1-m viewing distance, and are plotted for comparison.

The results from Experiment 2 are consistent with an increase in macular pigment density towards the foveola. The primary difference between the Judd (1951) 2° observer and the CIE (1964) 10° observer is in macular pigment density. The MacLeod–Boynton chromaticity diagram assumes an observer with the spectral sensitivity of the Judd (1951) 2° observer. We could however construct a chromaticity diagram that was analogous to the MacLeod–Boynton chromaticity diagram, but based on the CIE (1964) 10° Observer. Suppose that in the latter space, we establish the loci of physical lights, produced from our monitor primaries, that lie on a vertical line passing through the chromaticity of the background, that is, the tritan line of the 10° Observer. If now we represent these physical lights in the standard MacLeod–Boynton space, then it turns out that they fall on a straight line oriented at 30° clockwise from the vertical. It is consistent that our observers resemble more closely the 1964 Observer when detecting stimuli at >3° eccentricity, and the Judd observer when detecting stimuli presented around 1°.

The effect of filtering by macular pigment can be seen intuitively if we consider, not just the chromaticity of each stimulus, but its spectral composition, that is, for stimuli produced on a CRT, the relative contribution of each phosphor. Light from the blue phosphor is an effective stimulus for S- and M-cones and filtering by macular pigment will disproportionately reduce the energy available from this phosphor. Compared to the neutral background, our test stimuli contain a high proportion of light from the blue phosphor and they are therefore shifted to relatively lower L : M ratios when filtered by macular pigment. The test vector that is matched to the L : M ratio in the background must be further to the right in the array of candidates when the stimuli are filtered by macular pigment, than when they are not.

Conclusion

We propose transient tritanopia as an effective method for locating an individual's tritan line. The method has several practical advantages. Firstly, the procedure can be carried out using a CRT, without the need to construct a uniform auxiliary field (as is required for the method described by Webster *et al.* 1990). Secondly, it allows almost free choice of the spatial properties of the stimulus so that the experimenter can determine the tritan line for the exact retinal region to be used in a subsequent experiment. In preliminary experiments we have found that judgements of minimally distinct borders are extremely difficult to make non-foveally. We have also tested two further potential psychophysical methods, employing "small-field tritanopia" and reaction time, but neither produced precise and reliable results non-foveally (Sumner 2000). Further advantages over the minimally distinct border method are that the transient tritanopia method uses the observer's performance rather than subjective judgements, and that luminance noise may be employed so stimuli need not be precisely equiluminant.

The transient tritanopia method is a reliable means of locating an individual's tritan confusion line. In particular, the data we present here, confirm that this method is robust to moderate changes in the L/M component of adapting field chromaticity. We also show that the transient tritanopia method allows the experimenter to track successfully the rotation of the tritan line arising from changes in retinal location of the stimuli.

Acknowledgments

H. E. Smithson was supported by a BBSRC studentship and P. Sumner was supported by an MRC studentship. The work was additionally supported by MRC G9807068 to J. D. Mollon. We are grateful to Dr R. Sorensen for acting as an observer and to Prof J. Pokorny and Prof V. C. Smith for discussion.

References

Boynton, R. M. & Kaiser, P. K. (1978). Temporal analog of the minimally distinct border. *Vision Research, 18*(1), 111–3.

Dacey, D. M. (2000). Parallel pathways for spectral coding in primate retina. *Annual Reviews in Neuroscience, 23*, 743–75.

Derrington, A. M., Krauskopf, J., & Lennie, P. (1984). Chromatic mechanisms in lateral geniculate nucleus of macaque. *Journal of Physiology, 357*, 241–65.

Hammond, B. R., Jr., Wooten, B. R., & Snodderly, D. M. (1997). Individual variations in the spatial profile of human macular pigment. *Journal of the Optical Society of America A, 14*(6), 1187–96.

Krauskopf, J., Williams, D. R., & Heeley, D. W. (1982). Cardinal directions of color space. *Vision Research, 22*, 1123–31.

Mollon, J. D. & Polden, P. G. (1975). Colour illusion and evidence for interaction between cone mechanisms. *Nature, 258*, 421–2.

Moreland, J. D. & Bhatt, P. (1984). Retinal distribution of macular pigment. In G. Verriest (Ed.), *Colour Vision Deficiencies*, Vol. VII: Dr W Junk Publishers.

Pokorny, J., Smith, V. C., & Lutze, M. (1987). Aging of the human lens. *Applied Optics, 26*(8), 1437–40.

Pugh, E. N. & Mollon, J. D. (1979). A theory of the Pi 1 and Pi 3 colour mechanisms of Stiles. *Vision Research, 19*, 293–312.

Regan, B. C., Reffin, J. P., & Mollon J. D. (1994). Luminance noise and the rapid determination of discrimination ellipses in colour deficiency. *Vision Research, 34*, 1279–99.

Sumner, G. P. H. (2000). *The salience of colour: Studies in visual ecology and psychophysics*. Ph.D. thesis, University of Cambridge, UK.

Tansley, B. W. & Boynton, R. M. (1976). A line, not a space, represents visual distinctness of borders formed by different colors. *Science, 191*(4230), 954–7.

Webster, M. A., De Valois, K. K., & Switkes, E. (1990). Orientation and spatial-frequency discrimination for luminance and chromatic gratings. *Journal of the Optical Society of America A, 7*(6), 1034–49.

Webster, M. A. & Mollon, J. D. (1994). The influence of contrast adaptation on colour appearance. *Vision Research, 34*(15), 1993–2020.

CHAPTER 30

SOME PROPERTIES OF THE PHYSIOLOGICAL COLOUR SYSTEM

C. VON CAMPENHAUSEN AND J. SCHRAMME

Introduction to the Physiological Colour System

According to the Trichromatic Theory of Colour Vision a colour locus can be computed in colour space for each colour stimulus. The receptor absorption space, Fig. 30.1(a), is a colour space, in which absorption values S, M, and L of the s-, m-, and l-cones are plotted along the axes. If the intensity of the stimuli is varied, the colour loci are shifted up or down the straight lines originating in the origin of the coordinate system. At low intensities this corresponds roughly to colour appearance, since colour stimuli appear less different at low intensities, where they are close together and equally black in darkness. With growing intensities, on the other hand, the distances between the colour loci increase infinitely, whereas the appearance of coloured objects again becomes more similar and whitish at high intensities. Obviously, the distances between the colour loci do not correspond to perceptual differences, that is, the receptor absorption space is not uniform. Helmholtz (1891a,b) tried to overcome this deficit with Riemannian mathematics introducing a line element, which assigns new values to the distances between colour loci depending on the domains of colour spaces. The line element was developed further to improve uniformity of colour space by Schrödinger, Stiles and Walraven and others (Schrödinger 1984; Bouman and Walraven 1972; Wyszecki and Stiles 1982). Another line establishing uniform colour scales is based on empirical measurements such as the MacAdam Ellipses (MacAdam 1942; Wyszecki and Stiles 1982).

The Physiological Colour System (PCS) is an additional approach towards a uniform colour system. It was mentioned already in von Campenhausen and Schramme (2001) and Campenhausen (2001). The PCS is based on cone excitations as calculated by the Naka–Rushton relation, Fig. 30.1(b). If cone excitations Es, Em and El are plotted instead of the absorption values, the colour solid of the PCS is generated, Fig. 30.1(c). Because of the upper limitation in the Naka–Rushton relation the excitations do not increase proportionately with stimulus intensity. There is a point of maximal excitation of all cone types, which corresponds to the white pole of colour appearance systems. In Fig. 30.1(c) the meridians represent the colour loci of spectral stimuli of increasing intensity starting in the black pole and ending in the white pole. The three crossing lines are spectrum loci

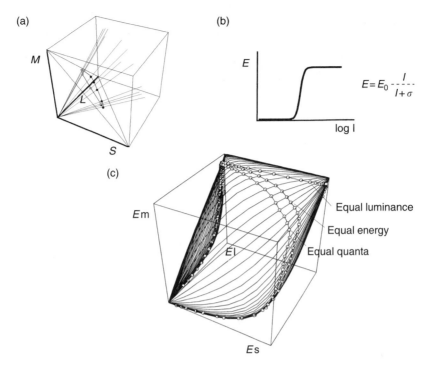

(a)

M

L

S

(b)

E

$E = E_0 \dfrac{I}{I + \sigma}$

log I

(c)

Em

Equal luminance

Equal energy

El

Equal quanta

Es

Figure 30.1 (a) Receptor absorption space with absorptions values S, L, and M of the three types of cones plotted along the axes. (b) Relation of the stimulus I and excitation E according to Naka and Rushton (1966). Horizontal shifts of the sigmoid curve caused by changes of σ represent changes of the state of adaptation. (c) Colour solid of the PCS with excitation values Es, El, and Em of the three types of cones plotted along the axes. Meridians represent color loci of spectral stimuli with increasing intensity connecting the black with the white pole. Three curves with open symbols represent colour loci of spectra (390–685 nm) defined as indicated.

for equal energy, equal quanta, and equal luminance spectra. The spectrum loci start and end in the black pole, because UV and IR do not generate excitations. However, we only calculated in a spectral range from 390 to 685 nm. At high intensities the excitation of this limited spectral range is located within the white pole.

Wavelength discrimination

If the principle of uniformity is fulfilled in the PCS, a certain distance within the colour solid of the PCS will represent a perceptual difference of a certain magnitude. The perceptual difference of this distance should be of the same magnitude in all spatial domains of the PCS. This should also apply to the infinitesimal distance representing the threshold of colour discrimination. If it were possible to predict the well-known wavelength discrimination curves by Euclidian metric in the PCS, the validity of uniformity in the PCS could be demonstrated.

(a)

(b)

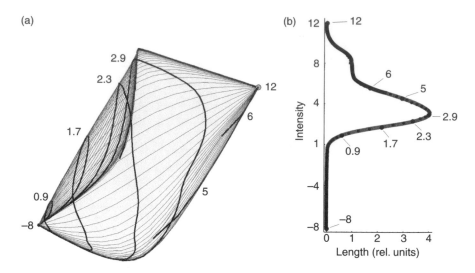

Figure 30.2 (a) Colour solid of the PCS with colour loci of equal energy spectra of different intensity levels, as indicated by the logarithmic factors. (b) The length of the spectrum curves in the colour solid of the PCS (abscissa) versus the intensity (ordinate).

In Fig. 30.2(a) equal energy spectra from 390 to 685 nm are plotted in the PCS for various levels of intensity, the logarithms of which are printed in the diagram. There is a maximal length of the spectrum locus at a medium intensity. This can also be seen in Fig. 30.2(b), where the spectrum locus length is plotted along the abscissa for the different intensities given at the ordinate. Wavelength discrimination should be best at the intensity producing maximal length of the spectrum locus and worse at higher and lower intensities. To test this, we divided the spectrum loci into short sections of equal length and computed the corresponding wavelengths. The length chosen for the sections should be proportional to the assumed threshold length for discrimination. At high and low intensities a smaller number of sections resulted from the division, because of the reduced length of the spectrum locus, indicating greater steps in the wavelength scale and hence higher thresholds of discrimination. The results can be plotted in the form of the well-known wavelength discrimination or $\Delta\lambda/\lambda$-curves.

At the greatest length (log intensity: 2.9) the computed threshold values $\Delta\lambda$ are smallest throughout the spectral range, as predicted, Fig. 30.3. But the threshold curve at this optimal intensity does not resemble the expected $\Delta\lambda/\lambda$-curve. This is understandable, since earlier investigators did not work in the optimal intensity range because of the limitations of their equipment. The curve computed for the lower intensity 1.7 fulfills the expectation much better, showing the minima above 600 nm and below 500 nm and even an indication of the short wave pessimum at 450 nm. The expected $\Delta\lambda/\lambda$-curve is just one of many other curves that may be recorded at other intensity levels.

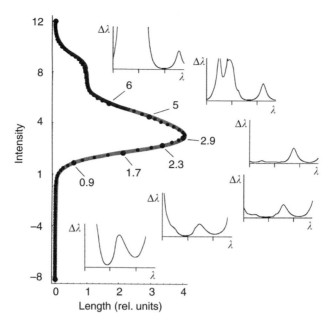

Figure 30.3 Intensity versus length of spectrum curves as in Fig. 30.2(b) and threshold curves for wavelength discrimination ($\Delta\lambda/\lambda$-curves) as computed for the intensity levels indicated by the numbers (logarithms of factors of intensity). Thresholds $\Delta\lambda$ are smallest in the spectral range where the length of the spectrum curve is longest. The curve computed for intensity 1.7 is enlarged in Fig. 30.5.

By varying the intensity in small steps in our calculations, we found curves resembling individual curves provided by earlier experimenters. Unfortunately, the experimental results are in general agreement only. The great variety is caused in part by different experimental parameters, such as stimulus field size or stimulus duration time, and methods, like stimulus adjustment or forced choice procedures, and last but not least different measures to avoid recording brightness instead of colour difference thresholds. It would be possible to fit our results more closely to selected empirical data by means of coefficients, but we prefer to look for general conformities first. There is agreement that with increasing intensity discrimination improves and declines again (Mollon *et al.* 1990; Reitner *et al.* 1992), as predicted in our computations. Since $\Delta\lambda/\lambda$-curves have been recorded for dichromats, we calculated these curves, as we did for the trichromats, and found good agreement again at the same intensity level (1.7) for protanopes, deuteranopes, and tritanopes, Fig. 30.4.

Our working hypothesis was that colour loci lying in a spherical surface around the origin of the PCS are equally bright. This is illustrated in the inset of Fig. 30.5. With modifications of this hypothesis we did not find discernibly better results. The dashed curve is taken from Wright and Pitt (1934). It should be kept in mind that no coefficients were introduced to improve the curve fit to this special case of an averaged curve.

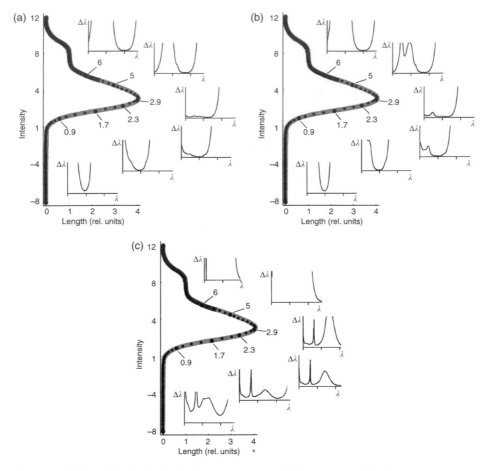

Figure 30.4 (a) Wavelength discrimination curves computed for protanopes, (b) deuteranopes, (c) tritanopes. Arrangement as in Fig. 30.3.

The calculation rests on receptor spectral sensitivity curves of the Smith–Pokorny type provided by Stockman and Sharpe (2000) and Stockman *et al.* (1999) and the Naka Rushton relation, only.

MacAdam ellipses

MacAdam ellipses demonstrate the lack of uniformity in the CIE 1931 (x, y)-chromaticity diagram, Fig. 30.6(a and b). They show the standard deviation (SD) of repeated colour matches in the chromaticity diagram. If the principle of uniformity were to apply to the chromaticity diagram, scatter and SD of matching experiments would form circles of equal size at all places of the chart. But mathematical transformation of the ellipses to the PCS should result in circles, if the PCS is uniform. We tested this assumption

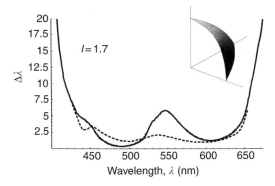

Figure 30.5 Wavelength discrimination curve computed for trichromats at the suboptimal intensity level 1.7, taken from Fig. 30.3. Dashed line: $\Delta\lambda/\lambda$-curve as measured and averaged by Wright and Pitt (1934). Inset: spherical surface on which the spectrum curve was projected to achieve equal brightness according to our working hypothesis.

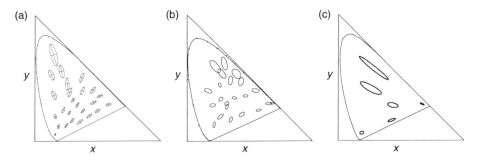

Figure 30.6 (a) MacAdam ellipses measured and computed by MacAdam (1942) for observer PGN. (b) MacAdam ellipses averaged from measurements with 12 subjects by Brown (1957). Data of (a) and (b) taken from Wyszecki and Stiles (1982). In (a) standard deviations of colour matches were recorded in the plane of the CIE 1931 (x, y)-chromaticity diagram. (b) Shows traces of the colour matching ellipsoids recorded in 3D-colour space. (c) MacAdam ellipses derived from the PCS. All ellipses shown are enlarged by a factor of ten.

starting with circles defined in the PCS. Again we stuck to the hypothesis that the sphere around the origin of the PCS colour solid represents colour of equal brightness. After transformation to the receptor absorption and CIE–XYZ space and calculation of the chromaticity coordinates these circles turned up as ellipses in the chromaticity chart, Fig. 30.6(c). Obviously, there is some agreement between the empirical (a, b) and the computed (c) MacAdam ellipses. The ellipses are longer in the green domain of the chromaticity chart and there is some correspondence of their direction in different domains.

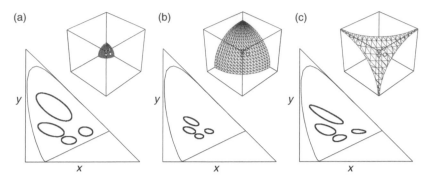

Figure 30.7 The computed MacAdam ellipses change with intensity. A set of four circles placed on spherical surfaces as shown in the insets, are mathematically transformed to the chromaticity chart. Ratios of radius of the spheres: 0.25 : 0.8 : 1.4. At medium brightness (b) the computed MacAdam ellipses are smaller than at lower and higher levels of brightness (a and c). Ellipses are not enlarged as in Fig. 30.6. Circles in the PCS are larger to show distortions due to nonlinearity of the mathematical transformation more clearly.

Both the empirical and the theoretical ellipses in Fig. 30.6 are ten times enlarged in the chromaticity diagram. The standard deviations in the experiments and the circles that we started with cover small colour differences only. The distortion of the circles due to the nonlinearity is only small, therefore, resulting in ellipses. Greater distortions can be observed if the calculation is started with larger circles in the PCS, so that no magnification is necessary after the mathematical transformation, Fig. 30.7. This figure shows that also the MacAdam ellipses depend on stimulus intensity. A pattern with four circles of equal size was placed on spherical surfaces with increasing distance from the origin of the PCS colour solid, as shown in the insets. The computed MacAdam ellipses are greater, more distorted and farther apart at higher and lower brightness. With threshold recordings which explore the infinitesimal neighbourhood around the colour loci, this nonlinearity is not demonstrated.

Final remarks

The PCS has a certain degree of uniformity as demonstrated by the computed wavelength discrimination curves and MacAdam ellipses, which blend with the experimental ones. Improvement of coincidence is principally difficult (a) because of the variation of the empirical data and (b) because of the Naka–Rushton relation, which cannot be assumed to be a perfect solution to the problem. The relation between light absorption in cones on the one hand, and excitation and adaptation on the other, rests on a network of molecular processes, the result of which will hardly be described adequately and exactly by one simple relation. Even if the Naka–Rushton relation is considered adequate, a solely unique uniform colour system cannot exist (c) because of the genetic polymorphism of the human rhodopsins. The merit of the PCS may be found in its simplicity.

References

Bouman, M. A. & Walraven, P. L. (1972). Color Discrimination Data. In Jameson, D. & Hurvich, L. M. (eds), Visual Perception. Vol. VII/4 of Autrum H *et al.* (ed.): Hdb. of Sensory Physiology, 484–516, Springer, Berlin.

Brown, W. R. J. (1957). Color discrimination of twelve observers. *J Opt Soc Am* 47, 137–43.

Campenhausen, C. von & Schramme, J. (2001). Three-dimensional interpretation of the color system of Auguilonius/Rubens 1613. *Color Res Application* 26(Suppl.), 17–19.

Campenhausen, C. von (2001). Eine Vorform der dreidimensionalen Farbensysteme in dem von Rubens illustrierten Lehrbuch des Franciscus Aguilonius (1613). *Med Hist J* 36, 32–72, in press.

Helmholtz, H. von (1891a). Versuch einer erweiterten Anwendung des Fechnerschen Gesetzes im Farbensystem. Z für Psychologie und Physiologie der Sinnesorgane 2, 1–30.

Helmholtz, H. von (1891b). Versuch, das psychophysische Gesetz auf die Farbenunterschiede trichromatischer Augen anzuwenden. *Z für Psychologie und Physiologie der Sinnesorgane* 3, 1–20.

MacAdam, D. L. (1942). Visual sensitivities to color differences in daylight. *J Opt Soc Am* 32, 247–74.

Mollon, J. D., Estèvez, O. & Cavonius, C. R. (1990). The two subsystems of colour vision and their roles in wavelength discrimination. In Blakemore C (ed), Vision, Coding and Efficiency. Cambridge University Press, 119–31.

Naka, K. I. & Rushton, W. A. H. (1966). S-potentials from luminosity units in the retina of fish (cyprinidae). *J Physiol* 185, 587–99.

Reitner, A., Sharpe, L. T., & Zrenner, E. (1992). Wavelength discrimination as a function of field intensity, duration and size. *Vis Res* 32, 179–85.

Schrödinger, E. (1984). *Gesammelte Abhandlungen.* Vol. 4. Friedr. Vieweg & Sohn, Braunschweig.

Stockman, A., Sharpe, L. T., & Fach, C. C. (1999). The spectral sensitivity of human short-wavelength cones. *Vis Res* 39, 2901–27.

Stockman, A. & Sharpe, L. T. (2000). Spectral sensitivities of the middle- and long-wavelength sensitive cones derived from measurements in observers of known genotype. *Vis Res* 40, 1711–37.

Wright, W. D. & Pitt, F. H. G. (1934). Hue discrimination in normal color vision. *Proc Phys Soc (London)* 46, 459–79.

Wyszecki, G. & Stiles, W. S. (1982). Color Science: Concepts and Methods, Quantitative Data and Formulae. 2nd edition, Wiley, New York.

INHERITED COLOUR DEFICIENCY: MOLECULAR GENETICS

CHAPTER 31

GENOTYPIC VARIATION IN MULTI-GENE DICHROMATS

S. S. DEEB, W. JAGLA, H. JÄGLE, T. HAYASHI, AND

L. T. SHARPE

Introduction

Normal color vision is trichromatic and is subserved by three different photopigments that are expressed in three separate classes of retinal cone: the short-wavelength sensitive (blue or B-), middle-wavelength sensitive (green or G-) and long-wavelength sensitive (red or R-) cones. The genes encoding the G- and R-opsins are arranged in a head-to-tail tandem array on Xq28 (Feil *et al.* 1990; Nathans *et al.* 1986a; Vollrath *et al.* 1988), which has been directly visualized by *in situ* hybridization (Wolf *et al.* 1999). A single R-photopigment gene is located at the 5′-position of the array followed by one or more G-photopigment genes. A locus control region (LCR), located upstream of the red photopigment gene, has been shown to be essential for cone photoreceptor-specific expression of all genes in the array (Wang *et al.* 1992). The R- and G-photopigment genes are highly homologous and encode opsins that differ in only 15 amino acids (Nathans *et al.* 1986a), seven of which are believed to be responsible for the approximately 31 nm difference in the peaks of the absorbance (λ_{max}) of the R- (532 nm) and G- (563 nm) cone photopigments (Asenjo *et al.* 1994; Merbs and Nathans 1992a; Sharpe and Volbrecht 1990).

The high degree of homology between the R- and G-pigment genes has predisposed the locus to illegitimate recombination between these two genes, resulting in deletions or the formation of red/green (R/G) or green/red (G/R) hybrid genes, and explains the genetic basis of the majority of color vision defects (Nathans *et al.* 1986b; Deeb *et al.* 1992). Exon 5 (which contains the 2 residues that account for two-thirds of the spectral difference between the red and green pigment) plays a major role in spectral tuning. The recombinational exchange of exon 5 produces hybrid pigments with large spectral shifts and corresponding effects on color vision. R/G hybrid genes are always associated with protan and G/R hybrid genes are usually associated with deutan color vision defects (reviewed in Motulsky and Deeb 2001). There is good evidence from studies of gene expression in the retina that only the two most proximal genes of the array are expressed (Winderickx *et al.* 1992; Yamaguchi *et al.* 1997). Studies of genotype–phenotype relationships also suggest that only the first two genes of the array play a role in color vision (Hayashi *et al.* 1999, 2001). Thus, deutan color vision results only if a

G/R hybrid gene occupies the second position in the array. Males who carry G/R hybrid genes that occupy the third or more distal positions in the array have normal color vision (Hayashi et al. 2001).

Severity of the color vision defect depends on the difference in absorption maxima between the pigments encoded by the first two genes of the array. The hypothesis is that if the first two genes of the array encode pigments with identical spectral sensitivity, the phenotype would be dichromacy, otherwise anomalous trichromacy is predicted. In this study we have tested this hypothesis by determining the sequence and order of genes in 50 dichromats (23 protanopes and 27 deuteranopes) whose arrays contain two or more genes. Of particular interest is the potential contribution of differences in amino acid sequence encoded by exon 2. It has been reported that such differences may contribute to color discrimination capacity, not because they cause spectral sensitivity differences, but by imposing differences in pigment stability that results in cones with different optical density (Neitz et al. 1999).

Subjects and methods

Subjects

Red-green colorblind young males were recruited in Freiburg im Breisgau (Germany), Tübingen (Germany) and Vienna (Austria) via word of mouth and by advertising in local newspapers and cinemas. Their color vision deficiencies were established by screening with the Ishihara pseudoisochromatic plates (Edition 5) and by the Rayleigh (red-green) color-matching equation measured on a Nagel Type I anomaloscope. Among these, 50 multi-gene dichromats (23 protanopes and 27 deuteranopes) were identified by Southern blot analysis (Sharpe et al. 1998).

Sequence and position of pigment genes

Details of all the experimental protocols are given elsewhere (Deeb et al. 2000). The total number of photopigment genes in the X-linked gene array, as well as the presence of hybrid genes and their sequence was determined by quantitative PCR amplification followed by single strand conformation polymorphism (SSCP) analysis. Long-range (LR) PCR amplification of a 15.8-kb DNA segment, using a unique forward primer in the LCR and a red or green-specific primers in exon 5, was used to identify the first gene of the array. To determine the nature of the 3′-terminal gene of the array, LR-PCR amplification of a 27.4-kb DNA segment was first performed, using a forward primer in exon 5 that matches both R and G sequences and a reverse primer in a unique sequence (TEX28 gene) located 3′ of the terminal gene of the array. A second round of amplification of exon 5 of the LR-PCR product, combined with restriction fragment analysis was used to determine whether the gene that occupies the 3′-terminal position in the array is G or a G/R hybrid. The nature of the genes located between the first and terminal genes of the array was determined by LR-PCR amplification using a forward primer in the promoter of G- pigment gene and a R- or G-specific primer in exon 5. Thus, the identity of the second gene in the array could be determined only for subjects with a total of three genes in the array. Identification of the second gene in the array is not feasible at this time since it would require amplification of an approximately 39-kb fragment.

The genotype with respect to the Ser180Ala polymorphism in each of the pigment genes of the array was first determined by amplification of exon 3 followed by digestion with *Fnu*4H. If both the Ser and Ala alleles were detected in the array, LR-PCR first was used to specifically amplify the first (R or R/G hybrid) gene or the downstream G- or G/R-pigment genes. Subsequently, exon 3 of each gene was amplified, digested with *Fnu*4H and the products resolved by electrophoresis on agarose gels.

Spectral sensitivities of the pigments

The predicted peak absorbances of the red, green, and hybrid photopigment spectra were inferred from published data on photopigments expressed *in vitro* (Asenjo *et al.* 1994; Merbs and Nathans 1992*a*) and *in vivo* (Sharpe *et al.* 1998).

Results and discussion

Gene arrays of protanopes

The array of each of the 23 protanopes contained a R/G hybrid gene in the first position, followed by one or more normal green pigment genes (Fig. 31.1a). Molecular analysis allowed inference of the λ_{max} of the visual pigments. The first two genes (a R/G hybrid and a normal G) of the arrays of 21 of the 23 protanopes encoded pigments predicted to have the same spectral sensitivity with a λ_{max} of approximately 532 nm, typical of a green pigment (Asenjo *et al.* 1994). This is consistent with the phenotype of protanopia. However, in two of the protanopes the first two genes encoded pigments that differed in λ_{max} by 2 nm which would have predicted protanomaly (Fig. 31.1b). These data indicate that R/G hybrid genes are the major cause of protanopia and imply that a separation by 2 nm in the λ_{max} of the two expressed pigments may not be sufficient to endow any color discrimination capacity, measured on a Nagel Type I anomaloscope. However, since there is some variability in the λ_{max} values determined by *in vitro* and *in vivo* methodologies (Asenjo *et al.* 1994; Merbs and Nathans 1992*b*; Sharpe *et al.* 1993), a difference of 1–2 nm may be within the error range of these measurements. These data also indicate that sequences of only exons 3, 4, and 5 contribute to the spectral separation that differentiates protanopia from protanomaly. It has been suggested that amino acid differences in exon 2 may play a role in stability of the pigments and, therefore in cone optical density (Neitz *et al.* 1999). As can be seen in Fig. 31.1, the first two genes of the array of a protanopes may (10/20) or may not (10/20) differ in exon 2.

Gene arrays of deuteranopes

The gene arrays of the 27 deuteranopic males are shown schematically in Fig. 31.2. Most (22/27) of the arrays comprised a normal R-gene in the first position followed by a G/R hybrid gene and one or more G-pigment genes (Fig. 31.2a). We determined the sequence

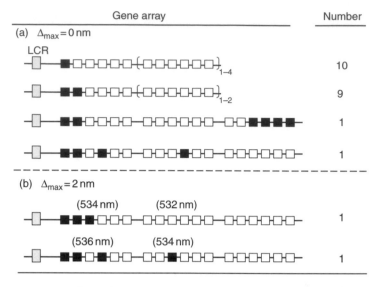

Figure 31.1 Gene arrays of 23 multi-gene protanopes. Shown are schematic representations of photopigment gene arrays deduced from molecular analyses of genomic DNA. LCR, locus control region which was shown to be necessary for expression of all genes of the array. Rectangles represent the six exons of the prototype R- (filled) and G- (open) pigment genes. The number of individuals carrying each class of array is given on the right. (a) Gene arrays in 22 males whose first two genes encode pigments with no separation in λ_{max} ($\Delta\lambda_{max} = 0$). The number of green pigment genes in the array is indicated as a subscript to the parentheses. (b) Subjects whose first two genes encode pigments that differ in λ_{max} by 2 nm, which would have predicted protanomaly. The inferred λ_{max} values are shown above the first two genes of the array.

of exon 5 of the gene that occupies the terminal position in the array. Of the 8 subjects who had a total of three genes, the normal G-gene occupies the third position in the array and, therefore, the hybrid gene occupies the second position. Thus far, a total of 25 subjects (20 deutans and 5 normals) whose R- and G-pigment gene arrays comprised one normal red, one normal green and one G/R hybrid gene have been studied in our laboratory. In all deutans, the G/R hybrid gene occupied the second position of the array, whereas in all subjects with normal color vision the G/R hybrid gene occupied the third (3'-terminal) position. This strongly suggests that the first two genes of the array determine the color vision phenotype, and that G/R hybrid genes are a major cause of deutan color vision. Consistent with this notion is that none of the other subjects with more than a total of three genes did the G/R hybrid gene occupy the terminal position. The normal G-pigment genes that occupy third or more distal positions from the LCR are apparently not sufficiently expressed in the retina to confer color discrimination capacity. This is consistent with our earlier results showing that only the first two genes of the array are expressed into mRNA in human retinae (Winderickx *et al.* 1992; Yamaguchi *et al.* 1997).

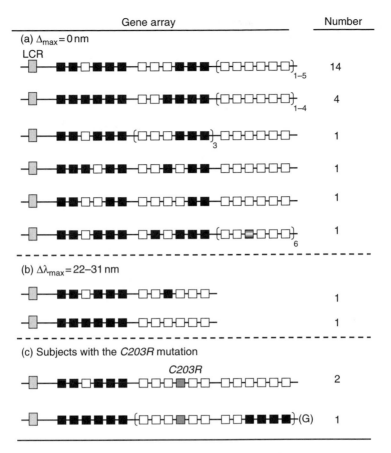

Figure 31.2 Gene arrays of 27 multi-gene deuteranopes. Shown are schematic representations of photopigment gene arrays deduced from molecular analyses of genomic DNA. Rectangles represent the six exons of the prototype R- (filled) and G- (open) pigment genes. (a) Gene arrays of subjects whose first two genes encode pigment with identical spectral sensitivity (exons 3, 4, and 5 are identical). In all subjects with a total of three genes, the third gene was shown to be a normal green. In none of the other subjects did a G/R hybrid gene occupy the terminal position in the array. The identity of the first and last genes of the array can presently be determined. Therefore, the gene order could be determined only in subjects with three genes (8/22). In subjects with more than a total of 3 genes, the G/R hybrid gene is assumed to occupy the second position, based on previous data (Hayashi *et al.* 1999, 2001; Winderickx *et al.* 1992; Yamaguchi *et al.* 1997). The dashed exon 3 in the subject with 6 G-genes indicates that both the Ser and Ala forms are encoded. (b) Two subjects who carry apparently normal gene arrays that would have predicted normal color vision. (c) Subjects with the C203R mutation in exon 4 (dotted box). The diagram at the bottom indicates that deuteranopia could have been caused by either the C203R mutation or the G/R hybrid gene in the second position. G, indicates the presence of a terminal normal green pigment gene.

Two of the twenty-seven deuteranopes had no hybrid genes. The sequence of the promoter, LCR, coding sequence and intron/exon junctions was determined to be normal. Therefore, there is still an unknown reason for these subjects to be dichromats. They may have a mutation in an intron of the G-pigment gene that contains a previously unrecognized regulatory element. We favor the alternative explanation that these two individuals have somatic mosaicism that resulted from unequal mitotic recombination between the R- and G-pigment genes on sister chromatids during embryonic development. Thus some of their tissues have the normal array whereas retinal photoreceptors have the array with the G/R hybrid gene. Since the DNA we analyzed was prepared from peripheral blood leucocytes, we may have missed detecting the hybrid genes. Analysis of DNA from other body tissues, such as hair or mouth may help resolve this issue.

Conclusions

The gene arrays of multi-gene dichromats are quite heterogeneous with respect to both the type of hybrid gene and the total number of genes. Hybrid genes play a major role in causing dichromacy (91 per cent of protanopia and 80 per cent of deuteranopia). The other cause of dichromacy is the C203R mutation in the green pigment gene, the frequency of which is surprisingly high in the German population. With few exceptions, dichromacy results if the two pigment encoded by the first two genes have identical or near identical (within 1–2 nm) spectral sensitivities. Contrary to what was claimed earlier, the difference in sequence of exon 2 does not confer any color discrimination capacity. Notably, in addition to being associated with subtle differences in color discrimination among males with normal color vision (Winderickx et al. 1992), the common Ser180Ala polymorphism in exon 3 of the red pigment gene contributes to the phenotype of dichromacy. There would have been a lower frequency of dichromacy had all R-pigment genes had Ser at position 180.

Prediction of dichromatic color vision from the genotype (more than one gene in the array) is still incomplete for two main reasons. First, there are a few dichromats who apparently have gene arrays that would be consistent with normal color vision. Second, in subjects with more than three genes, it is not possible with present technology to determine the nature of the second gene in the array and, therefore, to know for sure if the G/R hybrid gene is the cause of their color vision defect. However, based on our earlier results of retinal expression (Winderickx et al. 1992; Hayashi et al. 2001), and on earlier (Winderickx et al. 1992; Yamaguchi et al. 1997) and present results of genotype-phenotype relationships in deutans and normals with three pigment genes in the array, the most likely cause of deuteranopia in those with more than three genes is a G/R hybrid gene occupying the second position. The distal green pigment genes with normal sequence are most likely not expressed in these subjects.

Acknowledgments

This work was supported by a National Institutes of Health grant # EY08395 to S. Deeb, a travel grant from the Smith Kline Beecham-Stiftung to Wolfgang Jagla and by a grant from the Deutsche Forschungsgemeinschaft (Bonn-Bad Godesberg) SFB 430 (Tp A6) and a Hermann-und-Lilly-Schilling-Professur (Stifterverband, Essen) awarded to Lindsay T. Sharpe. We acknowledge the technical assistance of Lakshmi Goripathi.

References

Asenjo, A. B., Rim J., & Oprian D. D. (1994). Molecular determinants of human red/green color discrimination. *Neuron, 12*, 1131–8.

Deeb, S. S., Hayashi T., Winderickx, J., & Yamaguchi, T. (2000). Molecular analysis of human red/green visual pigment gene locus: relationship to color. *Methods in Enzymolgy, 316*, 651–70.

Deeb, S. S., Lindsey, D. T., Hibiya, Y., Sanocki, E., Winderickx, J., Teller, D. Y., & Motulsky, A. G. (1992). Genotype-phenotype relationships in human red/green color-vision defects: molecular and psychophysical studies. *American Journal of Human Genetics, 51*, 687–700.

Feil, R., Aubourg, P., Heilig, R., & Mandel, J. L. (1990). A 195-kb cosmid walk encompassing the human Xq28 color vision pigment genes. *Genomics, 6*, 367–73.

Hayashi, T., Motulsky, A. G., & Deeb, S. S. (1999). Position of a "green-red" hybrid gene in the visual pigment array determines colour-vision phenotype. *Nature Genetics, 22*, 90–3.

Hayashi, T., Yamaguchi, T., Kitahara, K., Sharpe, L. T., Jagle, H., Yamade, S., Ueyama, H., Motulsky, A. G., & Deeb, S. S. (2001). The importance of gene order in expression of the red and green pigment genes and in color vision. *Color Research and Application, 26*, S79–S83.

Merbs, S. L., & Nathans, J. (1992a). Absorption spectra of human cone pigments. *Nature, 356*, 433–5.

Merbs, S. L., & Nathans, J. (1992b). Absorption spectra of the hybrid pigments responsible for anomalous color vision. *Science, 258*, 464–6.

Motulsky, A. G. & Deeb, S. S. (2001). Color Vision and its Genetic Defects. In C. R. Scriver, A. L. Beaudet, W. S. Sly, and D. Valle (Eds). *The Metabolic and Molecular Bases of Inherited Disease*, Eighth Edition. (pp. 5955–76). (Vol. IV). New York: McGraw-Hill.

Nathans, J., Thomas, D., & Hogness, D. S. (1986a). Molecular genetics of human color vision: the genes encoding blue, green, and red pigments. *Science, 232*, 193–202.

Nathans, J., Piantanida, T. P., Eddy, R. L., Shows, T. B., & Hogness, D. S. (1986b). Molecular genetics of inherited variation in human color vision. *Science, 232*, 203–10.

Neitz, J., Neitz, M., He, J. C., & Shevell, S. K. (1999). Trichromatic color vision with only two spectrally distinct photopigments. *Nature Neuroscience, 2*, 884–8.

Sharpe, L. T., Fach, C. C., & Stockman, A. (1993). The spectral properties of the two rod pathways. *Vision Research, 33*, 2705–20.

Sharpe, L. T., Stockman, A., Jagle, H., Knau, H., Klausen, G., Reitner, A., & Nathans, J. (1998). Red, green, and red–green hybrid pigments in the human retina: correlations between deduced protein sequences and psychophysically measured spectral sensitivities. *Journal of Neuroscience, 18*, 10053–69.

Sharpe, L. T., & Volbrecht, V. J. (1990). Estimating middle-wavelength and long-wavelength cone sensitivity with large, long-duration targets and small, brief targets. *Perception, 19*, 745–57.

Vollrath, D., Nathans, J., & Davis, R. W. (1988). Tandem array of human visual pigment genes at Xq28. *Science, 240*, 1669–72.

Wang, Y., Macke, J. P., Merbs, S. L., Zack, D. J., Klaunberg, B., Bennett, J., Gearhart, J., & Nathans, J. (1992). A locus control region adjacent to the human red and green visual pigment genes. *Neuron, 9*, 429–40.

Winderickx, J., Battisti, L., Motulsky, A. G., & Deeb, S. S. (1992). Selective expression of human X chromosome-linked green opsin genes. *Proceedings of the National Academy of Sciences USA, 89*, 9710–14.

Winderickx, J., Lindsey, D. T., Sanocki, E., Teller, D. Y., Motulsky, A. G., & Deeb, S. S. (1992). Polymorphism in red photopigment underlies variation in colour matching. *Nature, 356*, 431–3.

Wolf, S., Sharpe, L. T., Schmidt, H. J., Knau, H., Weitz, S., Kioschis, P., Poustka, A., Zrenner, E., Lichter, P., & Wissinger, B. (1999). Direct visual resolution of gene copy number in the human photopigment gene array. *Investigative Ophthalmology and Visual Sciences, 40*, 1585–9.

Yamaguchi, T., Motulsky, A. G., & Deeb, S. S. (1997). Visual pigment gene structure and expression in human retinae. *Human Molecular Genetics, 6*, 981–90.

CHAPTER 32

HYBRID PIGMENT GENES, DICHROMACY, AND ANOMALOUS TRICHROMACY

WOLFGANG JAGLA, TANJA BREITSPRECHER, ITALA KUCSERA, GYULA KOVACS, BERND WISSINGER, SAMIR S. DEEB, AND LINDSAY T. SHARPE

Introduction

Human color vision is trichromatic owing to the existence of three different photopigments with distinct, spectral sensitivities expressed in three separate classes of photoreceptor cell: the short-wavelength sensitive (blue or S-), middle-wavelength sensitive (green or M-) and long-wavelength-sensitive (red or L-) cones. The L- and M-photopigment genes, each possessing a translated region of six exons, are highly homologous even in their intronic sequences. The L- and M-photopigments differ in only 15 amino acids (Nathans *et al.* 1986); 7 of which are believed to be responsible for the $\sim$32 nm difference in their wavelengths of maximal absorption (L = $\sim$528 nm and M = $\sim$560 nm) (Merbs and Nathans 1992; Asenjo *et al.* 1994; Sharpe *et al.* 1998).

The high degree of homology between the L- and M-photopigment genes and their juxtaposition in the head-to-tail tandem array (Nathans *et al.* 1986; Drummond-Borg *et al.* 1989), predisposed this locus to unequal crossing over, which results either in a change in gene number or in the formation of red/green (L/M) or green/red (M/L) hybrid genes, leading in some cases to color vision deficiencies (Nathans *et al.* 1986; Winderickx *et al.* 1992). Those deficiencies affecting the function of the L-cones are termed protan defects, with protanopia (a form of dichromacy) denoting the loss of L-cone function and protanomaly (or protanomalous trichromacy) denoting the alteration of M-cone function and associated with the presence of L/M hybrid genes which encode photopigments with anomalous spectral sensitivity (for reviews, see Sharpe *et al.* 1999; Motulsky and Deeb 2001). Similarly, those deficiencies affecting the function of the M-cones are termed deutan defects, with deuteranopia denoting the loss of M-cone function and deuteranomaly (or deuteranomalous trichromacy) denoting the alteration of M-cone function and associated with the presence of M/L hybrid genes that encode a photopigment with anomalous spectral sensitivity.

Clinically, the protan and deutan phenotypes are characterized by the types of Rayleigh (red–green) color matches (Rayleigh 1881) made on a small viewing field

(<2° in diameter) anomaloscope. The observer is required to match a spectral yellow (ca. 589 nm) primary light to a juxtaposed mixture of spectral red (ca. 679 nm) and green (ca. 544 nm) primary lights. Individuals with normal color vision choose a unique match between the red/green mixture ratio and the yellow intensity. By way of contrast, dichromats, because they possess only one functioning class of cone, L- or M- or a single hybrid pigment, are able to fully match the spectral yellow primary to any mixture of the spectral red and green primaries by merely adjusting the intensity of the yellow, regardless of the red-to-green ratio. And, anomalous trichromats, because they possess an anomalous L/M (protanomalous or green-shifted) or M/L (deuteranomalous or red-shifted) pigment instead of one of the normal (L or M) ones, have matching ranges that are intermediate between those of normals and dichromats; thus, signifying a less severe form of color vision deficiency (Pokorny et al. 1979; Sharpe et al. 1999). However, there is considerable variability in their Rayleigh matching ranges and midpoints. The variability is believed to be closely associated with the nature of the hybrid gene and the anomalous pigment it encodes, with smaller spectral separations (between the anomalous and remaining normal pigment) corresponding to greater severity. However, in some cases the same phenotype may be associated with different genotypes and, vice versa. Thus, other factors, such as cone pigment optical density, may influence the relationship between phenotype and genotype.

In the present study, we determined the variability in genotype among anomalous trichromats and dichromats and correlated this to their color vision phenotype. We wanted to establish which L/M and M/L hybrid genes in combination with normal genes engender dichromacy and which anomalous trichromacy. In particular, we asked the following question: what is the minimum difference between the spectral sensitivities of the normal L- (or normal M-) pigment and the anomalous pigment encoded by a M/L-hybrid gene (or by a L/M-hybrid gene) that confers some red-green color discrimination and allows an individual to be an anomalous trichromat rather than a dichromat? We already know that the primary determinants of the spectral shift are located in exon 5 (Neitz et al. 1991; Ibbotson et al. 1992; Williams et al. 1992; Merbs and Nathans 1992; Asenjo et al. 1994; Sharpe et al. 1998). The L/M sequence differences in exon 5—principally the residues at 277 and 285—result in spectral shifts of 15–25 nm, the exact value depending on sequences in exons 2–4. The in vivo measurements (Sharpe et al. 1998) suggest that substitutions at the sites confined to exons 2–4 produce much smaller spectral shifts. Exon 2 contributes 0–0.7 nm (for L2M3 versus M) or 1–3.6 nm (for L versus M2L3); exon 3, 1.0–4.0 nm; and exon 4, 2.4–4.0 nm. These results are in approximate agreement with the in vitro results (Merbs and Nathans 1992; Asenjo et al. 1994) and with inferences based on comparison of primate visual pigment gene sequences and cone spectral sensitivity curves (Neitz et al. 1991; Ibbotson et al. 1992; Williams et al. 1992). However, there is still considerable uncertainty about the actual degree of the spectral shift associated with sequence variations in each exon and about how the shifts implied by different sequence variations accumulate and interact.

Finally, in relation to the above issue, we wanted to take a closer look at the role of exon 2 in conferring color discrimination capacity and in influencing the optical density of photopigments. Codon differences in exon 2 between the L- and M-cone pigment genes are confined to three sites: codons 65, 111, and 116 (Nathans *et al.* 1986). *In vitro* (Merbs and Nathans 1992; Asenjo *et al.* 1994) and *in vivo* (Sharpe *et al.* 1998) data suggest that substitutions at these sites contribute very little (0.0–0.7 nm) to spectral tuning. However, recently it has been speculated that differences in the amino acids encoded by L and M exon 2 (in particular codon 65) are involved in determining the stability and, therefore, the optical density of the L and M cone photopigments, which might also contribute to red-green color discrimination capability (Neitz *et al.* 1999). This is because increasing the photopigment optical density broadens the relative sensitivity of the pigment away from the absorption peak. In particular, if two genes that differ only in their exon 2 sequences are expressed, then the resulting differences in the optical density of the pigments may engender some differences in spectral sensitivity that may be responsible for some residual red/green color discrimination (Neitz *et al.* 1999). If so, this would imply that multi-gene protanopic subjects would generally not be expected to have different exon 2 variants; whereas some protanomalous subjects, whose opsin genes are otherwise identical in their sequences, would.

Methods

Subjects

Fifty X-chromosome-linked (red–green) color deficient young males were recruited in Budapest (Hungary) and Tübingen (Germany). Their color vision deficiencies were established by Rayleigh (red–green) color-matching equation measured on an Oculus HMC Anomaloscope.

Molecular analysis

To determine the total number and ratios of photopigment genes in the X-linked gene array, the L and M photopigment gene promoter regions were amplified by competitive PCR using ^{32}P end-labeled primers and then subsequently analyzed by SSCP (Yamaguchi *et al.* 1997). The ratio of L and M photopigment genes and the total gene number was then evaluated by phosphoimaging. Details of the experimental protocols are given elsewhere (Deeb *et al.* 2000). Long-range (LR)-PCR using L-specific primers in the promoter and M-specific primers in exon 5 was used to determine if the first gene in the array was L or a L/M hybrid (Deeb *et al.* 2000). The amplified large fragments were then analyzed by internal PCR amplification followed by restriction analysis. LR-PCR using M-specific primers in the promoter and L- or M-specific primers in exon 5 was used to determine if the distal genes in the array were M- or a M/L hybrid or both (Deeb *et al.* 2000). The large fragments were then analyzed by internal PCR amplification followed by restriction analysis and/or sequencing. LR-PCR combined with restriction fragment analysis was used to identify the gene that occupies the 3′-terminal gene of the array (Deeb *et al.* 2000).

Results

Gene arrays of protan and protanomalous subjects

The Rayleigh match range and midpoint for each subject are given in Table 32.1 and Figure 32.1. Six subjects (Table 32.1, No. 1–6) were diagnosed to be protanopic. Two (No. 1 & 2) of them had single-gene arrays: one with a L2M3(A180)-hybrid gene; the other one with a L3M4(S180)- hybrid gene. The other four protanopic subjects had multi-gene arrays with two, three or four genes. Two (Nos 3 & 4) had arrays with a L1M2(A180)/L(A180) pairing, one (No. 5) with a L1M2(S180)/M(S180) pairing and one (No. 6) with a L2M3(A180)/M(A180) pairing. All the above genotypes are consistent with dichromacy since only a green pigment is encoded. Among the 18 protanomalous observers (Table 32.1, No. 7–24), No. 7 had a single L(S180)-gene in his array. However, his Rayleigh match range (70) is nearly that of a dichromat (73). All others had multi-gene arrays consisting of two, three, four and—in one case—six genes. There is considerable evidence that only the first two genes of the array are significantly expressed in the retina and contribute to color discrimination capacity (Winderickx *et al.* 1992; Yamaguchi *et al.* 1997, Hayashi *et al.* 2001). Based on this assumption, five different hybrid/M-gene pairs were found among the protanomalous observers: L2M3(A180)/M(A180) ($n =$ 7); L3M4(S180)/M(A180)($n = $ 1); L4M5(A180)/M(A180)($n = $ 5); L4M5(S180)/M(S180)($n = $ 1); and L4M5(S180)/M(A180)($n = $ 3). The first gene pair would predict protanopia or severe protanomaly since the difference in absorption maxima between the two encoded pigments is 0–0.7 nm. All other 4 gene combinations are consistent with protanomaly.

Gene arrays of deuteranopic and deuteranomalous observers

The four deuteranopic observers (Table 32.2, No. 1–4) had single L-genes (three with S180, one with A180). Among the 22 deuteranomalous observers (Table 32.2, No. 5–26), one (No. 5) had a single L(S180)-pigment gene and 21 had arrays consisting of one L-gene followed by one of five different types of ML-hybrid genes; and in most of them, by one or more normal M-genes. For those with a total of three genes, the normal M-gene was shown to occupy the third position in the array (i.e. the hybrid gene occupies the second position). The position of the hybrid gene in subjects with more than a total of three genes cannot be determined at this time. Based on present and previous findings (Winderickx *et al.* 1992; Yamaguchi *et al.* 1997; Hayashi *et al.* 2001), the hybrid gene was assumed to occupy the second position in arrays of subjects who had more than three genes. The following first-two-gene pairs that are assumed to contribute to the color vision phenotype were found: L(S180)/M1L2(S180) ($n = $ 2); L(S180)/M2L3(S180) ($n = $ 1); L(A180)/M2L3(S180)($n = $ 2); L(S180)/M3L4(A180)($n = $ 3); L(A180)/M3L4M(A180)($n = $ 8); L(A180)/M4L5(A180)($n = $ 4); L(S180)/M4L5(A180) ($n = $ 1). The first combination of two genes would predict dichromacy or severe anomalous trichromacy since there is no separation in the wavelength of maximum absorbance.

Table 32.1 Genotypes and color vision phenotypes among protans

No.	DNA ID	Age	Proximal gene	Distal gene(s)	Total gene number	Inferred spectral separation of photopigments (nm)			Oculus midpoints	Oculus ranges
						(Sharpe)	(Merbs)	(Asenjo)		
1	10259	21	L2M3/A180	None	1					73
2	10223	23	L3M4/S180	None	1					73
3	10090	52	L1M2/A180	M/A180	3	0.0	0	0		73
4	10094	23	L1M2/A180	M/A180	5	0.0	0	0		73
5	10261	28	L1M2/S180	M/S180	3		0	0		73
6	10193	47	L2M3/A180	M/A180	3	0.7	−0.2	0		73
7	10161	20	L2M3/A180	None	1					70
8	10209	32	L2M3/A180	M/A180 + (5′M − 3′L)	4	0.7	−0.2	0	35.35	59.3
9	10171	33	L4M5/S180	M/S180	3		1.9	4	34.5	47
10	10155	35	L2M3/A180	M/A180 + (5′M − 3′L)	4	0.7	−0.2	0	43	40
11	10169	25	L2M3/A180	M/A180	4	0.7	−0.2	0	54.5	23
12	10227	51	L2M3/A180	M/A180	5	0.7	−0.2	0	51.05	22.1
13	10106	48	L4M5/A180	M/A180	4	7.6	1.9		63.3	18.3
14	10191	25	L4M5/S180	M/A180	4	6.4	6.3	6	53.85	17.7
15	10257	26	L4M5/S180	M/A180	3	6.4	6.3	6	54	16
16	10221	26	L4M5/A180	M/A180	4	7.6	1.9		58	10
17	10229	51	L4M5/A180	M/A180	3	7.6	1.9		61.3	8.6
18	10219	42	L4M5/A180	M/A180	5	7.6	1.9		60.5	7
19	10108	23	L4M5/S180	M/A180	4	6.4	6.3	6	62	6
20	10183	24	L4M5/A180	M/A180	3	7.6	1.9		59	5.5
21	10159	19	L3M4/S180	M/A180	4	3.7	3.6	2	66.5	5
22	10185	28	L2M3/A180	M/A180	3	0.7	−0.2	0	50	4
23	10325	41	L2M3/A180	M/A180	4	0.7	−0.2	0	61	61
24	10181	18	L2M3/A180	M/A180	3	0.7	−0.2	0	65.5	3

Inferred spectral separations between the first gene and the second gene based on *in vitro* (Merbs and Nathans 1992; Asenjo *et al.* 1994) and *in vivo* data (Sharpe *et al.* 1998) and Oculus midpoints and ranges.

Table 32.2 Genotypes and colour vision phenotypes among deutans

No.	DNA ID	Age	Proximal gene	Distal gene(s)	Total gene number	Inferred spectral separation of photopigments (nm)			Oculus midpoints	Oculus ranges
						(Sharpe)	(Merbs)	(Asenjo)		
1	10179	21	L/A180	None	1					73
2	10055	21	L/S180	None	1					73
3	10225	37	L/S180	None	1					73
4	10263	31	L/S180	None	1					73
5	10187	24	L/S180	None	1					64
6	10088	23	L/A180	M4L5/A180	2	—	7.60	5.00	18	3.1
7	10173	25	L/S180	M3L4/A180 + M	3	—	7.90	8.00	19.5	1
8	10217	20	L/S180	M3L4/A180 + M	4	—	7.90	8.00	16.5	1
9	10211	49	L/A180	M4L5/A180 + M	3	—	7.60	5.00	18	2
10	10157	21	L/A180	M4L5/A180 + M	5	—	7.60	5.00	20.65	2.3
11	10265	30	L/S180	M2L3/S180 + M	5	—	3.70	4.00	12.15	3.7
12	10175	20	L/A180	M3L4/A180 + M4L5/A1	4	—	3.60	1.00	22.5	5
13	10151	51	L/S180	M4L5/A180	3	—	11.90	12.00	22.6	5.4
14	10086	24	L/A180	M4L5/A180 + M/A180	4	—	7.60	5.00	19	6
15	10207	28	L/A180	M3L4/A180 + M	4	—	3.60	1.00	14	6
16	10167	20	L/S180	M3L4/A180 + M	4	—	7.90	8.00	23.15	6.3
17	10215	24	L/A180	M3L4/A180 + M	4	—	3.60	1.00	23.25	7.5
18	10053	25	L/S180	M1L2/S180 + M/S180	5	—	0.00	0.00	24	8.1
19	10213	57	L/A180	M3L4/A180 + M	3	—	3.60	1.00	17.5	9
20	10163	49	L/A180	M2L3/S180 + M	3	—	−0.60	−3.00	34.6	12.6
21	10110	20	L/A180	M3L4/A180 + M/A180	4	—	3.60	1.00	22.3	18.9
22	10177	45	L/A180	M3L4/A180 + M	4	—	3.60	1.00	19.2	25.2
23	10165	21	L/A180	M3L4/A180 + M	4	—	3.60	1.00	24.05	27.5
24	10255	28	L/A180	M3L4/A180 + M	4	—	3.60	1.00	25	30
25	10153	53	L/A180	M2L3/S180 + M	4	—	−0.60	−3.00	27.05	41.5
26	10189	25	L/S180	M1L2/S180 + M	4	—	0.00	0.00	30.5	61

Spectral separation was inferred for the two pigments encoded by the L and M/L hybrid genes of each array. The M/L hybrid gene in the 5 subjects who have a total of 3 genes was experimentally shown to occupy the second position in the array. The M/L hybrid gene in those with more than three genes was assumed to occupy the second position in the array (see Discussion for justification). The *in vivo* spectral separation for deutans is not available.

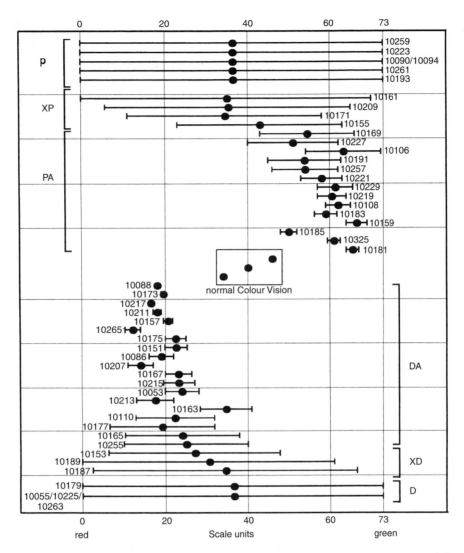

Figure 32.1 Rayleigh match midpoints and ranges of 50 observers with red/green colour vision defects. P = protanopic; PA = protanomalous; XP = extreme protanomalous; D = deuteranopic; DA = deuteranomalous; XD = extreme deuteranomalous. Subject numbers are given beside the ranges.

Two polymorphic variants in exon 4 were revealed by sequencing. In two subjects (Table 32.2, Nos 20 and 25) with a L(A180)/M2L3(S180)-pairing a V236M substitution was found in the ML-hybrid gene and in one subject (No. 24) with a L(A180/M3L4(A180)-pairing the V236M substitution was found in both the L- and the ML-hybrid gene. One S233A exon 4 polymorphic site was found in the LM-hybrid of a L(A180)/M3/L4(A180)-pairing (10175). Only one subject (10053) with an exon 2 polymorphic variant was observed in our population. He had a T651 substitution in the ML-hybrid gene of an L(S180)/M2L3(S180)-pairing.

Discussion

The great majority (>95 per cent) of the investigated anomalous trichromats had arrays with a hybrid pigment gene and at least one normal pigment gene. One protanomal and one deuteranomal had a single pigment gene. This was previously observed among subjects with severe deuteranomaly (Deeb et al. 1992). To explain this, we and others have shown that differences in cone pigment optical density are sufficient to allow for a small degree of chromatic discrimination (He and Shevell 1995; Sanocki et al. 1997; Neitz et al. 1999).

Among our 18 protanomalous subjects, we found four different types of LM-hybrid genes paired with one or the other of the two normal M-cone pigment genes. In total, five different pairings occurred. Predictions can be made about the spectral separation between the paired pigments on the basis of spectral sensitivity determinations. In vivo estimates of the peak absorbances of the normal and hybrid pigments are available from Sharpe et al. (1998), in vitro estimates from Merbs and Nathans (1992) and Asenjo et al. (1994). A scatter plot, indicating the correlation between the phenotype and genotype for the 18 protanomalous observers, is shown Fig. 32.2a. Generally, they fall into two groups. Large estimated spectral separations are associated with small matching ranges. And small estimated spectral separations are associated with large matching ranges. The most frequent arrangement in protanomals (seven subjects) was a L2M3-hybrid-gene followed by a normal M-gene. The spectral separation between the encoded pigments is estimated to be 0–0.2 (in vitro) and 0–0.7 nm from the in vivo measurements. This pairing involves only a difference in the sequence of exon 2 of the two genes and is obviously associated with a great variability in the matching range. The individuals can either have a small, a moderate, a large or even a fully extended matching range. It is remarkable that the same genotype is also frequently found in protanopic subjects (Jagla et al. 2002).

Among the 22 deuteranomalous subjects, five different ML hybrid genes were found paired with one of the two polymorphic variants of the L-cone pigment gene. The normal M-pigment genes that are present in the arrays are presumed to occupy third or more distal positions and are not sufficiently expressed in the retina to confer color discrimination capacity. Our earlier results showed that only the first two genes of the array are expressed into mRNA in the retina (Winderickx et al. 1992; Yamaguchi et al. 1997) and that deutan color vision defects arise only if the L/M hybrid gene occupies the second position in the array (Hayashi et al. 2001, Jagla et al. 2002). Thus far, a total of 30 subjects (20 deutans and 5 normals) whose arrays comprised one L, one M and one M/L hybrid gene have been studied in our laboratory. In all deutans, the M/L hybrid gene occupied the second position of the array, whereas in all subjects with normal color vision the M/L hybrid gene occupied the third (3′-terminal) position.

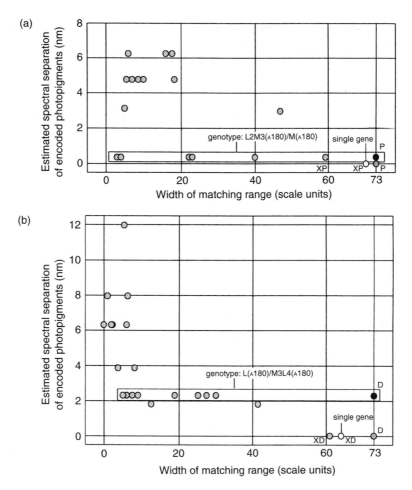

Figure 32.2 (a) Correlation between the estimated spectral separation, based on previous *in vitro* and *in vivo* determinations of peak absorbances of normal L and LM-hybrid pigments, and the ranges of Rayleigh matches obtained from observers with protan defects. The black filled circle represents 10 subjects with a protanopic phenotype and multi-gene arrays analyzed in a previous study (Jagla *et al.* 2002). (b) Correlation between the estimated spectral separation, based on previous *in vitro* determinations of peak absorbances of normal M and ML-hybrid pigments, and the ranges of Rayleigh matches obtained from observers with deutan defects. The black filled circle represents 15 multi-gene array deuteranopes analyzed in a previous study (Jagla *et al.* 2002).

Once again predictions can be made about the spectral separation between the pigment pairs on the basis of previous spectral sensitivity determinations. *In vitro* estimates of the peak absorbances are available from Merbs and Nathans (1992) and Asenjo *et al.* (1994). The most common occurrence found in deuteranomals (eight subjects) was an M3L4-gene paired with a normal L-gene. Intriguingly, this also involves only a difference in the sequence of exon 2 of the two genes. But here the separation between the pair is estimated to be 1.0–3.6 nm. The individual can either have a small matching range, indicating good red-green color discrimination or a moderate matching range, indicating poorer discrimination, or can be a complete dichromat (Jagla *et al.* 2002).

In conclusion, we find that the severity of anomalous trichromacy roughly correlates with the estimated spectral separation between the normal and the hybrid pigment. However, considerable phenotypic variability is associated with any given genotype. The variation found with L2M3 or M3L4-hybrid genes is greater than that found with other hybrids and cannot merely be associated with coding sequence differences in exon 2. These findings underscore an important issue in color vision: how spectral differences between two photopigments actually translate to color discrimination performance, and about how other retinal and cortical factors (such as individual variability in the gain of post-receptoral color-opponent channels) act upon the photopigment differences and influence discrimination.

Acknowledgments

This work was supported by a National Institutes of Health grant no. EY08395 to Samir S. Deeb and by grants from the Deutsche Forschungsgemeinschaft (Bonn–Bad Godesberg) SFB 430 (Tp A6) to Wolfgang M. Jagla and to Tanja Breitsprecher.

References

Asenjo, A. B., Rim, J., & Oprian, D. D. (1994). Molecular determinants of human red/green color discrimination. *Neuron 12*, 1131–38.

Deeb, S. S., Lindsey, D. T., Hibiya, Y., Sanocki, E., Winderickx, J., Teller, D. Y., & Motulsky, A. G. (1992). Genotype-phenotype relationship in human red/green color vision defects: Molecular and psychophysical studies. *American Journal of Human Genetics 51*, 687–700.

Deeb, S., Hayashi, T., Winderickx, J., & Yamaguchi, T. (2000). Molecular analysis of human red/green visual pigment gene locus: relationship to color vision. *Methods in Enzymology 316*, 651–70.

Drummond-Borg, M., Deeb, S. S., & Motulsky, A. G. (1989). Molecular patterns of X chromosome-linked color vision genes among 134 men of European ancestry. *Proceedings of the National Academy of Sciences, USA 86*, 983–87.

Hayashi, T., Yamaguchi T., Kitahara, K., Sharpe, L. T., Jägle, H., Motulsky, A. G., & Deeb, S. S. (2001). The importance of gene order in expression of the red and green visual pigment genes and in color vision. *Color Research and Application 26*, 79–83.

He, J. C. & Shevell, S. K. (1995). Variation in color matching and discrimination among deuter-anomalous trichromats: theoretical implications of small differences in photopigments. *Vision Research 35*, 2579–88.

Ibbotson, R. E., Hunt, D. M., Bowmaker, J. K., & Mollon, J. D. (1992). Sequence divergence and copy number of the middle- and long-wave photopigment genes in Old World monkeys. *Proceedings of the Royal Society of London B 247*, 145–54.

Jagla, W., Jägle, H., Hayashi, T., Sharpe, L. T., & Deeb, S. S. (2002). The molecular basis of dichromatic color vision in males with multiple red and green visual pigment genes. *Human Molecular Genetics 11*, 23–32.

Merbs, S. L. & Nathans, J. (1992). Absorption spectra of the hybrid pigments responsible for anomalous color vision. *Science 258*, 464–6.

Motulsky, A. G. & Deeb, S. S. (2001). Color Vision and its Genetic Defects. In *The Molecular and Metabolic Bases of Inherited Disease*, Eighth Edition. (Eds: Scriver, C. R., Beaudet, A. L., Sly, W. S., & D. Valle, D.) Vol. IV pp. 5955–76.

Nathans, J., Piantanida, T. P., Eddy, R. L., Shows, T. B., & Hogness, D. S. (1986). Molecular genetics of inherited variation in human color vision. *Science 232*, 203–10.

Neitz, M., Neitz, J., & Jacobs, G. H. (1991). Spectral tuning of pigments underlying red-green color vision. *Science 252*, 971–4.

Neitz, J., Neitz, M., He, J. C., & Shevell, S. K. (1999), Trichromatic color vision with only two spectrally distinct photopigments. *Nature Neuroscience 2*, 884–8.

Pokorny, J., Smith, V. C., & Verriest, G. (1979). Congenital color defects. In *Congenital and Acquired Color Vision Defects*. (Eds: Pokorny, J., Smith, V. C., Verriest, G., & Pinckers, A. J. L. G.), pp. 183–241. Grune & Stratton, New York.

Rayleigh, Lord (Strutt, R. J.) (1881). Experiments on colour. *Nature 25*, 64–6.

Sanocki, E., Teller, D. Y., & Deeb, S. (1997). Rayleigh match ranges of red/green color-deficient observers: psychophysical and molecular studies. *Vision Research 37*, 1897–907.

Sharpe, L. T., Stockman, A., Jägle, H., Knau, H., Klausen, G., Reitner, A., & Nathans, J. (1998). Red, green, and red-green hybrid pigments in the human retina: correlations between deduced protein sequences and psychophysically measured spectral sensitivities. *The Journal of Neuroscience 18*(23), 10053–69.

Sharpe, L. T., Stockman, A. Jägle, H., & Nathans J. (1999). Cone genes, cone photopigments, color vision and colorblindness. In *Color Vision: from genes to perception* (Eds: Gegenfurtner, K. & Sharpe, L. T.), pp. 3–52. Cambridge University Press, Cambridge.

Williams, A. J., Hunt, D. M., Bowmaker, J. K., & Mollon, J. D. (1992). The polymorphic photopigments of the marmoset: spectral tuning and genetic basis. *The EMBO Journal 11*(6), 2039–45.

Winderickx, J., Battisti, L., Hibiya, Y., Motulsky, A. G., & Deeb, S. S. (1992). Selective expression of human X chromosome-linked green opsin genes. *Proceedings of the National Academy of Science, USA 89*, 9710–14.

Yamaguchi, T., Motulsky, A. G., & Deeb, S. S. (1997). Visual pigment gene structure and expression in human retinae. *Human Molecular Genetics 6*(7), 981–90.

CHAPTER 33

MIDDLE WAVELENGTH SENSITIVE PHOTOPIGMENT GENE EXPRESSION IS ABSENT IN DEUTERANOMALOUS COLOUR VISION

MAUREEN NEITZ, KATHRYN BOLLINGER, AND JAY NEITZ

Introduction

The deutan-type colour vision deficiencies, deuteranopia and deuteranomaly, are the most common forms of colour blindness. In Europe and the United States, they affect 1 out of 17 males and 1 out of 280 females. A known cause of deutan colour vision defects is the loss of genes encoding the middle wavelength sensitive (M) photopigments (Deeb *et al.* 1992; Nathans *et al.* 1986). Deutan defects have also been found to be associated with a deleterious point mutation in the M photopigment genes (Bollinger *et al.* 2001; Winderickx *et al.* 1992a). However, these two gene defects account for only about one-fifth of deutan disorders.

Most people with deutan colour vision defects have both L and M genes (Deeb *et al.* 1992; Nathans *et al.* 1986; Neitz *et al.* 1996) and, thus, the cause of their colour vision defect is not apparent from their gene complement. The photopigment gene arrays in the majority of individuals with normal colour vision have one L gene followed by one or more M genes (Drummond-Borg *et al.* 1989; Nathans *et al.* 1986; Neitz and Neitz 1995). The L gene is found the furthest upstream or "first" in the 5′–3′ direction (Neitz *et al.* 1996; Vollrath *et al.* 1988). Figure 33.1 illustrates how a gene array like that commonly observed in deuteranomalous individuals is believed to have arisen by an unequal crossover between two normal arrays (Nathans *et al.* 1986); it contains two genes encoding pigments with maximum sensitivities in the long wavelength region of the spectrum and it has one additional gene compared to either parental array. The added gene is inserted between unaltered L and M genes displacing the M gene from its usual position as the second gene in the array. The inserted gene encodes an L-type pigment because it has exon 5 (which contains the critical spectral tuning sites) from a parental L gene (Asenjo *et al.* 1994; Merbs and Nathans 1992; Neitz *et al.* 1991a).

Presumably to be deuteranomalous as opposed to deuteranopic requires two genes to encode two slightly different pigments with spectral peaks in long wavelengths. The

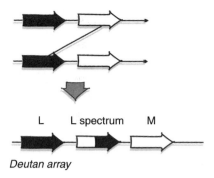

Figure 33.1 Schematic representation of how a deutan gene array has been proposed to arise from an unequal crossover between two normal arrays.

overwhelming majority of deutan individuals with gene arrangements like that shown in Fig. 33.1 are deuteranomalous as opposed to being deuteranopic. Deuteranomalous individuals have both the presence of two genes to encode L pigments and the absence of normal colour vision. The fact that some people have multiple L genes but normal colour vision and the fact that some cadaver eyes show expression of multiple L genes plus M genes had led us to suggest that the mutation that gives rise to the second L gene might be independent of the mutation that caused the colour vision defect. For example, in addition to the unequal crossover that produced the 5′M3′L "hybrid" gene, the M genes in deuteranomalous individuals might have specific mutations that interrupt expression or function of the M pigment or viability of the M cones (Sjoberg *et al.* 1998). Alternatively, it has been proposed that the addition of the second "L" gene and the loss of colour vision could be produced by a single mutational event, the unequal crossover. Two hypotheses have been proposed in this category.

The first hypothesis, originally proposed by Nathans and colleagues, assumed the existence of an L cone specific promoter upstream of the first gene in the array and the presence of an M cone specific promoter upstream of each normal M gene. Under this scenario, in the deuteranomalous array, a second L-pigment-encoding gene is in the normal M gene position, and it would be downstream of an M gene promoter (Nathans *et al.* 1986; Wang *et al.* 1999). If the promoters were L and M gene-specific, the presence of one M gene promoter associated with the 5′M 3′L "hybrid" gene and a second M promoter associated with a normal M pigment gene might result in co-expression of the two types of pigments in one population of cones leading to a colour vision defect. Against this hypothesis, we argued earlier that if deuteranomalous trichromats co-expressed normal M pigment they would be expected to have more normal relative sensitivity to green light in a Rayleigh match and choose a red/green mixture that is close to normal when tested on an anomaloscope; thus, it seemed more likely to us that M pigment expression is absent in deuteranomaly (Neitz *et al.* 1991*b*).

Recently, Nathans and colleagues have done experiments in transgenic mice, to test an alternative to their original hypothesis in which, rather than L and M pigments being directed into separate cone populations by the presence of cone-specific promoters (as discussed above), there is a stochastic process that randomly chooses a single gene from the array to be expressed in each L/M cone. This would imply that if both normal M and "anomalous" pigments are present in the deuteranomalous retina they reside in different cones (Wang *et al.* 1999).

Currently, the available evidence would seem to favour the idea that the identity of the L and M cones is determined by a stochastic process. Deeb and colleagues have proposed a hypothesis for deuteranomaly which is compatible both with there being a stochastic mechanism for determining cone identity and with deuteranomaly arising by a single mutational event. They have proposed that genes following the first two in the array are expressed either not at all or in a small number of cones (Hayashi *et al.* 1999; Yamaguchi *et al.* 1997*a,b*; Winderickx *et al.* 1992*b*). In support of this hypothesis, they found two men with normal colour vision who had an L gene last while deuteranomalous individuals had an M gene last. This demonstrates a correlation between gene order and colour vision phenotype (Hayashi *et al.* 1999); however, because these experiments were done on living individuals it was not possible to directly assay the M gene expression in the individuals known to be deuteranomalous. Thus, with regard to the theory that deuteranomaly is caused by a loss or reduction in M cones, a link that is missing in the causal chain between the genes and vision is a direct demonstration that M gene expression specifically in deuteranomalous individuals is low or absent compared to normal. From psychophysics we have argued that expression is functionally absent (Neitz *et al.* 1991*b*) and in support of the idea that M cones might be few or absent in deutan defects, Deeb and colleagues measured mRNA levels in cadaver eyes and found one example where an eye donor (colour vision phenotype unknown) had a gene arrangement similar to that of living deuteranomalous individuals and M pigment mRNA was not detected in his retina with their assay.

Attempts to understand gene expression of the M and L pigments are complicated by a number of factors. Both from results reported from our laboratories and those of Deeb and Motulsky it is certain that some of the human X-chromosome pigment genes are not expressed at detectable levels (Hayashi *et al.* 1999; Balding *et al.* 1998; Yamaguchi *et al.* 1997*a,b*; Winderickx *et al.* 1992*b*). However, it has been difficult for us to understand how the theory of Deeb and colleagues might be reconciled with our own results which demonstrate that more than two genes in the array can be expressed in some cases. A further complication is that there has recently been an increased appreciation for the fact that there is an enormous range in the ratio of L–M cones making it not unusual for people to have normal colour vision with only a very small proportion of either normal M or L cones (Carroll *et al.* 2000; Miyahara *et al.* 1998; Roorda and Williams 1999). This in combination with the fact that normal individuals can have gene arrangements similar to deuteranomals means that we cannot be completely certain that an isolated putative deuteranomalous eye donor with low expression of M genes was not a normal individual with an unusually small population of M cones, perhaps just a few per cent of the total, for which mRNA was not detected. Thus, at least in our minds, questions remain about the expression of M pigment genes in the most common occurrences of deuteranomaly. If a decrease in M cones is the cause of deuteranomaly, the important question arises of whether it is a reduction or complete absence of M cones that occurs.

Here, we report experiments to test the hypothesis that M gene expression is absent in all commonly occurring deutan defects. We used a sensitive assay to screen cadaver eyes from 150 males for the presence of M pigment mRNA. The frequency of deutan defects in the population is well known and the hypothesis that M gene expression is absent predicts that a number of eyes corresponding to the frequency of deutan defects in the population should be completely lacking mRNA for M pigment. Nine such eyes were found in the sample of 150, corresponding exactly to the predicted 6 per cent frequency of deutan defects in the population. Examination of genomic DNA from the 9 putative deutan donors revealed that all nine had photopigment gene arrays like those of living deutan men. Four of the putative deutan eye donors lacked M genes while the remaining five had normal appearing M genes. The five who had M genes were subject to further experiments using an ultrasensitive assay to determine the relative amount of M pigment mRNA in their retinas. In those experiments no M pigment mRNA was detected. These results are consistent with the hypothesis that the commonly occurring deutan defects in which individuals have normal appearing M genes, are caused by a failure to express M pigment. Moreover, it would appear that the failure is likely to be complete.

Materials and methods

Screen for putative deutan retinas

Human eyes from 150 male donors were obtained through the Wisconsin Lions Eye Bank. Male donors ranged in age from 3 to 91 years, with an average age of 66, a median age of 71, and a modal age of 77. Eyes were enucleated and refrigerated within 5.5 hours of death. An aliquot of retinal nucleic acid from each donor was used in a reverse transcriptase reaction (RT) followed by the polymerase chain reaction (PCR) to amplify L and M pigment cDNA containing exon 5. The reaction conditions and primers have been described elsewhere (Sjoberg *et al.* 1998). The forward PCR primer spans the exon 4–5 junction and thus will not amplify genomic DNA. The reverse primer corresponds to the 3′end of exon 5. The resulting PCR product was incubated with restriction endonuclease Rsa I which cleaves exon 5 of L pigment cDNA, but not M pigment cDNA. If a retina lacks M pigment mRNA, this assay will yield only the Rsa I cleaved exon 5 PCR product, and there will be no full-length PCR product.

Determination of the number and ratio of L/M genes by real-time quantitative PCR

A Sequence Detection System 7700 (Applied Biosystems, Foster City, CA) was used to estimate the ratio of L/M genes and the ratio of first/downstream genes according to a previously published protocol (Neitz and Neitz 2001).

Quantitative analysis of M gene expression using real-time quantitative PCR analysis

Nucleic acid was isolated from five presumably deutan retinas using a previously described method (Hagstrom *et al.* 2000). Quantitative, real-time RT-PCR was performed using probes specific for M and L cDNA. The protocol used was identical to that described for estimating the ratio of L:M genomic genes (Neitz and Neitz 2001) except that a different reverse primer was used. The reverse primer (5'TCGAAACTGCCGGTTCATAA) spans exons 5 and 6, and thus will amplify cDNA but not genomic DNA. Alternatively, RNA was reverse transcribed, exon 4 and part of exon 5 from both L and M cDNA was amplified and restriction digestion analysis was performed. Amplification was done with a forward primer (5'CATCTTTGGTTGGAGCAGGTACTGG) that spanned the junction between exons 3 and 4 and a reverse primer (5'GGGTTGGCAGCAGCAAAGCAT) to sequences within exon 5. The PCR product was end-labeled with P^{32} then incubated with restriction endonuclease Dde I, which cuts within the M gene-derived cDNA but not within the L gene-derived cDNA. The resulting fragments were separated by electrophoresis in an 8 per cent neutral polyacrylamide gel and visualized by phosphorimage analysis. The full-length PCR product was 323 base pairs (bp), whereas the products of the Dde I cleavage were 190 bp and 133 bp fragments.

Results and discussion

Identifying eye donors with deutan colour vision defects

Initial non-quantitative analysis of L and M gene expression was performed using nucleic acid preparations from foveal punches in a reverse transcriptase reaction followed by the polymerase chain reaction to amplify a segment of the L and M pigment cDNAs containing exon 5. There is an Rsa I restriction site in exon 5 of L pigment genes but not in M pigment genes. Donors whose retinas contained both L and M pigment mRNAs had fragments corresponding to uncut (M pigment cDNA) and cut (L pigment cDNA) PCR product, while those donors who lacked M pigment cDNA displayed only cut product. Out of a population of 150 male eye donors, we identified nine who lacked detectable M photopigment gene expression.

For each of the 150 eye donors, including the nine who lacked detectable M gene expression, the number and ratio of L:M genes was determined using two real-time quantitative PCR assays (Neitz and Neitz 2001). One assay estimated the relative ratio of first to downstream genes and provides an estimate of the number of genes in each array. The second assay estimates the ratio of L:M genes. Four of the nine donors who lacked detectable M gene expression lacked M genes. The remaining five donors had M photopigment genes as well as two L genes. These latter five donors were analysed further with the goal of determining whether M pigment mRNA was completely absent.

M gene expression in deutan colour vision defects

Real-time PCR was performed on nucleic acid preparations derived from 6 mm diameter foveal punches. Reverse transcription and PCR were performed sequentially in the same tube and probes specific for M and L cDNA were used to quantitate each species. Quantitation of L versus M cDNA for the five donors having two L and one M genes is shown in Fig. 33.2. No amplification of M pigment cDNA was detected from any of the identified deutan eye donors. Since probes for the L and M cDNAs are present in the same tubes it is possible to estimate the absence of M mRNA relative to the amount of L mRNA that was present in the retina. On most runs of the quantitative PCR assay, relative fluorescence intensity from the L cDNA specific probe rose above background fluorescence between 21–22 PCR cycles (Fig. 33.2). The PCR process is very efficient and until reagents become limiting the amount of product approximately doubles with every cycle. Fluorescence from the M cDNA-specific probe did not rise above background until after 37 PCR cycles, which is 15–16 cycles after the L-specific probe fluorescence exceeded background. Since during each cycle the amount of PCR product is doubled, this means that M cDNA was present at a level of less than one copy of M in 2^{15} or 2^{16} copies of L or less than about one copy in 50,000. A normal donor who had been previously characterized as having approximately 10 per cent M mRNA was used as a positive control and to demonstrate that low levels of M gene expression, when present, are easily detected with this assay.

Of course not being able to detect M pigment mRNA does not rule out that it could be present at an exceedingly low level. We note that the human fovea contains about

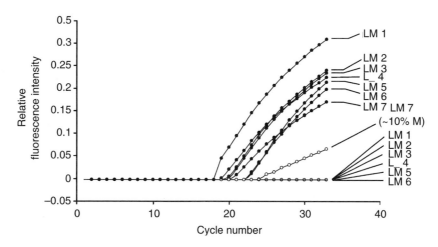

Figure 33.2 Real-time quantitative RT-PCR amplification plots. Closed circles indicate fluorescence intensities from the L-cDNA specific probes; open circles indicate fluorescence intensities from the M-cDNA specific probes. Curves labelled LM 1, LM 2, LM 3, LM 5, and LM 6 are from deutan retinas from donors with genomic M genes. L_4 is from a deutan retina, from a donor lacking genomic M genes. LM 7 is a control retina, previously estimated to have 10 per cent L mRNA.

100,000 cones. The sensitivity of these experiments (1 in 50,000) is equivalent to being able to detect the presence of just two M cones if all the other foveal cones were L. From this it seems very likely that M cones are completely absent from the eyes of deuteranomalous men. The fact that M gene expression seems to be completely silenced is an important clue towards ultimately elucidating the mechanism that controls expression of the X-chromosome pigment genes.

As introduced above, the current evidence seems to favour the hypothesis that a stochastic mechanism determines the identity of the L and M cones. The general idea of a stochastic process can be separated from theories of the specific mechanisms that make the random choice. Both Nathans' and Deeb's groups have forwarded a theory for a specific mechanism in which the choice is made by binding via intermediate proteins of the single locus control region (LCR) to the promoter region of one of the pigment genes in the array. At least in its present form, this specific mechanism does not seem to fully explain many of the observations about the expression of the genes. In a simple version of this theory the probability of a gene being expressed is related to its distance from the LCR so that "transcriptionally active complexes between the LCR and promoters of pigment genes located downstream of the first two proximal pigment genes are less likely" (Yamaguchi *et al.* 1997*a*). Distance is envisioned to affect gene expression in a probabilistic manner, accordingly, the third gene *is* expressed but the probability of any one cone expressing it is lower. In whole retinas of individuals with one L, one M and a hybrid gene Yamaguchi *et al.* (1997*b*) report the "average ratios of expression of these genes (exon 4 in this particular experiment), as estimated by mRNA, was 200(red) : 50(green) : 1(hybrid)". In contrast to what Deeb and colleagues have predicted for deuteranomaly, we do not find such a gradient of expression among the genes. Instead, expression seems to be completely interrupted for the M genes in deuteranomalous individuals. The results of Deeb and colleagues are strong evidence for a relationship between a gene's position in the array and its level of expression. However, consideration of all available data, including that presented here, indicates that the relationship is a complicated one. The evidence favours the hypothesis that deuteranomaly is caused by a one-step mechanism in which an M gene is displaced to a downstream position as proposed by Deeb. Our present results suggest that the downstream M genes are completely excluded from expression in deuteranomalous individuals. It does not appear that the regulation of expression can be purely a simple effect in which probability of expression is inversely proportional to the distance from the LCR. The relative expression of L and M cones in normal humans is hugely variable and some people have more M than L cones even though they have an L gene first in the array. In those cases, a distal gene is expressed with a higher probability than one more proximal to the LCR. In deuteranomaly genes after the first two appear to be completely silent, however, in some individuals, who presumably have normal colour vision, genes after the first two escape being silenced (Sjoberg *et al.* 1998).

The LCR is a DNA element that is required for expression of the X-chromosome pigment genes and it has the characteristics of an enhancer. Its relationship to the photopigment genes differs from the simple cases where there is a 1 : 1 relationship between enhancer and gene. The photopigment genes must share the one enhancer and there is little doubt that this means that only one pigment gene from the array can be active at any one time. However, usually interactions between enhancers and promoters via their intermediate proteins are considered to be dynamic processes. Thus, there is no known biological reason why the presence of a single enhancer for an array of genes would by itself restrict the expression to just one gene per cell. If the interaction was dynamic, the enhancer could switch between the genes so that, over time, more than one pigment would be produced in each cell. The idea that the enhancer binds permanently to one gene provides a simple explanation for why only one gene would be expressed in each cell. However, we are not sure that this hypothesis can explain many of the other facts of photopigment gene expression. We find the idea very attractive that the identity of an L versus an M cone is determined by a stochastic process. However, it seems possible that the exact mechanism that makes the random choice is different from what has so far been envisioned. Ultimately, a truly satisfying theory, whether it involves a permanent bond between a promoter and the LCR or not, will have to explain the variability across individuals both in the total number of genes that are expressed from an array and in the relative numbers of L and M cones. It will also have to explain the variability in cone ratio within an eye, in which the L : M cone ratio rises sharply in the far periphery (Hagstrom *et al.* 1998). A final piece of evidence that would seem to argue against the idea that presence of a single LCR is what is responsible for directing a single pigment into each cone is that the howler monkey has an LCR for each gene (Dulai *et al.* 1999). We presume that these monkeys have separate populations of L and M cones, but in the context of these questions about mechanisms for photopigment gene expression it would be interesting to know for sure.

Acknowledgments

This work was supported by an unrestricted RPB grant, NEI grants EY09303, EY01931 & EY09620 and the David & Ruth S. Coleman Charitable Foundation. The authors would like to thank P. M. Summerfelt and C. Bialozynski for technical assistance. M. N. is the recipient of the RPB Lew Wasserman Merit Award.

References

Asenjo, A. B., Rim, J., & Oprian, D. D. (1994). Molecular determinants of human red/green color discrimination. *Neuron 12*, 1131–8.

Balding, S. D., Sjoberg, S. A., Neitz, J., & Neitz, M. (1998). Pigment gene expression in protan color vision defects. *Vision Research 38*, 3359–64.

Bollinger, K., Bialozynski, C., Neitz, J., & Neitz, M. (2001). The importance of deleterious mutations of M pigment genes as a cause of color vision defects. *Color Research and Application 26*, S100–5.

Carroll, J., McMahon, C., Neitz, M., & Neitz, J. (2000). Flicker-photometric electroretinogram estimates of L:M cone photoreceptor ratio in men with photopigment spectra derived from genetics. *Journal of the Optical Society of America A 17*, 499–509.

Deeb, S. S., Lindsey, D. T., Hibiya, Y., Sanocki, E., Winderickx, J., Teller, D. Y., & Motulsky, A. G. (1992). Genotype-phenotype relationships in human red/green colour-vision defects: molecular and psychophysical studies. *American Journal of Human Genetics 51*, 687–700.

Drummond-Borg, M., Deeb, S. S., & Motulsky, A. G. (1989). Molecular patterns of X-chromosome-linked color genes among 134 men of European ancestry. *Proceedings of the National Academy of Sciences USA 86*, 983–7.

Dulai, K. S., von Dornum, M., Mollon, J. D., & Hunt, D. M. (1999). The evolution of trichromatic color vision by opsin gene duplication in New World and Old World primates. *Genome Research 9*, 629–38.

Hagstrom, S. A., Neitz, J., & Neitz, M. (1998). Variations in cone populations for red-green color vision examined by analysis of mRNA. *Neuroreport 9*, 1963–7.

Hagstrom, S. A., Neitz, M., & Neitz, J. (2000). Cone pigment gene expression in individual photoreceptors and the chromatic topography of the retina. *Journal of the Optical Society of America A 17*, 527–37.

Hayashi, T., Motulsky, A. G., & Deeb, S. S. (1999). Position of a "green-red" hybrid gene in the visual pigment array determines colour-vision phenotype. *Nature Genetics 22*, 90–3.

Merbs, S. L., & Nathans, J. (1992). Absorption spectra of the hybrid pigments responsible for anomalous color vision. *Science 258*, 464–6.

Miyahara, E., Pokorny, J., Smith, V. C., Baron, R., & Baron, E. (1998). Color vision in two observers with highly biased LWS/MWS cone ratios. *Vision Research 38*, 601–12.

Nathans, J., Piantanida, T. P., Eddy, R. L., Shows, T. B., & Hogness, D. S. (1986). Molecular genetics of inherited variation in human color vision. *Science 232*, 203–10.

Neitz, J., Neitz, M., & Kainz, P. M. (1996). Visual pigment gene structure and the severity of human color vision defects. *Science 274*, 801–4.

Neitz, M., & Neitz, J. (2001). A new test for mass screening of school age children for red-green color vision defects. *Color Research & Application 26*, S239–S249.

Neitz, M., & Neitz, J. (1995). Numbers and ratios of visual pigment genes for normal red-green color vision. *Science 267*, 1013–16.

Neitz, M., Neitz, J., & Jacobs, G. H. (1991a). Spectral tuning of pigments underlying red-green color vision. *Science 252*, 971–4.

Neitz, M., Neitz, J., & Jacobs, G. H. (1991b). Relationship between cone pigments and genes in deuteranomalous subjects. In B. Drum, J. D. Moreland, and A. Serra (Eds), *Colour Vision Deficiencies X*, Kluwer Academic Publishers.

Roorda, A., & Williams, D. R. (1999). The arrangement of the three cone classes in the living human eye. *Nature 397*, 520–2.

Sjoberg, S. A., Neitz, M., Balding, S. D., & Neitz, J. (1998). L-cone pigment genes expressed in normal colour vision. *Vision Research 38*, 3213–19.

Vollrath, D., Nathans, J., & Davis, R. W. (1988). Tandem array of human visual pigment genes at Xq28. *Science 240*, 1669–72.

Wang, Y., Smallwood, P. M., Cowan, M., Blesh, D., Lawler, A., & Nathans, J. (1999). Mutually exclusive expression of human red and green visual pigment-reporter transgenes occurs at high frequency in murine cone photoreceptors. *Proceedings of the National Academy of Sciences, USA 96*, 5251–6.

Winderickx, J., Sanocki, E., Lindsey, D. T., Teller, D. Y., Motulsky, A. G., & Deeb, S. S. (1992*a*). Defective color vision associated with a missense mutation in the human green visual pigment gene. *Nature Genetics 1*, 251–6.

Winderickx, J., Battisti, L., Motulsky, A. G., & Deeb, S. S. (1992*b*). Selective expression of human X chromosome-linked green opsin genes. *Proceedings of the National Academy of Sciences, USA 89*, 9710–14.

Yamaguchi, T., Motulsky, A. G., & Deeb, S. S. (1997*a*). Visual pigment gene structure and expression in human retinae. *Human Molecular Genetics 6*, 981–90.

Yamaguchi, T., Motulsky, A. G., & Deeb, S. S. (1997*b*). Levels of expression of the red, green and green-red hybrid pigment genes in the human retina. In C. R. Cavonius (Ed.), *Colour Vision Deficiencies XIII*. Dordrecht: Kluwer Academic Publishers.

INHERITED COLOUR DEFICIENCY: PSYCHOPHYSICS AND TESTS

PRELIMINARY NORMS FOR THE CAMBRIDGE COLOUR TEST

D. F. VENTURA, L. C. L. SILVEIRA, A. R. RODRIGUES,
J. M. DE SOUZA, M. GUALTIERI, D. BONCI, AND
M. F. COSTA

Introduction

Normal colour vision is trichromatic and can be assessed by different tests (Lakowski 1969; Pokorny *et al.* 1979; Birch 1993). There are basically two functions that are tested: matching and discrimination (Committee on Vision 1981).

Colour matching can be precisely tested using the Rayleigh equation for the red–green system (or the Moreland equation for the blue–yellow system). The equipment used is an anomaloscope, in which the subject is required to match a field produced by a mixture of red and green to another produced by spectral yellow. The subject varies the relative amounts of red and green in the mixture until a match is achieved. Trichromatic subjects equate the two fields with a known proportion of red and green, while for colour deficient observers the proportion varies according with the type of loss. A deuteranomalous requires more green light while a protanomalous requires more red (Pokorny *et al.* 1979; Committee on Vision 1981).

Other tests measure discriminative capacity. This is the case for the Farnsworth–Munsell 100 Hue Test (FM100), an arrangement test in which the subject orders colour objects—plastic caps covered with Munsell papers of different hues. The amount and type of errors made in this task indicate the severity and type of loss (Pokorny *et al.* 1979).

In both matching and discrimination, the result is the range of colours in which there is confusion or lack of discrimination. In trichromatic subjects this range is very narrow, while in the pathological cases it is wider and varies in location according with the type of deficiency.

Discriminative capacity can also be inferred from the popular Ishihara plates, a traditional test, built in a way that eliminates luminance or contour cues. The test consists of printed plates presenting a figure (a number) to be distinguished from a background. Both figure and background are composed by small circles of different sizes and luminances with the figure in a given hue and the background in another, in such a way that the discrimination cannot be made on the basis of intensity or contour (Regan *et al.* 1994).

The idea of measuring hue discrimination in a spatial and luminance noise situation inspired the recent development of the Cambridge Colour Test (CCT) (Reffin *et al.* 1991;

Mollon and Reffin 1989; Regan *et al.* 1994), whose target is a Landolt C presented on a computer display. Since the CCT is a computerized test, its construction allows easy change in stimulus parameters and permits threshold determination of the discrimination between any pair of target and background hues. It presents a rapid testing procedure in which three thresholds are obtained, respectively in a protan, a deutan and a tritan line, called Trivector, and a longer testing procedure in which three MacAdam ellipses are determined, either along a tritan line or along a deutan–protan line, the Ellipses test. The latter is used for tritanopic subjects.

Normative data for the CCT are not available since both the original (Regan *et al.* 1994) and the commercial versions (Mollon and Reffin 2000) of the test are rather recent developments. Thus, the present study presents preliminary norms and compares a self-built and the commercial version of the test. The results are compared with the Farnsworth–Munsell 100 Hue test.

Methods

Subjects

The subjects, aged 18–30 years old with at least 20/20 Snellen acuity and no known colour vision deficiency were tested in São Paulo, SP at the Universidade de São Paulo (45 subjects, 22.5 ± 2.74 years old) and in Belém, PA at the Universidade Federal do Pará (30 subjects, 21.82 ± 2.88 years old). They were recruited among students. Inclusion criteria were absence of reported ophthalmologic and neurophthalmologic pathologies. A third inclusion criterion was based on performance in the Trivector test (see below). Informed consent was obtained from all subjects, in accordance with the Declaration of Helsinki determinations.

Equipment

The São Paulo group used the commercial version of the test, the Cambridge Colour Test, CCT v2.0, with VSG 5 card and Sony FD Trinitron colour monitor (from Cambridge Research Instruments). The Belém group used a self-built system for an IBM RISC 6000 workstation and an IBM 6091 19i colour monitor, with a graphics board IBM POWER GT4-24bits-3D and software programmed by author ARR.

Procedure

Tests were performed mono- or binocularly in a darkened room, with the computer monitor screen off or dimmed and with the subject positioned at 3 m from the stimulus monitor. The subject was instructed to indicate the position of the Landolt C opening by pressing the corresponding button in a response box (São Paulo) or the respective keyboard arrows (Belém).

The short test version, the Trivector, was determined first, for screening purposes. Subjects that exceed the values of $100 \times 10^{-3} \, u'v'$ units in either the deutan or protan axis or $150 \times 10^{-3} \, u'v'$ units in the tritan axis were excluded.

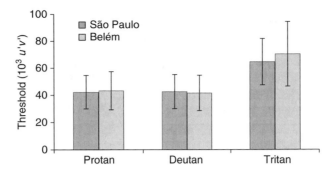

Figure 34.1 Averages and standard deviations of colour discrimination thresholds in the protan, deutan and tritan axis obtained in the Trivector Test by the groups from São Paulo and Belém.

Eight-vector or twenty-vector ellipses were determined in the São Paulo and Belém set-ups, respectively for all subjects that passed the Trivector test. The $u'v'$ coordinates for the centres of the three ellipses lay along the tritanopic confusion axis and were: Field 1: 0.197, 0.469; Field 2: 0.193, 0.509; Field 3: 0.204, 0.416. They constituted the background colour against which hues corresponding to equally spaced vectors were tested (see Regan *et al.* 1994, Figs 34.1 and 34.2).

Psychophysical procedure

The test uses the staircase psychophysical method to measure threshold discrimination, presenting two staircases in random alternation. In each staircase, testing begins with a saturated hue and proceeds to a less saturated hue every time the subject makes a correct response. Incorrect responses or no responses are followed by presentation of hues with higher saturation value. Step size is halved or doubled, following correct or incorrect responses respectively. After a criterion of six incorrect responses or six reversals, the series is terminated and a threshold is computed. In succession, testing on a new pair of hues is begun. The results are expressed in $u'v'$ coordinates in CIE colour space.

Results

Testability

Instructions were easily understood and the subjects required no practice in the test. Sessions lasted around 40 min, with 3–4 min for the Trivector test and 30 min for the three 8-vector ellipse determinations. The experimenter always remained in the testing room with the subject.

The Trivector test

The Trivector test was a rapid procedure that required 3–4 min after the S received the instructions.

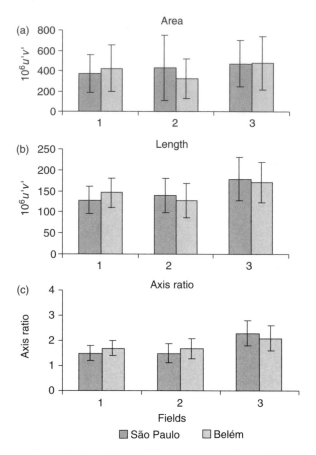

Figure 34.2 Averages and standard deviations of ellipse parameters obtained by the São Paulo and Belém groups in the Ellipses Test. (a) ellipse area, (b) length of longer axis, (c) ratio between the long and the short diameters.

Trivector discrimination thresholds for all subjects tested were below the Cambridge Colour Test Manual limits of $100 \times 10^{-4} u'v'$ units for the protan and deutan lines and of $150 \times 10^{-4} u'v'$ units for the tritan line (Table 34.1, Fig. 34.1).

The Ellipses test

The ellipse parameters—area, long diameter, and the ratio of long and short diameters—obtained for the São Paulo and for the Belém groups are presented in Fig. 34.2. Average areas are presented in Table 34.2. Ellipses from trichromatic subjects had very small areas and axis ratios compared to those of congenital and acquired colour defective subjects, who present very elongated or much broader ellipses (Regan *et al.* 1994; Ventura *et al.* Chapter 42, this volume).

Table 34.1 Averages, Standard deviations and tolerance limits for the CCT Trivector test*

	Protan	Deutan	Tritan
Data type			
São Paulo	42.3 (12.3)	42.6 (12.6)	64.7 (17.2)
Belém	44.9 (13.1)	56.5 (16.7)	73.8 (23.4)
Combined data	43.2 (11.4)	47.3 (15)	67.7 (19.6)
Tolerance limit			
Upper limit	69.3	82.4	113.4
Lower limit	25.2	24.7	37.3

* in $10^{-4} u'v'$ units.

Comparison between the São Paulo and Belém data

There were no significant differences in the Mann-Whitney rank sum test between the São Paulo and Belém sets of data. Therefore, the results of the two groups were combined. The combined averages and standard deviations are based on the total n of 72 Ss and are presented in Table 34.1.

Intra-subject reliability

The ellipse areas obtained for each of the fields were compared to verify the Ss consistency in this test. Highly significant positive correlations ($p < 0.001$ except where noted) were obtained comparing the areas of: Fields 1 and 2 (Belém A: $R = 0.77$; São Paulo: $R = 0.70$), Fields 1 and 3 (Belém: $R = 0.78$; São Paulo: $R = 0.74$) and Fields 2 and 3 (Belém: $R = 0.66$, $p < 0.01$; São Paulo: $R = 0.81$).

Tolerance limits for the CCT

Tolerance limits describe the range in which a given percentage of a normally distributed population is found, with a given probability. The number of subjects in our data allows the use of tolerance limits for 90 per cent of the population with 95 per cent probability (Dixon and Massey 1957), for the Trivector and the Ellipses test parameters (Tables 34.1 and 34.2, Fig. 34.3). A base 10 logarithmic transformation was applied to normalize the data. The results are expressed as the corresponding antilog in the same base.

Comparison with the Farnsworth–Munsell 100 Hue test

Subjects were tested with the FM 100 for comparison with the CCT. Their scores ranged from superior to average discrimination but the FM 100 error score had none or very low positive correlation correlation with the CCT Trivector. There was also no significant correlation for any of the CCT Ellipse parameters ($p > 0.05$).

Table 34.2 Averages, SDs, and tolerance limits for the Ellipses tests

	Area[a]			Length[b]			Axis Ratio		
	Field 1	Field 2	Field 3	Field 1	Field 2	Field 3	Field 1	Field 2	Field 3
Data									
São Paulo	368.6 (187.9)[c]	426.6 (233.4)	473 (231.5)	127.7 (32.4)	138.8 (41.4)	178.9 (50.9)	1.5 (0.3)	1.5 (0.4)	2.3 (0.5)
Belém	422.3 (227.2)	319.9 (193.1)	477.4 (259.4)	145.5 (34)	127.3 (41.1)	170.4 (48)	1.7 (0.3)	1.7 (0.4)	2.1 (0.5)
Combined data	337.3 (166.9)	418 (200)	465.8 (233)	127.7 (35.8)	142.1 (38.7)	174.9 (47.7)	1.6 (.3)	1.6 (.4)	2.2 (.5)
Tolerance limits									
Upper Limit	746.1	901	1004.9	209.3	226.9	286.1	2.4	2.4	3.4
Lower Limit	122.3	158	174.8	72.2	83.1	99.4	1.1	1	1.3

[a] $10^{-6}\,u'v'$ units.
[b] $10^{-5}\,u'v'$ units.
[c] average (SD).

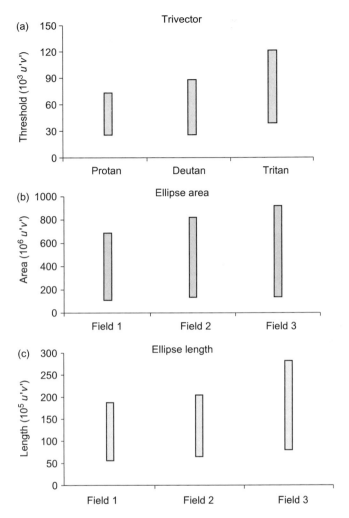

Figure 34.3 Tolerance Limits for 90 per cent of the population with 95 per cent probability for subjects aged 18–30-years-old for (a): Trivector Protan, Deutan, and Tritan thresholds ; (b) Ellipse area and (c) Ellipse length of Fields 1, 2, and 3, based on the combined data from the São Paulo and Belém groups.

Age

Subjects ranged in age from 18 to 30 years old. Within this range no trend in CCT results was observed. Correlation between age and CCT results was absent or very low for both the Trivector thresholds and the Ellipse parameters.

Discussion

The assessment of colour discrimination with the Ellipses CCT is easy to perform and reproducible in different setups. The fact that the test refers to CIE colour space and is very precisely quantifiable makes it potentially an important instrument for testing acquired colour defect as well as small degrees of congenital colour anomaly.

The need to establish norms for the CCT cannot, therefore, be underrated. In a test that may be used by clinicians or could have practical applications in industry for personnel selection, a set of norms is an obvious asset. In the clinical setting it is frequently not possible to invest in determination of norms as is often done by research groups, which usually define their own norms for each test.

The present results offer these norms for the 18–30-year-old range and are part of a study that extends them to other ages. It should be stressed that the present norms are based on data collected in two different centres, with different equipment and software. The absence of statistical difference between the two sets of data is an indication of the reliability and robustness of the CCT.

Tolerance limits have been used as a convenient statistical definition of norms (Salomão and Ventura 1995). They bracket a percentage of the population with a given probability. The upper and lower tolerance limits for colour discrimination defined here are for 90 per cent of the population with 95 per cent probability.

The Trivector upper tolerance limits are lower than the recommendation made by the CCT instruction manual and could be rounded up to 70×10^{-4} $u'v'$ for protan, $85 \times 10^{-4} u'v'$ for deutan and $115 \times 10^{-4} u'v'$ for tritan threshold.

Lower limits are also described. The values of $25 \times 10^{-4} u'v'$ for protan and deutan and $40 \times 10^{-4} u'v'$ for tritan define the lower limit of the norms. Individuals presenting scores at or below these values have superior discrimination. There are professional situations in which these skills are useful or even required (Birch 1993).

The MacAdam ellipse parameter values, obtained for the same subjects, are used to define ellipse norms, not available previously, also establishing tolerance limits. The area of colour space where there is no discrimination is probably the most useful parameter to describe acquired dyschromatopsia since colour vision loss is frequently diffuse. In these cases ellipse length and diameter ratio might not be revealing of the losses. Upper tolerance limits for ellipse area, lie around 750 to 1010×10^{6} $u'v'$ for the three fields tested, while the corresponding lower limits range from 125 to 175×10^{6} $u'v'$. Classification of losses in specific directions of colour space are best described by the ellipse length. Upper tolerance limits for the length of the long diameter range from about 210 to 290×10^{5} $u'v'$ for Fields 1 to 3 and the lower tolerance limits ranged from about 75 to 100×10^{5} $u'v'$.

Since no other norms are available for the CCT, we compare here the values of the scores reported by Regan et al. (1994) in their first extensive use of the test. All subjects considered by them as normal trichromats fall within the tolerance limits defined by the present norms. The fields they used had slightly different position in the CIE space but this does not seriously affect the results since MacAdam ellipses in these regions are very similar for trichromats (Birch 1993).

Acknowledgements

This work was supported by FAPESP #0030/00-98, FINEP #66.95.0407.00, CNPq #523303/95-5 and CAPES-PROCAD grants to DFV; CAPES-RENOR, IBM, JICA, PRONEX, FINEP-PNOPG/FADESP #090/00-99, CNPq-PNOPG #550663/2001-0, and #521640/96-2, and UFPa-PROINT #372/2001 grants to LCLS Authors DFV, LCLS, and JMS are CNPq research fellows. MFC and ARR have graduate fellowships from CAPES, whilst DB and MG have undergraduate fellowships from CNPq. LCLS was a Visiting Professor supported by USP-PRPG. We thank Claudiel Luiz dos Santos for administrative assistance and Alexandre M. Braga for helping in the software development. We are also indebted to Prof José de Oliveira Siqueira from the Universidade de São Paulo for statistical advice.

References

Birch, J. (1993) *Diagnosis of Defective Color Vision*, Oxford University Press, New York.

Dixon, W. J. & Massey, F. J. (1957) *Introduction of Statistical Analysis*, McGraw-Hill, New York.

Committee on Vision (1981) *Procedures for Testing Color Vision*, National Academy Press, Washington DC.

Lakowski, R. (1969) Theory and practice of colour vision testing: a review. *British Journal of Industrial Medicine*, 26, 173–89; 265–88.

Mollon, J. D. (1997) 'aus dreyerley Arten von Membranen oder Molekülen': George Palmer's legacy. In *Colour Vision Deficiencies XIII*, Ed: Cavonius, C. R., Kluwer, Dordrecht, pp. 3–20.

Mollon, J. D. & Reffin, J. P. (1989) A computer-controlled colour vision test that combines the principles of Chibret and Stilling. *Journal of Physiology*, 414, 5P.

Mollon, J. D. & Reffin, J. P. (2000) *Handbook of the Cambridge Colour Test*. Ed: Cambridge Research Systems, London, UK (www.crsltd.com).

Pokorny, J., Smith, V. C., Verriest, G., & Pinckers, A. J. L. G. (1979) *Congenital and Acquired Colour Vision Defects*, Grune & Stratton, New York.

Reffin, J. P., Astell S., & Mollon, J. D. (1991) Trials of a computer-controlled colour vision test that preserves the advantages of pseudoisochromatic plates. In *Colour Vision Deficiencies X*, pp. 69–76, Eds: Drum, B., Moreland, J. D., and Serra, A., Kluwer, Dordrecht.

Regan, B. C., Reffin, J. P., & Mollon, J. D. (1994) Luminance noise and the rapid determination of discrimination ellipses in colour deficiency. *Vision Research*, 34, 1279–99.

Salomão, S. R. & Ventura, D. F. (1995) Large-sample population age norms for visual acuities obtained with Vistech/Teller acuity cards. *Investigations in Ophthalmic Vision Science*, 36(3), 657–70.

CHAPTER 35

EVALUATION OF "COLOUR VISION TESTING MADE EASY"

STEPHEN J. DAIN

Introduction

"Colour Vision Testing Made Easy" is a colour vision test specifically designed for children and based on the pseudo-isochromatic (PIC) principle. There has been one evaluation of the test (Cotter *et al.* 1999) in which 2 of 21 CVD (colour vision deficient) adults passed and 5 per cent of boys (age 5–7 years) failed. No definitive diagnoses were available. In designing a test for children, there are two issues that merit specific attention, in addition to colorimetric design.

Cognitive demand

Children must understand what is expected of them. In PIC tests this may be the naming of relatively simple shapes (they will need to know the names of the shapes), the identification of numbers (they will need to know their numbers) or they will need to point to other examples, like symbols (they will need to understand the concept of same and different).

Perceptual demand

In order to perceive a shape in the PIC plate, they will need to assemble the individual dots into the shape or symbol. The shape or symbol will need to be sufficiently delineated in colour from the background. The shapes or symbols will need to be sufficiently different from one another.

In many PIC tests letters with serifs are used and may be confusing. In Fig. 35.1, for instance, the numeral 1 may, not unreasonably, be seen as a 7. Given the random dot nature of PIC tests, a circle and square are quite similar whereas a cross, triangle, and circle (or a square) are much more easily distinguished.

Colour vision demands

The lesser cognitive and perceptual abilities of a child might be compensated for by increasing the colour differences, but this begs the question "what colour difference does a normal child need as distinct from an adult?" Raising the colour difference to accommodate these issues may lead to a loss of sensitivity in the test performance.

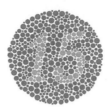

Figure 35.1 Layout of a PIC test plate with numerals incorporating a serif. This is intended to illustrate the possibility of interpreting the "1" as a "7".

The colour vision design is the core activity. In this aspect, the issues of test design do not differ from adults. Differences in spectral sensitivity in children are unlikely to be sufficient to destroy equiluminance (which is not exact anyway). The PIC design for evaluating protan deficiencies must account for the clues due to losses of red luminosity, so equiluminance may not be optimal anyway.

"Colour Vision Testing Made Easy"

The test uses symbols throughout. The first set of plates contains simple shapes (circle, square, and star) with a luminance contrast defined symbol often present in addition to the colour difference defined. A second set of three plates uses cognitively more complex symbols (stylized outlines of a sailing boat, balloon and string, and dog). Examples in black and white are given for the child to point to. There are only colour-defined shapes in this series. In principle, given the advantage of the cognitive and perceptual task in the first series, the second series is not investigated here since this study is, essentially, an evaluation of the colorimetric design before proceeding to specific tests on children.

Evaluation—Colorimetric assessment

Individual elements of each plate type were measured using a Topcon SR-1 telespectroradiometer in the range 400–760 nm in 10-nm steps with a spectral half band width of 5 nm. The plates were illuminated with quartz halide tungsten filament lamp supplied from a stabilized power supply (0.1 per cent current regulation). Initial calibration was done using freshly pressed barium sulphate for which the manufacturer (Kodak) provides batch spectral reflectance data. The system was further calibrated using a set of 12 British Ceramic Research Association tiles for which spectral reflectance data had been obtained from National Physical Laboratory, UK (NPL) in 1986 and 1997. Note, there are differences in the NPL data due to NPL changing the spectral reflectance scale. This results in no significant change in chromaticity but a uniform increase in luminous reflectance.

Chromaticities were calculated using the CIE (1931) standard observer and CIE Illuminant C.

Table 35.1 Description of the plate construction in the first 9 plates

Plate	Background	Colour-defined figure	Non-confusion defined figure	Distracters
1	Olive-green	One yellow-brown	One yellow	Blue-green
2 & 4	Yellow-brown	One olive-green	One blue-green	
3	Yellow-brown	One olive-green	One blue-green	Yellow
5 & 6	Olive-green	One yellow-brown	One yellow	
7 & 9	Yellow-brown	Two olive-green		Yellow
8	Olive-green	Three yellow-brown		Blue-green

Results—Colorimetric assessment

There are 9 plates with 5 different designs, plus a demonstration plate. The demonstration plate is not reported on except in that the shapes are defined in both chromaticity and luminous reflectance difference. The luminous reflectance difference ($\Delta L^* = 10.2$) is typical, in the author's experience, of similar demonstration plates. The plates all have common features. All have a figure defined by colour difference. Some have a luminous reflectance and colour-defined figure. Some have additional colours distributed through the background and colour-defined figure which are termed "distracters" for the present purpose. The construction is summarized in Table 35.1. It may be seen that the colorimetric task is always the discrimination of yellow-brown from olive-green, although they alternate as the figure and background colours.

Colorimetrically, therefore, the discrimination task is the same in all the plates. In addition some plates include yellow or blue-green dots which appear to act only as distracters or to mask any luminance clues between the figure and the background. As a consequence, the colours of all of the tests are plotted in a single figure (see Fig. 35.2).

Discussion—Colorimetric assessment

The representation of the colours and the colorimetric analysis use the CIE 1976 Luv system (CIE 1977). Given that the figure and background of PIC plates are, at least nominally, equiluminant, the L^* value is not used and the analysis is in terms of chromaticity difference alone. In Fig. 35.2 it may be seen that the chromaticity difference is a little better aligned with the deutan rather than protan confusion lines. A similar effect may also be seen in Ishihara's test (Dain *et al.* 1993). The mean chromaticity difference is a little larger than that in Ishihara's test: mean (of all the colours represented in Fig. 35.2) $\Delta u'v' = 0.047$ compared with the Ishihara mean of the same task and representative set of $\Delta u'v' = 0.035$. This would be consistent with, but not necessarily predictive of, an observation that CVTME would generate more false negatives. Since performance on colour vision tests is also affected by non-colour factors (as discussed above), the significance of the larger colour difference can only be evaluated by clinical studies.

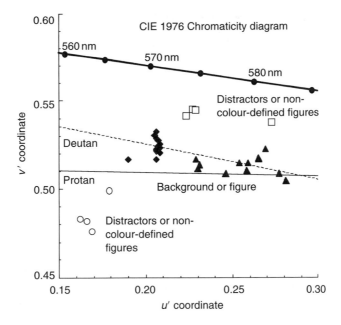

Figure 35.2 Chromaticities of the four groups of colours used in CVTME comprising two groups used for the colour discrimination process in a background/symbol pair and the two groups used for luminous reflectance defined symbols and distracters.

The chromaticities of the three editions were measured and the inter-edition variation is no more than the intra-edition variations ($\sigma = 0.04 \, \Delta u'v'$ in both cases).

The colorimetric design is typical of PIC tests. The observation that the colour task is the same in each plate but that the provision of distracters, different symbols and, sometimes, luminous reflectance defined symbols provides the opportunity to look at non-colour issues in plate design.

Evaluation—Performance assessment

Subjects:

- 10 protanopes
- 6 protanomals
- 14 deuteranomals
- 11 deuteranopes
- 42 normals

The subjects were obtained from the clinic patients and Optometry students, School of Optometry, UNSW. A diagnosis of colour-normal colour vision or the type of colour vision deficiency was made on the on basis of a Rayleigh equation anomaloscope

(Nagel, Neitz OT or Heidelberg Mk I). The colour deficient subjects also undertook at least;

- Ishihara (24 plate) and SPP-1 PIC tests
- Farnsworth–Munsell D-15 test
- Farnsworth lantern

The tests were carried out under daylight fluorescent tubes at 220 lux.

Results

The pass/fail performance for each plate for normal and colour vision deficient subjects was assembled into overall performance of the three PIC tests, in Fig. 35.3 and, for each plate, values of sensitivity and specificity which were combined to give Youden's Index (Youden 1950) (YI) where YI = sensitivity + specificity − 1.

   These YIs are set out in Table 35.2. There is no published method of assigning confidence limits to YI. Those in Table 35.1 have been calculated as follows. Specificity and sensitivity are binomial measures and the 95th percentile confidence limits have been applied to each of these measures given $n = 39$ colour vision deficient subjects and $n = 42$ normals (Pearson and Hartley 1954). The confidence limits of YI are then derived as the root mean square of the confidence limits of specificity and sensitivity since specificity and sensitivity are uncorrelated variables (ISO 1995). The confidence limits

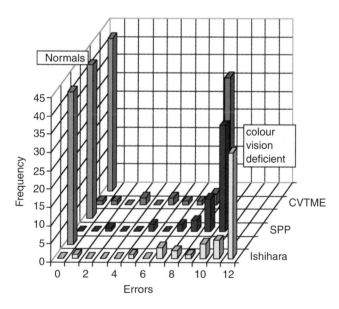

Figure 35.3 Distribution of errors made in the Ishihara, SPP-1 and CVTME tests.

Table 35.2 Youden's Index for each plate of CVTME, mean of the plates and the test as a whole. The limits are the 95 percentile confidence limits (see text for further details)

Plate	Ishihara	SPP	CVTME
1	0.83 + 0.08 − 0.15	0.92 + 0.05 − 0.11	0.88 + 0.08 − 0.13
2	0.85 + 0.08 − 0.13	0.92 + 0.05 − 0.11	0.95 + 0.06 − 0.11
3	0.93 + 0.05 − 0.11	0.79 + 0.10 − 0.14	0.90 + 0.07 − 0.12
4	0.89 + 0.07 − 0.12	0.87 + 0.08 − 0.13	0.90 + 0.07 − 0.12
5	0.93 + 0.05 − 0.11	0.90 + 0.07 − 0.12	0.88 + 0.08 − 0.13
6	0.96 + 0.05 − 0.11	0.90 + 0.07 − 0.12	0.83 + 0.08 − 0.15
7	0.89 + 0.07 − 0.12	0.90 + 0.07 − 0.12	0.93 + 0.05 − 0.11
8	0.87 + 0.08 − 0.13	0.92 + 0.05 − 0.11	0.90 + 0.07 − 0.12
9	0.91 + 0.05 − 0.11	0.90 + 0.07 − 0.12	0.88 + 0.08 − 0.13
10	0.87 + 0.08 − 0.13	0.97 + 0.02 − 0.10	
11	0.85 + 0.08 − 0.13		
12	0.98 + 0.02 − 0.10		
Mean	0.90 + 0.02 − 0.03	0.90 + 0.02 − 0.03	0.89 + 0.02 − 0.03
Whole test	1.00	1.00	0.97 − 0.10 + 0.03

of the combined plates of each test are derived using the total number of observations (number of subjects × number of plates in the test).

Discussion

Overall CVTME passes one subject with a colour vision deficiency who is failed by the other tests. Taken with the data of Cotter *et al.* (1999) and the larger colour difference in the plates reported here, this indicates a tendency to pass very mild deuteranomals. While it might be argued that these are very mild deficiencies and of little educational or career significance, it might be avoidable in the design of the test.

Given the same colorimetric task, it is of interest to look at the other aspects of the plate construction. The following were considered as factors in the validity of each plate type by comparing the mean and confidence limits of the YI of plates groups as follows;

Symbol used (square, star, or circle)

Number of confusion symbols in the plate (1–3)

Use of distracters

Use of a non-confusion symbol

Colour of background.

No factor was shown to have a significant effect (the difference in YI for the group was always less than the confidence interval, $p > 0.05$). Given the limited number of plates, N is, of necessity, small and significant effects would not be easily shown.

Conclusions

The colorimetric design of CVTME is reasonable and CVD adults are, with one exception, identified. Colorimetrically, the task is less demanding than Ishihara's and this is consistent with the, previously identified, propensity to pass very mild deuteranomals. The perception task of the simple symbols is, from a child's point of view, less demanding than numerals but there is no evidence that any of the symbols used were a better choice.

Acknowledgment

To Dr Terrace Waggoner for supply of the tests for evaluation.

References

CIE (1978). *Recommendations on Uniform Color Spaces, Color-Difference Equations, Psychometric Color Terms.* Supplement No 2 of CIE Publication No. 15 (E-1.3.1) 1971. Paris. Bureau Central de la Commission Internationale de l'Éclairage.

Cotter, S. A., Lee D. Y., & French A. L. (1999). Evaluation of a new color vision test; "Color Vision Testing Made Easy". *Optom Vis Sci* 76(9): 631–6.

Dain, S. J., Honson, V. J., & Curtis, C. (1993). Suitability of fluorescent tube light sources for the Ishihara test as determined by colorimetric methods. In Drum, B. (Ed.) *Colour Vision Deficiencies XI.* Netherlands. Kluwer. pp. 327–33.

ISO (1995). Guide to the expression of uncertainty. International Organisation for Standardization. Genève.

Pearson, E. S. & Hartley, H. O. (1954). *Biometrika Tables for Statisticians.* London. Cambridge University Press, table 41.

Youden, W. J. (1950). Index for rating diagnostic tests. *Cancer* 3: 32–5.

CHAPTER 36

SURVEY OF THE COLOUR VISION DEMANDS IN FIRE-FIGHTING

STEPHEN J. DAIN AND LAURA E. HUGHES

Background

The setting of colour vision standards requires

1. Knowledge of colour vision deficiencies.
2. Knowledge of the colour-contingent decisions of the specific job.
3. Understanding of the consequences of error.

These aspects are unlikely to be within one person's expertise. In individual cases it also requires a full colour vision diagnosis. In the New South Wales Fire Brigades (NSWFB) the previous colour vision standard was to pass Ishihara's test or, if fail, then pass the Lanthony Desaturated D15 test. More recently the requirement became to pass Ishihara's test or, if fail, then pass the Farnsworth–Munsell Standard D15 test (FMD-15). The change was based in the work of Margrain and Birch (1994) and Margrain *et al.* (1996). Fire-fighters are also required not to be protan. This, more recent, requirement comes from the Australian national commercial drivers standard which excludes protans. The NSWFB requires recruits to hold a rigid truck licence. However, the relevance of the FMD-15 to real tasks has been challenged by NSWFB Union. There is also an issue with long term "retained" fire-fighters. In country areas, retained fire-fighters are paid a retainer and then a fee per incident attended while maintaining other part or full-time employment. They have no medical standards to meet (including colour vision). Some may subsequently apply for full time positions (sometimes after many years apparently incident-free service). They must then comply with the medical standards, and some fail.

We undertook a survey of colour contingent tasks with regard to colours used, redundancy of coding and significance of error, both safety and financial. From this were identified the most critical issues on the basis that the worst case sets the colour vision testing and pass criteria needed. This was carried out at the NSWFB Training College and selected fire stations in Sydney with the assistance of the fire-fighters at those locations. The training college also houses the communications room for the Sydney area.

Results of survey

Examples of the more critical colour coding

Hydraulic and pressure hoses used for cutting, spreading, and lifting

Hydraulic lines and air bag hoses are coded various colours. The newer hydraulic lines are coded red and blue, which obviates the problem, but older colour codes are more complex. The colours also vary between manufacturers. The codes allow fire-fighters using the equipment to communicate which line is of interest to the person controlling the power. Errors may result in serious injury or damage.

Triage labels

Triage Tags are also used by fire fighters in multiple services incidents. They are used to denote "Dead" (white with a black border), "Walking" (fluorescent yellow-green), "Priority #1" (fluorescent red-pink) and "Priority #2" (fluorescent orange). The tags are labelled in writing but, particularly at a distance, their fluorescent colour is the indicator of the severity of injury. Only the "Dead" label is effectively non-colour coded, having a printed border.

Immobilisation devices

In the rescue service the Kendrick Extrication Device and the Paraguard immobilisation devices are used. Both have colour coded straps, which assist with fitting and buckling correctly. Although the position of the straps is a good indicator of accuracy, colour codes may play a significant role, especially when used in awkward and complex surroundings.

Computer displays in Communications Unit

The communications centre also relies on colour codes. Fire-fighters working here receive emergency calls and communicate these to the relevant stations. Much of the display screen used for this purpose is colour coded and owing to the nature of the work, speed is critical and errors are potentially disastrous. For example, the red and green phosphors are used to denote available and unavailable vehicles.

Gas detectors

Gas detector tubes include a CO_2 detector, oil detector, and CO detector. These change shades of colour according to the level of gas present.

Indicator papers

These are essentially the same as seen in any chemical laboratory. The colour(s) involved depends on the analysis being undertaken.

Building evacuation and fault indicator systems

Fire alarm panels play a vital role in identifying the location of a fire. The panels are clearly labelled to identify different zones and each zone has a light emitting diode (LED), which lights up red when there is an alarm. An amber/yellow LED lights up if there is a fault and a green LED may also be lit to indicate an "OK" status. These colours are specified in the Australian Standards AS 4428.1-1998.

Fire extinguishers

Portable fire extinguishers are colour coded to indicate the type. The specific colours are listed in the Australian Standards AS/NZS 1841.1:1997. Fire-fighters need to be able to recognize the type of extinguisher and do so primarily by the colour although it may be possible to identify each by the nozzle; in particular the carbon dioxide extinguisher (black) has a large nozzle, which means it is easy to identify.

Gas cylinders

Industrial gas cylinders are also colour coded to identify their contents. The colour codes are listed in the Australian Standards AS 4484-1997. Rapid and accurate identification is required in order for the fire-fighters to deal with each cylinder appropriately. Gas cylinders are identified mainly by their colour although other clues may be present. Cylinders are usually labelled, but in certain situations, such as identifying the cylinders from a distance, the labels are not easily read. Different sizes and nozzle shapes may be further clues to identification. LPG and refrigeration gases are similar in shape, but are a different size to other gas cylinders. Acetylene tends to be in a wider shorter cylinder but may not be easily differentiated under adverse conditions. Helium and carbon dioxide have a different nozzle, but again this may not always be easily identifiable.

Pipes and ducts

Water, steam, oil and combustible liquids, gases, vapours and dusts, acids and alkalis, air, other fluids, and electricity each have a colour code for the pipes or ducts carrying them.

Smoke and flames

The colour of smoke and flames give clues to the substances burning and whether a building may be entered. There are no standard charts and the classification is by colour name.

Colour as an issue in detection

When fighting bush fires, fire-fighters must be able to locate and identify the, primarily red, vehicles and their colleagues amongst the green and brown bush. A major factor in fire-fighter deaths in bush fires is loss of visual contact with the fire service vehicle. The NSWFB has independently made the decision that vehicles would remain red and white rather than the yellow favoured in some countries (Solomon 1990).

Colorimetric survey—measurement of more critical tasks

The more critical colour contingent decisions (on the advice of NSWFB personnel) were surveyed colorimetrically and documented. The full documentation included the colours used, significance of colour coding and consequence of error. Measurements were made with a Minolta P503I spectrophotometer with a wavelength range 400–10–700 nm 10-nm half spectral bandwidth and 0°/total geometry. The spectrophotometer was calibrated using set of 12 British Ceramic Research Association tiles for which calibration data had been provided by the National Physical Laboratory calibration 1986 and 1997 and also freshly pressed barium sulphate with reflectance data provided by Kodak. The chromaticities of the colours were calculated using CIE Standard Illuminant D_{65} and the CIE 1931 Standard Observer.

Results—colorimetric

Figures 36.1–36.3 show examples of the chromaticities of the colours used in fire extinguishers, gas cylinders and pipes and ducts respectively plotted in CIE 1976 colour space.

Table 36.1 then sets out the significant issues in each of these colour coding systems.

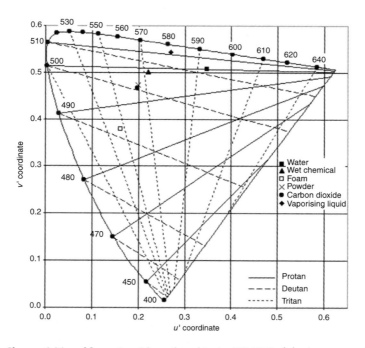

Figure 36.1 Chromaticities of fire extinguishers plotted in the CIE 1976 $u'v'$ colour space with the confusion lines for congenital colour vision deficient subjects superimposed.

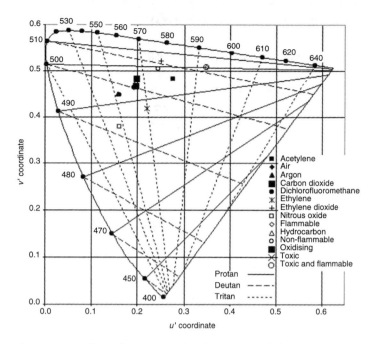

Figure 36.2 Chromaticities of gas cylinders plotted in the CIE 1976 $u'v'$ colour space with the confusion lines for congenital colour vision deficient subjects superimposed.

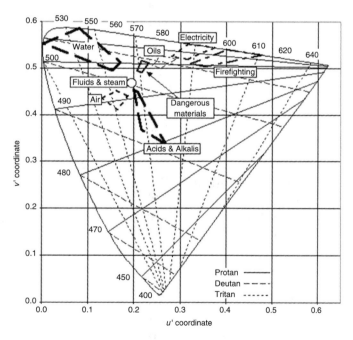

Figure 36.3 Chromaticities of pipes and ducts plotted in the CIE 1976 $u'v'$ colour space with the confusion lines for congenital colour vision deficient subjects superimposed.

Table 36.1 Colour coded Fire Brigade equipment, the colours used and the likely issues for colour vision deficient users

Equipment	Colours used	Equipment likely to be confused		
		Protans	Deutans	Tritans
Hydraulic lines and air bag hoses	Variety, including red, green, blue, white, and yellow. The new colours implemented on the hydraulic lines are red and blue.	The lines and hoses	The lines and hoses	The lines and hoses
Triage tags	Walking—green Dead—black 1st Priority—pink-red 2nd Priority—orange	Walking & 2nd Priority	Walking, 1st & 2nd Priority	
Communications	Red, Green, Magenta, Yellow, Black, White, Blue	Red, Green, Magenta, Black	Red, Green, Magenta	Blue, Yellow
LED displays on emergency fire panels	Fire—red Area Safe—green Malfunction—yellow/amber	Area Safe & Fire	Area Safe & Fire	
Industrial pipes	Water—Green, Steam—Silver, Oils—Brown, Gas—Yellow, Acids—Violet, Air—Light blue, Other Fluids—Black, Fire-Fighting—Red, Electricity—Orange, Communications—White	Water, Oils, electricity & Fire Fighting Air & Acids	Water & Oils	Water & Air Oils, & Acids
Gas cylinders	Acetylene—claret, Peacock blue—Argon, dichlorodifluoromethane; aqua ethylene—Violet; ethylene oxide—Buff, Flammable—Signal Red; Hydrocarbon—Silver; Nitrogen—Pewter; Nitrous oxide—Ultramarine, Non-flammable—Brown, Oxygen—Black, Toxic—Golden yellow.	Flammable, acetylene & Non-flammable	Nitrous Oxide & Ethylene	Nitrous Oxide, Argon, & Dichlorodifluoromethane
Sprinkler heads	White, Blue, Yellow, Red, Orange, Green, Blue, Mauve, and Black	Red, Orange, Green, Mauve, & Black	Red, Orange, Green, & Mauve	Blue, Yellow, Green, & Red

Discussion

Figures 36.1–36.3 and Table 36.1 demonstrate the complexity of the colour codes used and illustrate the propensity for error. In a qualitative way they demonstrate the need for a colour vision standard. While non-colour clues are sometime present, inadequate redundancy of coding from other clues point to the reliance on colour and the consequential need to frame a colour vision standard.

Conclusion

The critical tasks may be summarized as

1. Categorical colour coding of pipes, ducts, and gas cylinders.
2. LED signals on fire and evacuation panels.
3. Detection of fire service vehicles in a bush scene.

Acknowledgments

Dr Maryanne Dawson, NSWFB Chief Medical Officer, Trevor Dunn, NSWFB Medical Section, Jay Brand, NSWFB Fire-fighters Union and staff of the NSWFB and NSWFB Training College.

References

Margrain, T.H. & Birch, J.A. (1994). A suitable study to evaluate colour vision requirements for firefighters? *Occupational Medicine* (London) **44**(5): 257–8.

Margrain, T.H. Birch, J.A. & Owen, C.G. (1996). Colour vision requirements of firefighters. *Occupational Medicine* (London) **46**(2): 114–24.

Solomon, S. S. (1990). Lime-yellow as related to reduction of serious fire apparatus accidents: The case for visibility in emergency vehicle accident avoidance. *Journal of American Optometrical Association* **61**(11): 827–31.

CHAPTER 37

LANTERN COLOUR VISION TESTS: ONE LIGHT OR TWO?

JEFFERY K. HOVIS

Introduction

Shortly after the Second World War Neubert (1947) summarized a number of studies in which he compared the clinical efficacy of pseudoisochromatic plates and lantern colour vision tests. One of the interesting findings in his paper was how the pass rate of a lantern test was inversely related to the number of test lights displayed. He reported that 31 per cent of the subjects passed the lantern when the test lights were presented individually, 17 per cent passed when the lights were presented in pairs, and 6.6 per cent passed when the lights were presented as a triplet. Neubert attributed the higher failure rates to changes in the test lights' appearance as a result of simultaneous contrast affects. This result suggests that care should be taken in using lantern tests as an occupationally related colour vision test when there is a disparity in the number of lights displayed by the lantern and the actual task.

Although the number of lights in the lantern display appear to be an important performance parameter in Neubert's study, there were a few design and protocol issues that could have also contributed to his findings. First, each subject set the intensity of the lights by adjusting a rheostat so that the lights were easily seen. This means that the intensity and chromaticity coordinates of the test lights may not have been constant across conditions or subjects. Second, it is not clear whether the total number of presentations was equated in each display condition. If the total number of lights is less on the single light presentations, then observers who were "guessing" on some presentations would be more likely to pass the test because the total probability of making a single error is lower compared to trials where more test lights are presented. Finally, the lantern in Neubert's study used a yellow test light instead of white along with green and red so that the results may not be valid for aviation and maritime signal light colours.

Because it appears that the performance on lantern tests depends on the number of test lights displayed, this study investigates how the pass/fail results are affected when one or two test lights are displayed at each presentation.

Methods

Lantern

The lantern used in this study was a prototype to be used for the civilian maritime industry. It displayed either one light or two horizontally separated lights. The basic design of this prototype lantern was similar to the Holmes–Wright B lantern except that the prototype lantern test lights were dimmer in the single aperture mode and brighter in double aperture mode (Holmes and Wright 1982).

The individual test lights subtended an angle of 26-s arc at the 4.6-m test distance and the pair was separated by 20-min arc. There were 4 red lights, 3 green lights and 4 white lights presented in the single light sequence. Figure 37.1 shows the chromaticity coordinates and point brilliance of the test lights used in this study. The single red colour was presented at one of three different intensities. The point brilliance of the lights was calculated from the luminance measured with a Minolta LS-100 with a 10× close-up lens attached and the 4.6-m viewing distance.

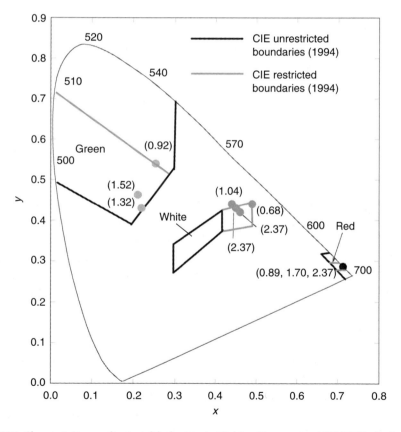

Figure 37.1 Chromaticity coordinates of the lantern test lights with respect to 1994 CIE limits for signal lights (CIE 1994). Values listed in the parentheses are the point brilliances of the test lights in μlux.

Table 37.1 Frequencies of the different types of congenital red–green colour vision deficiencies participating in the study and the prevalences in the Caucasian population for comparison (Pokorny *et al.* 1979).

Type of defect	Per cent in study ($N = 62$)	Per cent in Caucasian colour-defective population
Deuteranomalous	32	64
Protanomalous	15	12
Deuteranope	33	12
Protanope	21	12

Subjects

One hundred colour-normals and 62 colour-defectives participated in the study. Subjects were recruited through advertisements in local papers, electronic bulletin boards and flyers. They all reported that they were in good health. The only visual problems reported were refractive errors, amblyopia due to strabismus, colour vision deficiencies, or any combination of the three conditions. Corrected acuities were at least 6/9 in the better eye and 6/18 in the worse eye. The better eye acuity limit was based on the visual acuity standard for Canadian civilian maritime personnel. The mean age of the colour-normal group was 30 years (SD $\pm$ 10) and the mean age of the colour-defectives group was 31 years (SD $\pm$ 14). The difference in mean ages was not significant (t-test; $p \leq 0.05$).

Table 37.1 shows the frequencies of the different types of red-green colour vision deficiencies within the sample. Relative to the expected prevalence in the Caucasian colour-defective population, there was a higher frequency of deuteranopes and protanopes with a corresponding lower frequency of deuteranomalous individuals (Pokorny *et al.* 1979). These differences were significant (χ^2; $p < 0.05$). The result that the sample had a larger proportion of individuals with the more severe deficiencies was probably due to the degree of self selection created by the recruitment processes. The experiment protocol was reviewed and approved by the University of Waterloo Office of Research Ethics.

Testing procedure

Subjects were administered a variety of colour vision tests in this study. This paper will present only the results of the Nagel Anomaloscope and the one lantern test. The anomaloscope was administered before the lantern using the white adaptation mode. The anomaloscope findings were used to classify the colour vision of all subjects.

The lantern test was administered in a dark room after 9 min of adaptation to this light level. Stray light falling in the plane of either the observer or the lantern was no greater than 0.01 lux. Subjects were informed that there would be either one or two small coloured lights presented. They were to identify the colours as red, green, or white. After examples of each were shown, 11 single test lights were presented followed by 11 paired lights for practice. No feedback was given about their performance on the practice series. The trial was then repeated, with the single lights presented before the paired lights. There was no time limit for the presentation, but subjects were prompted for a response after 5 s. If a subject used a colour name that was not one of the acceptable responses, then s/he was reminded of the possible answers and the presentation was repeated.

Results

Pass/fail

The single (S-series) and double (D-Series) light test series were scored separately. Scoring was based on the worst performing colour-normal individual (worst-normal) on each series. The worst-normal criterion was used because the intended purpose of the lantern was to administer it to only those individuals who fail a colour vision screening test. All colour-normals also passed the Ishihara screening test.

The maximum number of errors made by any colour-normal was one. One individual made an error on the S-Series and another individual had a single error on the D-Series. None of the colour-normals made an error on both the S- and D-Series and so the failing score was more than one error for each series.

Twenty-two per cent of the colour-defectives passed the S-Series and 5 per cent passed the D-Series. Figure 37.2 shows the percentages for each type of defect who passed each series. Note that all the deuteranomalous individuals who passed the D-Series also passed S-Series. These deuteranomalous individuals all had a mild defect with a range on the Nagel anomaloscope that was no larger than 10 units. There were no colour-defective

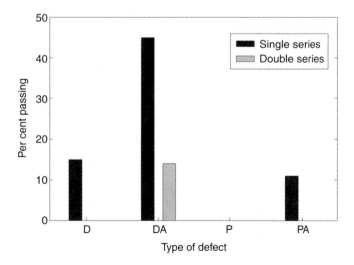

Figure 37.2 Percentages of the various types of colour vision defectives who passed on the single and double light presentations. D corresponds to deuteranopia, DA corresponds to deuteranomaly, P corresponds to protanopia and PA corresponds to protanomaly.

individuals who failed S-Series and then passed the D-Series. This includes the practice trial.

Number and types of errors

The colour-defective group was subdivided into those who passed the S-Series ($P_{S\text{-Series}}$) and those who failed the S-Series ($F_{S\text{-Series}}$) in order to determine the reason for the difference in performance on the two displays. Figure 37.3 shows the mean percent errors made by the each subgroup for each condition. The figure shows a number of trends that are expected based on the subject stratification. These are the differences in errors for the two groups for the S-Series and the increase in the percent errors on the D-Series for the $P_{S\text{-Series}}$ group. The unique feature of the results is the interaction between the groups and test conditions. The $P_{S\text{-Series}}$ group percent errors increased on the D-Series, whereas the percent errors for the $F_{S\text{-Series}}$ group did not change with the number of lights displayed. That is, the performance for the $F_{S\text{-Series}}$ did not worsen when the number of lights increased or with the addition of an adjacent light. The main effects and interaction were significant (ANOVA with subjects nested within display; $p \leq 0.05$ rejection level).

Figure 37.4 shows the frequency of the different errors made on the individual lights for each display and group. Both groups showed some similar trends in types and number of errors they made. These trends were that errors on the red test lights were infrequent and the frequency was not affected by the display; errors on the green lights were more frequent; the most common green error was misnaming it white; the white test light was misnamed frequently in both displays. Differences between the groups include the result

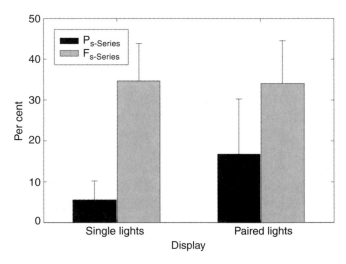

Figure 37.3 Mean of the total errors (in percent) made by the group who passed on the S-Series and those who failed on the S-Series for the single and paired light displays. Error bars represent one standard deviation.

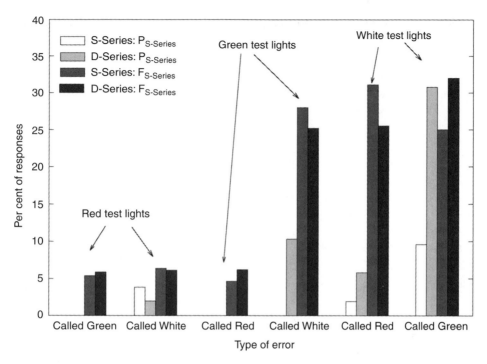

Figure 37.4 Percentages of the different types of incorrect responses made by the $P_{S\text{-Series}}$ and $F_{S\text{-Series}}$ subjects on the single light display (S-Series) and paired light display (D-Series).

that errors made by the $P_{S\text{-Series}}$ subjects on the S-Series display were relatively infrequent for all colours, but their errors increased on the white and green lights in the D-Series. In contrast, the number of errors made on the D-Series by the $F_{S\text{-Series}}$ group remained relatively constant across displays. The difference between the S-Series and D-Series for this latter group was that the nature of the errors changed. For example, the majority of errors on the individual white lights were misnaming it as red, but the majority of the mistakes on the white lights in the paired display was misnaming it as green.

Discussion

The major finding of this study was that the lantern was easier to pass for some colour-defectives when only one light was displayed. The pass rate for a single light display was 22 per cent as compared to 5 per cent for the paired-light display. This result confirms Neubert's earlier findings (Neubert 1947). This study also showed that the group who passed the single light display was fairly heterogeneous in terms of the severity of the defect, while it appears that only individuals with mild colour vision defects can pass the paired-light display. This finding could explain some of the variability in correlations between lantern tests and field trials when the number of lights displayed differ in the two tests. (Hovis and Oliphant 1999; Sloan-Rowland 1943; Kinney *et al.* 1979; Steen *et al.* 1974) Of course, there were other factors in these studies that could have also contributed to the variability. These factors include differences in brightness and colour between the lantern and field trial displays.

The result that dichromats were present in the $P_{S-Series}$ group suggests that the correlation between a lantern that presents single lights and clinical colour vision tests will be relatively lower than with lanterns that present pairs of test lights.

The issue that these results cannot directly address is whether the increase in the errors on the D-Series for the $P_{S-Series}$ group was due to the increase in the total number of lights or to the contrast effects of an adjacent light. We believe that, for the majority of the $P_{S-Series}$ subjects, the increase in errors was due to the contrast affects. Support for this conclusion comes from pooling the first and second S-Series trials. This would be equivalent to presenting the same number of test lights as a single D-Series. The mean percent errors for the pooled $P_{S-Series}$ group increased slightly to 8.7 per cent (SD : ±6.8) versus 5.6 per cent for the second S-Series shown in Fig. 37.2. However, the pooled value for the S-Series remained significantly lower than the percent error on the second D-Series for this group. This indicates that the difference in the total number of lights presented in the S-Series and D-Series did not account for the increase in errors on the D-Series for $P_{S-Series}$ group.

The increase in the mean percentage of errors when the practice session was included was obviously due to the fact the $P_{S-Series}$ subjects had more errors on the practice session. However, the mean percent errors for the two S-Series were not significantly different (paired *t*-test; $p < 0.05$). The $F_{S-Series}$ group exhibited a small nonsignificant decrease in errors on the second trial. Although there was not a significant difference in the percent of errors made by the colour-defectives on the two S-Series trials, the reduction in the mean percent errors on the second trial indicates that there was learning present even without feedback.

Despite the fact that the increase in errors on the D-Series was probably due to contrast effects and not due to a probability summation effect for the majority of subjects, there was one exception. A protanomalous subject actually passed on the first S-Series, but failed the second presentation. He also failed on both D-Series. This result suggests that there is a minority of colour-defectives who will do worse if more test lights are presented based on probability summation or perhaps a fatigue effect. This last result is also consistent with the previous studies which showed that a small number of colour-defectives can pass the Holmes–Wright Type A lantern when the minimum number of test lights is presented, but did not pass when the number of lights are increased or the test is repeated (Hovis and Oliphant 1998; Birch 1999).

Figure 37.4 shows the frequency of the different types of errors made by the two groups on the coloured test lights for the two displays. The types of errors made by both groups on the test lights follow the trends shown in previous studies. Errors on the red lights are extremely infrequent if the lights are visible and confusing green and white lights with each other are the most common errors (Kinney *et al.* 1979; Birch

1999) The difference between the groups is that the $P_{S\text{-Series}}$ group made more errors on the D-Series, particularly on the white test lights, whereas the frequency of errors on the different test lights for the $F_{S\text{-Series}}$ group showed minor changes on the two displays.

The nature of the errors made by the $P_{S\text{-Series}}$ on the D-Series white lights was generally consistent with simultaneous colour contrast effects. That is, white-called-green responses tended to occur when the white light was paired with a red light and white-called-red errors tended to occur when the white was paired with a green light. In all cases, the red and green coloured light were identified correctly by the subjects. The one result that is more difficult to explain is that these subjects misnamed a dim white light green when it was paired with another white light, regardless of whether or not the brighter white light was identified correctly. This suggests that the brightness difference between the two whites were being interpreted as a hue difference, with the dimmer white mistaken for green. One might expect predominantly green error responses because the majority of subjects in $P_{S\text{-Series}}$ group were deutan. However, this was also the most common error on this white-white pair for the protans. This type of behavior may be due to experience. In general, a green signal light would appear dimmer than a white light and colour-defectives have associated this brightness difference with the colour difference.

Consistent with the idea that $P_{S\text{-Series}}$ subjects were interpreting dim lights as green was the result that errors on green lights were lower when it was the dimmer member of the green-white pair (11.3 per cent errors) than when it was the brighter member of the pair (31 per cent errors). Thus, the brightness differences, which were probably more obvious in simultaneous presentation, confounded their hue judgements with the dimmer light identified as green and the brighter light identified as white.

The errors made on the white lights by the $F_{S\text{-Series}}$ group also showed some contrast effects despite the fact that there was a more equal representation of protans and deutans. The most common error on a single dim white light was red for both protans and deutans. However, when the dim white light was paired with either a white or red light, the errors changed to green. This is why the most frequent type of white light error changed from red on the S-Series to green on the D-Series.

Errors on the green lights were also similar between the protan and deutans in the $F_{S\text{-Series}}$ group. The most common error on the green light in the S-Series was misnaming it as white. However, when the same light was paired with a red light, then the green light was identified correctly as expected based on the contrast effects. This decrease in errors on the green lights when presented with red lights has been reported previously; particularly when the green is dimmer (Heath and Schmidt 1959; Chapanis 1949). When a green light was paired with a white light, then the frequencies of both types of errors increased slightly. However, because there were more pairs of red-green lights in the D-Series, the net result was little change in the total number of errors on the green lights in D-Series display.

One may find it surprising that the percentage of errors on the D-Series display did not increase for the $F_{S\text{-Series}}$ group. There are at least three reasons for this result. First, as mentioned previously, there was actually decrease in errors made on the green lights when they were paired with a red light. This decrease in mistakes counteracted the increase in mistakes on other green lights in the D-Series. Second, there may have been a ceiling effect on the errors made on dim white test lights. These lights were the ones most often missed by all colour-defectives, but mean percentage of errors on these dim lights for the $F_{S-Series}$ group when presented individually was slightly over 65 per cent with 76 per cent of the subjects making errors on both the S-Series and D-Series. Thus, it would be difficult for the number of errors to increase since it was already near the maximum for S-Series. Third, not every possible combination of the 11 test lights was presented in the pair displayed. In particular, green–green and red–red pairs were not presented. This was due to a design limitation of the lantern and probably affects the overall error rate. Although the simultaneous contrast effects may not have affected the percentage of errors made by the $F_{S-Series}$ group, these effects did influence the nature of their errors.

Conclusion

This study demonstrates that the number of lights displayed in a lantern test is another important design consideration, along with intensity, size and colour, to consider when validating lantern tests against a field test. Generally, increasing the number of lights increases the failure rate. This difference in the pass rates for the single and paired light displays suggests that some of the variability reported in the studies correlating lantern tests to field tests may be due to the difference in the number of lights presented in the different displays. The increased failure rate is probably due to a combination of simultaneous contrast effects and simultaneous comparison of the adjacent lights. The simultaneous contrast effects could be either in terms of chromatic effects or brightness effect. Simultaneous comparison makes any brightness or hue differences more obvious which may confound the observers' judgements. White lights are most susceptible to contrast effects especially if the observer relies on brightness clues to help in colour discrimination.

Acknowledgements

I thank Steven Gibson and Richard Samuell for their assistance in this project. This work was carried out under contract with Transport Canada, Marine Safety.

References

Birch, J. (1999). Performance of red–green color deficient subjects on the Holmes–Wright Lantern (Type A) in photopic viewing. *Aviation Space and Environmental Medicine*, 70, 897–901.

Chapanis, A. (1949). Simultaneous chromatic contrast in normal and abnormal color vision. *American Journal of Psychology*, 62, 526–39.

Commission Internationale de l'Eclairage (1994). *Review of the Official Recommendations of the CIE for the Colours of Signal Lights* CIE 107-1994. Vienna, Austria.

Heath, G. G. & **Schmidt, I.** (1959). Signal color recognition by color defective observers. *American Journal of Optometry Archives of the American Academy of Optometry,* 36, 421–37.

Holmes, J. G. & **Wright, W. D.** (1982). A new color-perception lantern. *Colour Research and Application,* 7, 82–8.

Hovis, J. K. & **Oliphant, D.** (1998). Validity of the Holmes–Wright lantern as a color vision test for the rail industry. *Vision Research,* 38, 3487–92.

Kinney, J. S., Paulson, H. M., & **Beare, A. N.** (1979). The ability of colour defectives to judge signal lights at sea. *Journal of the Optical Society of America,* 69, 106–13.

Neubert, F. R. (1947). Colour vision in the consulting room. *British Journal of Ophthalmology,* 31, 275–88.

Pokorny, J., Smith, V. C., Verriest, G., & **Pinckers, A. J. L. G.** (1979). *Congenital and Acquired Colour Vision Defects.* New York: Grune and Stratton.

Sloan-Rowland, L. (1943). *Selection and validation of tests for color vision—Relationship between degree of color deficiency and ability to identify signals from a biscuit gun.* Army Air Forces School of Aviation Medicine Project No 137 Report No 7, Randolph Field, Texas.

Steen, J. A., Collins, W. E., & **Lewis, M. F.** (1974). Utility of several clinical tests of color defective vision in predicting daytime and night time performance with the aviation signal light gun. *Aerospace Medicine,* 45, 467–72.

CHAPTER 38

EXTREME ANOMALOUS TRICHROMATISM

JENNIFER BIRCH

Introduction

A spectral anomaloscope is the reference test for identifying and diagnosing different types of congenital red–green colour deficiency. The Nagel anomaloscope presents a Rayleigh colour match in a 3° circular bipartite field. The reference colour is a monochromatic yellow wavelength (589 nm), which can be altered in luminance. An exact match must be obtained in the other half of the field of view with a suitable mixture of monochromatic red and green wavelengths (670 and 546 nm). Normal trichromats make precise colour matches within a small range of red/green mixture ratios. The normal matching range, mean match and standard deviation must be established for a particular instrument. The matching ranges of protanomalous and deuteranomalous trichromats form two separate distributions (Birch 1983). Protanomalous trichromats require significantly more red in their mixture ratio and deuteranomalous trichromats require significantly more green. The extent of the matching range varies individually and demonstrates the severity of the discrimination deficit. Some severe deuteranomalous trichromats are able to match all red/green ratios from pure green to the short wavelength limit of the normal matching range. Protanomalous trichromats never match pure red but part of the long wavelength portion of the normal matching range may be included in the matching range. Protanopes and deuteranopes are able to match all red/green mixture ratios with yellow, including pure red and pure green, by altering the luminance of the yellow reference field. When a match is made, the yellow luminance setting provides information about the relative luminous efficiency of the eye. Protanopes and protanomalous trichromats have reduced sensitivity to long wavelengths and the match at the long wavelength limit of the matching range is always made with low yellow luminance. Deuteranopes and deuteranomalous trichromats make matches at the limits of the matching range with approximately the same yellow luminance value.

Careful examination of individual matching ranges with the Nagel anomaloscope shows that some colour deficient subjects are able to match with both an excess of red and an excess of green but are unable to match all red/green mixture ratios. The term extreme anomalous trichromatism was proposed by Walls (1959) for these colour deficient people. This paper describes anomaloscope and clinical colour vision test results for 27 extreme anomalous trichromats.

Subjects and methods

A review was made of records obtained for 781 people with red–green colour deficiency (759 males and 22 females). All subjects were identified by failure of the Ishihara plates and diagnosis of the type of colour deficiency was made with the Nagel anomaloscope (Birch 1997a). There were 471 anomalous trichromats (454 males and 17 females). In this group, 27 unrelated subjects (24 males and 3 females) were diagnosed as extreme anomalous trichromats. In each case, the limits of the matching range were determined to an accuracy of 2 scale units on the red/green mixture scale. The yellow luminance scale value was recorded at these limits. Pure green is at 0 and pure red at 73 on the red/green mixture scale. The mean yellow luminance for a match with pure red was found to be 2 scale units (SD+/−0.6) in protanopia and 15 scale units (SD+/−2.5) in deuteranopia. The mean yellow luminance for a match with pure green was found to be 29 scale units (SD + / − 4.0) in protanopia and 16 scale units (SD + / − 1.8) in deuteranopia. The mean normal match is at 44 (SD + / − 2 scale units). In addition to the Ishihara plates, all 27 subjects completed the American Optical Company (Hardy, Rand, and Rittler) plates (HRR plates) and the Farnsworth D15 test (D15). Classification of protan and deutan deficiency is more reliable with the HRR plates than with the Ishihara plates (Birch 1997b). The Farnsworth–Munsell 100 hue test (F–M 100 hue) was completed by 15 subjects (13 males and 2 females). Classification of the type of colour deficiency was recorded with both plate tests and estimated by visual inspection of the D15 and F–M 100 hue results diagrams. Severity of colour deficiency was estimated with the HRR grading plates, failure of the D15 test and the F–M 100 hue error score. Failure of the D15 test was one or more isochromatic colour confusions demonstrated across the hue circle in the results diagram (Birch 1997b). All pigment tests were illuminated with the MacBeth Easel lamp (Source C, 350 lux).

Results

Results are summarized in Table 38.1. Twelve subjects (11 males and 1 female) matched red/green mixture ratios which included pure green, 0 on the mixture scale, and extend almost to pure red at seventy-three on the mixture scale. Pure red was invariably described as "too red" to obtain a match with the reference yellow. The yellow luminance for a match with full green varied between 35 and 15 scale units. These values included typical values obtained by protanopes (high values) and deuteranopes (low values). The yellow luminance at the red limit of the matching range was between 2 and 13 scale units for subjects who matched full green and between 5 and 25 scale units for the remaining subjects. These values also include typical values obtained by protanopes (low values) and deuteranopes (high values) for these red/green mixture ratios. In Table 38.1, a yellow luminance setting at the green limit of the matching range is recorded as "High" if within 2SD of the protanopic mean value and "Low" if within 2SD of the deuteranopic mean value. At the red limit of the matching range, the yellow luminance is recorded as "Low"

Table 38.1 Summary of clinical test results for 27 extreme anomalous trichromats diagnosed with the Nagel anomaloscope

| Sub. | M/F | Nagel anomaloscope | | | Ishihara plates | AO HRR plates | | D15 | F-M 100 hue | |
		Match Range	Green limit Lum.	Red limit Lum.	Class	Class	Grade	Class	Error score	Class
1	M	0–70	High	Low	Protan	Protan	Severe	Pass	104	Protan
2	M	0–70	Low	Low	Red–green	Deutan	Severe	Red–green	480	None
3	F	0–70	High	Low	Protan	Protan	Severe	Red–green	252	None
4	M	0–68	High	Low	Protan	Protan	Severe	Red–green	—	—
5	M	0–65	High	Low	Protan	Protan	Severe	Protan	208	Protan
6	M	0–65	High	Low	Protan	Protan	Severe	Protan	92	Protan
7	M	0–65	Equal		Red–green	Protan	Severe	Red–green	92	None
8	M	0–65	Low	Low	Protan	Protan	Severe	Red–green	364	Deutan
9	M	0–65	High	Low	Protan	Protan	Severe	Protan	—	—
10	M	0–65	High	Low	Red–green	Protan	Severe	Red–green	—	—
11	M	0–62	High	Low	Protan	Protan	Severe	Protan	—	—
12	M	0–62	High	Low	Protan	Protan	Slight	Protan	128	Deutan
13	M	0–62	Low	Low	Deutan	Deutan	Severe	Red–green	—	—
14	M	0–60	Equal		Deutan	Deutan	Severe	Pass	136	Deutan
15	M	0–60	High	Low	Deutan	Protan	Severe	Pass	—	—
16	M	0–60	Equal		Deutan	Deutan	Severe	Deutan	—	—
17	M	0–60	High	Low	Protan	Protan	Severe	Protan	—	—
18	M	0–60	High	Low	Protan	Protan	Severe	Protan	—	—
19	F	0–58	High	Low	Red–green	Deutan	Severe	Protan	—	—
20	F	2–54	Equal		Protan	Pass	—	Pass	176	None
21	M	6–68	Equal		Red–green	Deutan	Slight	Pass	144	Deutan
22	M	10–70	High	Low	Red–green	Protan	Severe	Pass	112	Protan
23	M	15–60	High	Low	Red–green	Red–green	Slight	Red–green	168	Deutan
24	M	15–60	High	Low	Protan	Protan	Slight	Protan	84	Protan
25	M	25–60	High	Low	Protan	Protan	Severe	Protan	104	Protan
26	M	25–60	High	Low	Protan	Protan	Severe	Protan	—	—
27	M	30–60	Low	Low	Protan	Protan	Severe	Red–green	—	—

if within 2SD of the protanopic mean value and "High" if within 2SD of the deuteranopic value. The yellow luminance values at the matching limits were approximately equal in five subjects and were typical of deutan luminance values.

Protan/deutan classification was obtained for 20 subjects with the Ishihara plates and for 25 subjects with the HRR plates (Table 38.2). The HRR plates mainly obtained a classification when the Ishihara did not and was different for only one person (subject 15). One female subject was classified as protan by the Ishihara plates but passed the HRR plates and the D15 without error. One male subject was not classified by the Ishihara plates and made an equal number of protan and deutan errors on the HRR plates. The HRR test graded colour deficiency as severe in 22 subjects and slight in four subjects.

The D15 test was failed by 21 subjects indicating significant colour deficiency. Only 1 of the 5 subjects who passed the D15 was graded as slightly colour deficient by the HRR plates. The D15 error pattern was typically protan for 11 subjects, deutan for one subject and equivocal for nine subjects. One female subject was classified as protan by the D15 and deutan by the HRR plates. Error scores obtained by the 15 subjects who completed the F–M 100 hue test varied between 84 and 480. The axis of confusion was protan for six subjects and deutan for 5 subjects. The remaining four subjects demonstrated poor overall hue discrimination. The F–M 100 hue classification differed from the HRR classification for five subjects. A summary of the classification results is shown in Table 38.3.

The normal matching range for the Nagel anomaloscope is 44 (SD + / − 2 scale units), pure green is a 0 and pure red at 73 on the red/green mixture scale. Individual matching ranges and the yellow luminance setting at the extremes of the matching range are shown. Protan /deutan classification with the Ishihara plates, classification and grading of severity with the American Optical Company (Hardy, Rand, and Rittler) plates and

Table 38.2 Classification of the type of colour deficiency obtained with individual clinical tests

	Number of subjects	Protan	Deutan	Red–green
Ishihara plates	27	16	4	7
AO HRR plates	26	19	6	1
Farnsworth D15	21	11	1	9
F–M 100 Hue test	15	6	5	4

Table 38.3 Classification of the type of colour deficiency obtained for 27 extreme anomalous trichromats from all clinical tests failed

	Protan	Protan and red–green	Deutan	Deutan and red–green	Mixed protan, deutan, and red–green
Number of subjects	10	7	2	4	4

classification results for Farnsworth D15 tests and the Farnsworth–Munsell 100 Hue test (and the error score) are also shown.

Discussion

Progress in the molecular genetics of colour vision deficiency relies on matching phenotype with genotype. It is therefore essential that accurate diagnosis of the type of red–green colour deficiency is obtained and that unusual phenotypes, such as extreme anomalous trichromatism, are identified. Accurate diagnosis is obtained by careful determination of the limits of the red–green matching range on a spectral anomaloscope. Extreme anomalous trichromats make matches with a significant excess of both red and green light but are unable to match all red–green mixture ratios.

Extreme anomalous trichromatism is a heterogenous type of colour deficiency but, as in protanomalous and deuteranomalous trichromatism, some unrelated subjects obtain identical anomaloscope matching ranges (Table 38.1). Protanomalous and deuteranomalous trichromats who obtain the same anomaloscope matching range also set the same yellow luminance values suggesting that the genotype is the same. However, some extreme anomalous trichromats obtain identical matching ranges but the range of yellow luminance scale values show that there are large differences in relative luminous efficiency. Luminance values at the limits of the matching range include both typical protan and deutan characteristics. Protan luminance values, with characteristic reduced sensitivity to long wavelength red light, predominate in this group of subjects. Differences in relative luminous efficiency may result from variations in expression of the same abnormal cone photopigments with the photopigment expressed at the highest level having the major influence. Alternatively, differences in relative luminous efficiency may result from expression of a range of different abnormal photopigments which coincidentally produce the same hue discrimination deficit.

In the present study, protan/deutan classification with clinical tests was unusually variable, and inconsistent, both for individuals and for the group as a whole. This is not found in groups of protanomalous and deuteranomalous trichromats. Only 12 of the 27 subjects were classified unequivocally by all the tests completed, 10 as protan and 2 as deutan. The 10 subjects classified as protan all made anomaloscope matches with typical protan luminance values and the two subjects classified as deutan both made anomaloscope matches with typical deutan (equal) yellow luminance values at the limits of the anomaloscope matching range. Classification was equivocal (red–green colour deficient) or inconsistent for the remaining 15 subjects. These results support the observations made by Walls (1959) that extreme anomalous trichromatism is a "mixed" type of protan/deutan colour deficiency and that protan/deutan classification is "unstable" with clinical tests. Walls (1959) also noted that most extreme anomalous trichromats have reduced sensitivity to long wavelength red light and suggested that mis-diagnosis as protanomalous trichromats, or protanopes, may occur in large population studies if the anomaloscope matching range is not fully explored.

The finding of three extreme anomalous trichromats in a group of twenty-two colour deficient females was unexpected. It was not possible to obtain information on inherited X chromosome genotypes because no colour deficient male relatives were available for examination. The mechanism governing expression of abnormal X chromosome photopigment genes is likely to be more complex in women than in men. Women who are compound mixed heterozygotes, for protan and deutan colour deficiency, are usually reported to have clinically normal colour vision. Some female heterozygotes can be identified from slightly abnormal anomaloscope matches. These findings suggesting that photopigment genes from both X chromosomes can be expressed in different cone receptors in the form of a retinal mosaic (Jordan and Mollon 1994). Heterozygotes for protan deficiency are more easily identified than heterozygotes for deutan deficiency because the anomaloscope mean match is slightly displaced towards red (Schmidt's sign).

The prevalence of anomalous trichromatism has been estimated to be approximately 6 per cent in the UK male population. Identification of 24 extreme anomalous trichromats from 759 anomalous trichromats suggests that the prevalence of this type of inherited colour deficiency is about 0.25 per cent of the male population.

References

Birch, J. (1997a) Efficiency of the Ishihara plates for identifying red–green colour deficiency. Ophthal. Physiol. Opt. 17: 403–8

Birch, J. (1997b) Clinical use of the American Optical Company (Hardy, Rand and Rittler) pseudoisochromatic plates for red–green colour deficiency. Ophthal. Physiol. Opt. 17: 248–54

Birch, J. (1983) Diagnosis of defective colour vision using the Nagel anomaloscope. Doc. Ophthalmol. Proc. Series 33, Ed. G. Verriest. Junk: The Hague; pp. 231–5

Jordan, G. and Mollon, J. D. (1993) A study of women heterozygous for colour deficiencies. Vision Res. 33: 1495–508

Walls, G. L. (1959) How good is the HRR test for color blindness? Amer. J. Optom. Archiv. Amer. Acad. Optom. 36: 169–93

COLOUR NAMING, COLOUR CATEGORIES, AND CENTRAL COLOUR-CODING IN A CASE OF X-LINKED INCOMPLETE ACHROMATOPSIA

J. B. NOLAN, M. A. CROGNALE, AND M. A. WEBSTER

Introduction

We have previously described the extent and molecular basis of colour vision deficits in a case of X-linked incomplete achromatopsia (Crognale *et al.* 2000). In the previous study we presented determinations of equiluminance as a function of light level, unique hue settings, colour discrimination ellipses, and electrophysiological findings. The psychophysical results revealed rod-based luminosity under all light levels and incomplete achromatopsia. Surprisingly, there was also a marked improvement along the tritan axis for discrimination ellipses (as measured by the Cambridge Colour test—a computer version of pseudoischromatic plate tests) (Regan *et al.* 1994) after a rod bleach. ERG recording of 30 Hz flicker failed to reveal evidence of cone function. VEP responses showed prolonged response latencies and abnormal waveforms for tritan, L–M cone isolation, and achromatic stimuli. In addition, molecular genetic results revealed an absence of L pigment genes and an inactivating mutation (C203R) (Nathans *et al.* 1989; Winderickx *et al.* 1992) in a subset of his M-pigment genes including the first gene in the array. The molecular results suggest that the subject's residual colour capacities were based largely upon rods and S-cone signals with a possibility of residual M-cone signals. The present study was conducted to examine categorical colour perception and the nature of central processing of colour in this individual. We also wished to extend our investigation of rod contribution to this subject's colour discrimination and colour categorization. Here, we present data from colour naming and categorization, colour contrast adaptation, and a battery of standard colour tests performed with and without a rod bleach.

Methods

Subject

The subject (JN) was a 33-year-old male with X-linked incomplete achromatopsia. Best-corrected visual acuities were 20/200 in both eyes. His threshold visual fields showed some areas of reduced macular sensitivity. Fundus examination showed both optic nerves with hazy, ill-defined borders. There appeared to be some optic disc elevation with no cupping. ERG measures revealed severely reduced photopic ERGs and no recordable 30 Hz flicker responses.

His pupillary reflexes were normal. His extraocular muscle movements were full and smooth in all fields of gaze. There was also some micronystagmus with slit lamp observation. A photostress recovery test appeared normal; 40 s (OD), 50 s (OS). The anterior segments of both eyes were normal. His intraocular pressures were normal.

Colour screening tests

A battery of standard clinical screening tests was used to measure colour discrimination including: the Farnsworth panel D-15, Ishihara (38-plate edition), Farnsworth Lantern test, and the FM 100 Hue test. Plate and arrangement tests were administered under standard lighting (Verilux). The subject was previously unaware that he had unusual colour vision and attributed most of his vision problems to his reduced visual acuity.

Colour categorizing

The procedures for colour categorizing were similar to those of previous studies (Berlin and Kay 1969). JN and control subjects were shown the full palette of maximum saturation Munsell chips (Fig. 39.1) and outlined which regions corresponded to each of the 11 basic colour names (white, black, pink, orange, yellow, red, brown, green, blue, purple, and gray).

Colour naming

A colour-naming task was conducted on J. N. and 2 control subjects using the OSA colour chip set and procedures similar to Boynton and Olson (1987). In this case, the subject provided colour names for the chips viewed in isolation and in a randomized sequence. Colour names were restricted to basic categories (red, green, blue, yellow, orange, brown, pink, gray, purple, and white). The chips were presented two times each to the controls and three times each for subject J. N.

Chromatic contrast adaptation

The contrast adaptation procedures followed those described previously (Webster and Mollon 1991). Briefly, stimuli were generated using a Cambridge Research graphics board and presented on a Sony Monitor. The subject viewed a fixation cross in the center of the display. The subject adapted for 3 min to a 5° square uniform region centered 3° above the fixation. During adaptation, colours in this region were modulated sinusoidally (1 Hz)

No rod bleach

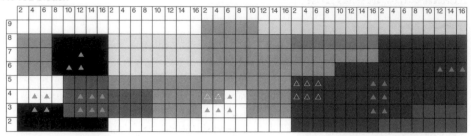

After rod bleach

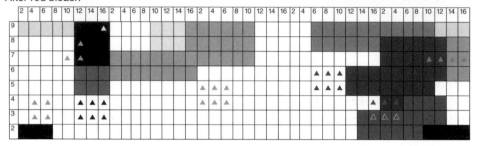

Figure 39.1 See colour plate section. Colour categories of J. N. and a control with and without a rod bleach. The array represents the palette of Munsell chips varying in lightness and chroma. Cell colours indicate the range of chips that subject J. N. chose for each colour term before (top) and after (bottom) rod bleach. Filled triangles indicate the corresponding range for a control subject. Open triangles indicate agreement between J. N. and the control.

along different directions in a two-dimensional receptor-based colour space defined by the achromatic axis and the equiluminant S-cone axis as defined by the observers luminosity function (the constant rod axis for J. N., or the constant L + M axis for the control). Following adaptation, the observer was then presented with a brief (0.5 s) test colour in the same region as the adaptation. The subject adjusted the luminance and/or chromaticity of a comparison field centered 3° below fixation to match the appearance of the test field. Adjustments were made during a 6-s "top up" period between test presentations. Since J. N. had difficulty adjusting both hue and contrast simultaneously, two conditions were run wherein adjustments were restricted to either hue or contrast for both subjects. Points plotted were based on the mean of four settings for each subject.

Rod contribution

The colour screening tests and colour categorization tasks were repeated after a 5-s exposure to an adapting light (4×10^7 scotopic trolands) chosen to strongly bleach the rods. The subject was tested between 2 and 6 min post adaptation and readapted every 6 min to maintain adaptation.

Results and discussion

Colour categorization

The results from the colour categorization of the Munsell palette for J. N. and a representative control can be seen in Fig. 39.1. The regions chosen by J. N. for the basic colour names without a rod bleach are quite large but were in rough agreement with those of the control subject. The control subject's categories were consistent with previous data from normal subjects. There are specific changes in J. N.'s categories consistent with his colour deficiencies (e.g. black for red consistent with a protan loss and enlarged colour regions consistent with reduced colour discrimination).

The colour regions chosen by J. N. after a rod bleach are significantly smaller than those without a bleach, in agreement with his subjective report of increased colour saturation and objective improvements on the Cambridge Colour test (Crognale *et al.* 2000). This reduction following a rod bleach may be further evidence for antagonistic rod input in this subject. This antagonism could take the form of inhibitory influence or a veiling noise corrupting the signals mediating his colour vision. After a bleach J. N.'s colour regions show similar mean differences from the control as before the bleach (red and yellow and orange towards green), but with additional shifts towards lighter values. In comparison, the control subject's settings are virtually identical before and after a bleach. That J. N. can continue to set consistent and reasonable values for colour categories despite his profound loss of colour vision suggests that the colour categorization task may depend strongly on learning of subtle cone-based cues and perhaps reveals little about his phenomenal experience of colour.

Colour naming with OSA chips

The results from the OSA colour naming are in general agreement with those from the Munsell palette with subject J. N. showing consistency in naming colours as well as characteristic shifts and confusions similar to those seen in the Munsell task. Table 39.1 shows results from a small sample of chips nearest to the centroids of colour regions from Boynton and Olson. Notably, J. N. is in agreement with the controls for most of these chips (shaded rows) even for yellow, which was shifted in the Munsell categorization task. Again purple, blue, and pink were confused. Consensus in naming was best near these chips and was somewhat worse in desaturated or dark regions. Pink was sometimes called white or blue by J. N. Yellows and oranges were sometimes called green, and purples were sometimes called blue. These data suggest that colour naming is largely intact in J. N. despite his inability to pass most colour vision tests. Again this suggests that J. N. is utilizing varied and subtle cues in order to produce fairly accurate colour naming from weak chromatic signals. Note that both the naming and categorization tasks do not necessarily rely on colour vision capabilities since other cues such as luminance differences could provide a basis for judging the chips. In the following experiments we therefore tested colour sensitivity directly.

Table 39.1 Colour naming for OSA chips near centroid values from Boynton and Olson. Shaded rows show focal colours which J. N. labelled consistently with controls

Colour	OSA chip			Subject						
	L	g	j	J. N.	J. N.	J. N.	A	A	R	R
red	−4	2	−8	pur	red	pur	red	red	pur	pur
green	0	4	2	grn	grn	grn	grn	grn	grn	grn
orange	0	6	−8	org	org	org	org	org	org	org
purple	−3	−3	−1	blu	pin	blu	pin	pin	pur	pin
gray	−1	1	−1	gry	pin	pin	gry	wht	brn	brn
pink	1	1	−5	blu	gry	blu	pin	pin	pin	pin
white	4	2	0	wht	wht	grn	wht	wht	wht	grn
brown	−3	3	−3	org	brn	brn	org	brn	brn	brn
yellow	3	9	−1	yel	yel	yel	yel	yel	yel	yel
blue	−1	−3	3	blu	blu	blu	blu	blu	blu	blu

Chromatic contrast adaptation

Contrast adaptation is believed to affect colour sensitivity at a cortical locus (Webster 1996). We therefore used this adaptation to explore central mechanisms of colour-coding in J. N. Contrast matching for a range of test contrast after adaptation showed similar *magnitudes* of adaptation for J. N and controls (Fig. 39.2(e) and (f)). However he showed less evidence for *selective* changes in adaptation—that is his settings showed less dependence on the particular adapting axis than the controls' (Fig. (39.2(a)–(d)). For J. N., when contrast was adjusted while hue was fixed, there was little evidence that the changes in perceived contrast were selective for either the S or Luminance axis (a) or along either intermediate directions (b) (i.e. along axes where rod and S signals varied in phase or in antiphase). In contrast the control subject (c and d) showed selective adaptation along all of these directions as indicated by the contours of the matches that were always oriented away from the adapting axis (because the largest contrast losses were along the adapting axis (Webster and Mollon 1991).

When contrast was fixed and hue was adjusted however, there were small but reliable shifts in the direction predicted by adaptation of selective mechanisms for both "cardinal" and intermediate adaptation axes for subject J. N. and for the control. For example adapting to the S axis rotated the perceived test angle toward the achromatic axis (filled triangles) or vice versa (unfilled triangles). Similarly, adapting to the +45° axis biased both the pure S and pure achromatic test toward the −45° axis or vice versa. While the shifts were small, for J. N. all 8 intermediate pairs shifted in the direction predicted by selective adaptation, a pattern that would be expected by chance with a probability of $1/2^8$ or <0.005.

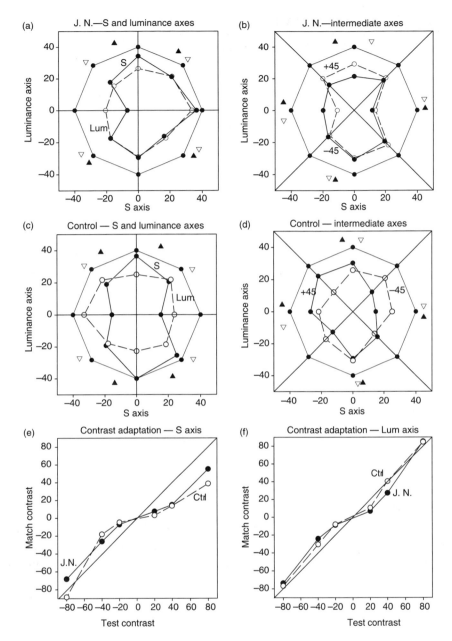

Figure 39.2 Chromatic contrast adaptation for J. N. and a control subject. Adaptation along S and luminance axes are shown in panels (a) and (c) while adaptation along the ±45°-intermediate axes are in panels (b) and (d) (upright filled triangles—S or +45° adaptation hue-angle matches; inverted open triangles—luminance or −45° adaptation hue—angle matches; open circles—pre-adaptation contrast matches; filled circles— post-adaptation contrast matches). In the panels (e) and (f) matching contrast is plotted as a function of test contrast for S and luminance conditions (open circles—control; filled circles—J. N.).

Table 39.2 Results of colour vision tests before and after a rod bleach

Test	Before bleach	After bleach
Ishihara	0/25 correct	0/25 correct

FM-100	TES = 708
	    low discrimination (no axis)
		TES = 796;
		    low discrimination (no axis)

D-15	Fail—protan and deutan errors	Fail—largely deutan errors
FALANT	Fail—1/9, 2/9 correct	Fail—4/9, 2/9 correct

The results from chromatic contrast adaptation thus suggest that J. N.'s central repres- entation of colour has mechanisms that can be weakly selective for modulations along a luminance and tritan axis. Residual M-cone function (which we did not test for) may provide further input to these mechanisms.

Rod influence

None of the standard colour tests performed in the present study revealed a change in colour discrimination after a strong rod bleach (Table 39.2). Of these tests, only the FM-100 and the D-15 could reveal tritan improvement after a bleach as was found previously with the Cambridge Colour test. However, the FM-100 failed to show any improvement after the rod bleach. The D-15 test showed initially a mixed deutan/protan axes of error. Performance on the D-15 showed no improvement after the rod bleach but the deutan error axis became more prominent (Smith and Pokorny 1980). Since a tritan axis is not observed in the unbleached condition, an improvement along the tritan axis could not be evaluated. Thus far, only discrimination measured with the Cambridge Colour test and our results from colour categorization support J. N.'s verbal report that colour vision appears improved after a rod bleach.

Conclusions

Despite profound colour deficiencies, the subject demonstrates consistent but shifted colour category and naming behavior, while showing weak evidence for selectively tuned central chromatic mechanisms. Results from colour categorization and discrimination, but not standard colour tests support antagonistic rod influences on colour vision.

References

Berlin, B. & Kay, P. (1969). *Basic Color Terms: Their Universality and Evolution.* Berkeley: University of California Press.

Boynton, R. M. & Olson, C. X. (1987). Locating basic colors in the OSA space. *Color Research and Application, 12*(2), 94–105.

Crognale, M. A., Nolan, J. B., Webster, M. A., Neitz, M., & Neitz, J. (2000). Color vision and genetics in a case of cone dysfunction syndrome. *Color Research and Application, 26,* S284–7.

Nathans, J., Davenport, C. M., Maumenee, I. H., Lewis, R. A., Hejtmancik, J. F., Litt, M., Lovrien, E., Weleber, R., Bachynski, B., Zwas, F., *et al.* (1989). Molecular genetics of human blue cone monochromacy. *Science, 245*(4920), 831–8.

Regan, B. C., Reffin, J. P., & Mollon, J. D. (1994). Luminance noise and the rapid determination of discrimination ellipses in colour deficiency. *Vision Research, 34*(10), 1279–99.

Smith, V. C. & Pokorny, J. (1980). Cone dysfunction syndromes defined by colour vision. In G. Verriest (Ed.), *Colour Vision Deficiencies V* (pp. 69–82). Bristol: Hilger.

Webster, M. A. (1996). Human colour perception and its adaptation. *Network: Computation in Neural Systems, 7*, 587–634.

Webster, M. A. & Mollon, J. D. (1991). Changes in colour appearance following post-receptoral adaptation. *Nature, 349*(6306), 235–8.

Winderickx, J., Sanocki, E., Lindsey, D. T., Teller, D. Y., Motulsky, A. G., & Deeb, S. S. (1992). Defective colour vision associated with a missense mutation in the human green visual pigment gene. *Nature Genetics, 1*(4), 251–6.

ACQUIRED DEFICIENCIES OF COLOUR VISION

EFFECTS OF RETINAL DETACHMENT ON S AND M CONE FUNCTION IN AN ANIMAL MODEL

GERALD H. JACOBS, JACK B. CALDERONE,

TSUTOMU SAKAI, GEOFFREY P. LEWIS, AND

STEVEN K. FISHER

Introduction

Detachment can physically damage the retina and disrupt the normal metabolic traffic between photoreceptors and the choroidal blood supply. These changes initiate a series of cellular and molecular events in the retina that can lead to profound retinal remodeling (Fisher and Anderson 2001). Among the many functional changes that may ensue are alterations in color vision. Nearly a century ago Köllner reported that blue–yellow defects are characteristic of patients with retinal detachment (Köllner 1907). Although subsequent research has revealed a more complex picture of color vision change than he described, the generalization that retinal detachment often leads to blue–yellow color defects remains intact (Pokorny *et al.* 1979; Fletcher and Voke 1985). Recent investigators have sought indications of detachment-induced changes in the retina that might correlate with the onset of blue–yellow color vision defects. Two such effects have been reported. First, the relative contributions from S and M/L cones of patients who had undergone reattachment surgery were assessed through measurement of the amplitudes of different waveform components of the electroretinogram (ERG). A lowered ratio of signals from S versus M/L cones was inferred suggesting that S cones were relatively more vulnerable to the damaging effects of detachment (Hayashi and Yamamoto 2001). Second, histochemical staining of human retinas that had suffered recent detachment indicated that S cones were almost entirely lost from the detachment zone while M/L cones were still abundantly present (Nork *et al.* 1995). Both of these outcomes imply that blue–yellow color defects following retinal detachment may result from alterations in the photoreceptors themselves and that, specifically, S cones are more susceptible to change under these conditions than M/L cones.

There are obvious limitations imposed on attempts to understand the biological basis of change induced by retinal detachment in clinical patients. Consequently, researchers have often turned to animal models in which the details of detachment can be controlled, their consequences can be more directly studied, and various therapeutic interventions can be evaluated. We have recently been examining the dynamics of retinal detachment and reattachment in ground squirrels. These rodents have cone-rich retinas and therefore offer an especially favorable context for studies of the influence of retinal detachment on contributions from S and M/L cone populations.

Methods

Subjects

Adult California ground squirrels (*Spermophilus beecheyi*) of both sexes were used. An abundance of information about retinal organization and vision in this species has been accumulated. The features that make this animal an attractive target for studies of cone-based vision are summarized elsewhere (Jacobs *et al.* 2002). For present purposes the most important of these is that the retina of the California ground squirrel contains two classes of cone totaling about 7.5 million receptors with M cones ($\lambda_{max} = 518$ nm) outnumbering S cones ($\lambda_{max} = 436$ nm) by an overall ratio of about 14 : 1.

Apparatus and procedures

ERGs were differentially recorded from contact lens electrodes installed on the eyes of ground squirrels anesthetized with a mixture of xylazine (9 mg/kg) and ketamine (70 mg/kg). Through a dilated pupil the animal viewed the screen of a computer-controlled color monitor (Radius, Intellicolor) positioned to subtend a rectangular area of 116 × 101 deg. The stimulus was a spatially uniform field, temporally modulated as a 37.5 Hz square wave (mean luminance = 50 cd/m^2). The control software was written in Matlab using extensions as described earlier (Brainard *et al.* 1999).

Stimuli modulating the contrast seen by either the S or the M cones were designed based on estimates of the spectral absorption properties of the ground squirrel cones as modified by measurements of absorption by the lens of this species (Jacobs *et al.* 2001). The maximum contrasts were 63.1 per cent for M cone stimulation and 76 per cent for S cone stimulation. The procedures for stimulus calibration and the recording apparatus have been described in detail (Jacobs *et al.* 1996; Brainard *et al.* 1999). In brief, analog hardware was used to window the amplified ERG signal with a sinusoid set to the frequency of the stimulus train (37.5 Hz). For each stimulus sequence the position of the window was shifted to maximize its correlation with the ERG signal. The window positions could then be used to extract information about the relative phases of the cone signals. Responses were averaged over the last 50 of a total of 70 stimulus sequences and these amplitudes were recorded from a computer display. For S and for M cone modulation, the contrast level was varied from the maximum available downward in nine or ten steps to levels as low as 0.7 per cent. Five complete stimulus sequences were recorded at each contrast level and these values were averaged.

ERG contrast-response functions were obtained from normal animals, from animals 24 hours following experimental retinal detachment, and at various time points following retinal reattachment. Retinal detachments were created by infusing sodium hyaluronate (0.25 per cent) in a balanced salt solution from a glass micropipette inserted through the sclera at the region of the pars plana to a site between the neural retina and the pigment epithelium (Anderson *et al.* 1986). For a subset of animals, the retinas were subsequently reattached by injecting a 0.2 ml mixture of sulphur hexafluoride (20 per cent) and room air (80 per cent) following parcentesis to control intraocular pressure. At the end of the experiment animals were killed with an overdose of pentobarbitone, the retina was removed and flattened, and the size and position of the detached region was measured. From maps of the density distributions of S and M cones in the ground squirrel retina (Kryger *et al.* 1998) the number of receptors of each type that lay in the zone encompassed by the detachment could be determined.

Results

As documented elsewhere, ground squirrels give large and reliable ERG responses to fast flicker (Jacobs *et al.* 2002). Over the contrast range examined, ERG amplitude increases linearly with increasing contrast. Figure 40.1 (top) illustrates this relationship for both M and S cone isolation. Note that intersubject variability is relatively small. By convention, the slope of the fitted line defines the contrast gain for each mechanism (Kremers *et al.* 1999). For data from a large sample ($N = 41$) of ground squirrels the mean ratio of M and S contrast gains was 21.4 (SD = 8.0). The retinas were subsequently detached in a number of these animals and then, 24-hours following surgery, a second set of ERG measurements were made. As illustrated by the M-cone contrast/response functions shown for two animals in Fig. 40.1 (bottom), detachment reduces the amplitude of the ERG. These functions are also well captured by linear regressions so that the magnitude of the loss engendered by detachment is reflected in a lowered contrast gain relative to the normal. The results obtained for S-cone isolation were similar in nature. For a subset sample of 22 ground squirrels, the mean M/S contrast gain ratio prior to detachment was 25.79 (SD = 8.62), while following detachment the corresponding value was 18.66 (SD = 12.55). These values are reliably different (paired samples $t = 2.359$; d.f = 21; $p < 0.03$). Note that for this comparison the detachment appears to have had a proportionally larger impact on M-cone than on S-cone signals.

The lower M/S contrast gain ratio detected by this comparison could have a number of interpretations. For one thing, detachments can obviously vary from animal to animal. The retinal distributions of different cone types are heterogeneous so, for example, detachments of equal size but varying locations can potentially have unequal impacts on the different cone types. Consequently, a better evaluation of the differential effects of detachment on cone function requires an accurate mapping of the detached area and a determination of the cone populations in this region. To accomplish this, we examined 11 animals that were tested prior to surgery and then again 24 hours following detachment. In this experiment an attempt was made to systematically vary the size of the detached region. Following the procedures described above, an indication of the

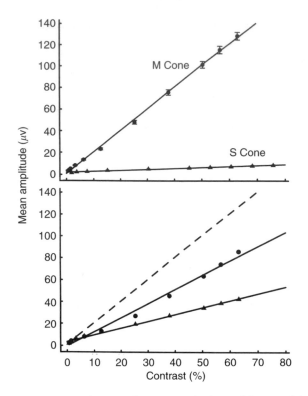

Figure 40.1 Top: Contrast response functions for ERG signals obtained from modulation of S and M cones in the ground squirrel. The plotted points are mean values obtained for S cone isolation ($N = 25$) and M cone isolation ($N = 35$). Error bars show −1 SEM. Bottom: Contrast response functions obtained for M cone isolating stimuli in normal animals (dashed line is the average taken from the top panel) and two animals whose retinas had been detached (continuous lines).

number of S and M cones that lay in the zone of the detachment was retrieved from anatomical examination of a flat mount of the retina. From this information we could make comparisons between the proportions of receptors of each type in the detachment zone and the ERG results.

Figure 40.2 summarizes the relationships that emerge from this experiment. The open circles indicate for each animal the numbers of both types of cone (expressed as a percentage of the total in the normal retina) located outside of the detachment zone. It can be seen that the detachments covered almost the full span of potential sizes including both very small and very large portions of the retina. The dashed line is a linear regression providing the best fit to these size measurements. The excellent fit of this line ($r^2 = 0.987$) shows that detachments varying greatly in size always include the same proportion of S and M cones, but since the slope of this line is less than 1, the proportion of receptors in the detached region is always somewhat smaller for S than for M cones. The second set of data shown in Fig. 40.2 (solid circles) is the contrast gains for M and S cone stimulation,

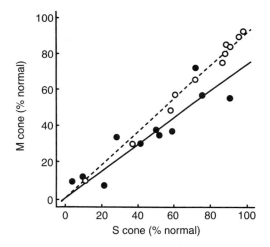

Figure 40.2 Effects of retinal detachment on receptor and contrast gain loss in 11 ground squirrels. The open circles plot the proportion of the total cone population for both S and M cones that fell outside of the detachment zone. The dashed line is the best fitting linear regression (slope = 0.916, r^2 = 0.987). The solid circles show the contrast gains measured for both S and M cone stimulation, each plotted as a percentage of its pre-detachment value. The best fitting linear regression (continuous line) has a slope of 0.739 and an r^2 = 0.801. See text for further discussion.

again specified as a percentage of their pre-detachment values. Across the sample there is a large variation in the size of the reduction in contrast gain produced by detachment. These data too are well fit with a linear regression (r^2 = 0.801) indicating that the loss of contrast gain following detachment is directly proportional to the magnitude of the detachment. If the loss in contrast gain engendered by detachment were the same as the relationship between the proportions of S and M cones affected, the slopes for the two functions should be the same; alternatively, a proportionally greater effect on S than on M function would predict a steeper slope. In fact, although the differences are not statistically reliable (t = 1.329; d.f. = 18; ns), what is observed is a shift in the opposite direction, that is, the slope for contrast gain is shallower than that predicted based on a greater vulnerability of S cones.

ERGs were also recorded from animals following reattachment of the retina. Reattachment leads to at least a partial recovery of the ERG response in all animals, the details of which are currently under study. Of interest here is whether the recovery triggered by reattachment is different for signals originating from the two classes of cone. To examine this, eight animals were tested prior to detachment and then at 24 hours following detachment. Just after this second recording session the retina was reattached and the recordings were repeated an additional three times at test intervals spanning the range from 7–42 days. As noted above, detachment causes a drop in the M/S contrast/gain ratio. Following reattachment, however, we detected no further change in the contrast/gain ratio even though the actual contrast gain values for both S and M cone activation improved by a factor of about 1.5–2 over the examination period.

Discussion

ERGs recorded from the cone-rich retina of the ground squirrel can be used to accurately assess the consequences of retinal detachment while the use of cone-isolating stimuli permits examination of signals originating from independent activation of the S and M cone classes. This study was motivated by the classic result that retinal detachment in human patients often leads to blue–yellow color vision defects and by recent observations suggesting that these color vision changes may be the direct result of a greater susceptibility of S cones to the effects of detachment. Our experiments show quite plainly that retinal detachment in the ground squirrel model does not have a larger impact on S cone than on M cone function as indexed by signals originating in the outer retina. To the contrary, to the extent there is any differential effect of detachment on function subserved by the two cone types the results here suggest the loss may be slightly in the opposite direction, that is, a proportionally greater effect of detachment on M than on S cone function.

The results reported here appear contradictory to the claim that there is a selective loss of S cones in retinal detachment, but there are obvious differences in the nature and duration of detachment in that study (Nork *et al.* 1995) and the present one and, of course, they involve different species and different indicators for inferring cone function. The earlier study involved examination of ten human eyes taken at 2.5–11 days following traumatic detachments. Our choice of a relatively shorter detachment time (24 hours) was predicated on the observation that photoreceptor degeneration in the ground squirrel is quite rapid following detachment far faster, for instance, than that seen in the cat, a standard model for studying retinal detachment (Linberg *et al.* 2000). Nork *et al.* (1995) used histochemical and immunocytochemical staining in conjunction with light microscopic observations to assess photoreceptor changes. Carbonic anhydrase (CA) staining served as a principal marker to separately assess the presence of S and M/L cones. In normal retinas M/L cones stain positively for CA while S cones do not stain. In the detached human retinas, unstained cones showed a virtually total dropout and they were completely absent from two retinas that were detached and subsequently reattached (Nork *et al.* 1995). Although that result seems clear cut, there are several reasons to suggest that it may not represent the final word. First, another study of human retinal detachment that utilized a range of different cellular markers found that at least some S cones in fact survive even long-term detachments (Charteris *et al.* 2000). Second, some M/L cones are observed to become CA negative following injury (Nork *et al.* 1995) which suggests the need for caution in using CA labeling as a sole indicator of cone identity. Finally, although ground squirrels are clearly not humans, our results are apparently not just species specific since a study of the rod-dominated cat retina has also failed to show any differential impact of detachment on the subsequent relative numbers of S and M cones (Rex 2001).

Our results are more directly contradictory to the earlier ERG study done on human patients (Hayashi and Yamamoto 2001). While there is no obvious resolution of the two studies, it can be noted that, unlike the present experiment, the human study provided no compelling way of isolating contributions from the different cone classes to the recorded ERG.

If, as our results might suggest, S cones are not inherently more vulnerable to damage associated with retinal detachment, then what is the basis for the observation that blue–yellow color vision defects are frequently documented in cases of retinal detachment? An earlier research summary shows there are in fact quite a number of potential mechanisms that might explain why S cone related visual losses are common in cases of retinal damage (Mollon 1982). These include factors associated with differences in the relative numbers of S and M/L cones, the distinctive pathways through which these different cone classes transmit information into the central visual system, the possibility that diagnoses of blue/yellow defects from standard color vision tests are prone to artifact, as well as the prospect that S cones are inherently more vulnerable to damage. Our results would argue against this last possibility. Paradoxically, in this experiment outer retinal signals from the M cones actually appear somewhat more susceptible to loss than were corresponding signals from S cones and one should note that their preferential loss would also alter the nature of blue/yellow spectral opponency and this too could lead to the appearance of a blue/yellow color vision defect.

Acknowledgements

This research was supported by grants from the National Eye Institute (EY02052 and EY00888).

References

Anderson, D. H., Guerin, C. J., Erickson, P. A., Stern, W. H., & Fisher, S. K. (1986). Morphological recovery in re-attached retina. *Investigative Ophthalmology and Visual Science, 27*, 168–83.

Brainard, D. H., Calderone, J. B., Nugent, A. K., & Jacobs, G. H. (1999). Flicker ERG responses to stimuli parametrically modulated in color space. *Investigative Ophthalmology and Visual Science, 40*, 2840–47.

Charteris, D. G., Sethi, C. S., Lewis, G. P., Leitner, W. R., & Fisher, S. K. (2000). Intraretinal and peri-retinal pathology in complex human retinal detachment. *Investigative Ophthalmology and Visual Science, 41*, S664.

Fisher, S. K., & Anderson, D. H. (2001). Cellular effects of detachment on the neural retina and the retinal pigment epithelium. In C. P. Wilkinson (Ed.), *Surgical Retina* (3rd edn, Vol. 3, pp. 1961–86). St. Louis: Mosby.

Fletcher, R., & Voke, J. (1985). *Defective Colour Vision: Fundamentals, Diagnosis and Management.* Bristol: Adam Hilger Ltd.

Hayashi, M., & Yamamoto, S. (2001). Changes of the cone electroretinograms to colour flash stimuli after successful retinal detachment surgery. *British Journal of Ophthalmology, 85*, 410–13.

Jacobs, G. H., Calderone, J. B., Sakai, T., Lewis, G. P., & Fisher, S. K. (2002). An animal model for studying cone function in retinal detachment. *Documenta Ophthalmologica, 104,* 119–32.

Jacobs, G. H., Neitz, J., & Krogh, K. (1996). Electroretinogram flicker photometry and its applications. *Journal of the Optical Society of America A, 13,* 641–8.

Köllner, H. (1907). Untersuchungen über die Farbenstörung bei Netzhautablosung. *Zeitschrift für Augenheilkunde, 17,* 234–58.

Kremers, J., Usui, T., Scholl, H. P. N., & Sharpe, L. T. (1999). Cone signal contributions to electroretinograms in dichromats and trichromats. *Investigative Ophthalmology and Visual Science, 40,* 920–30.

Kryger, Z., Galli-Resta, L., Jacobs, G. H., & Reese, B. E. (1998). The topography of rod and cone photoreceptors in the retina of the ground squirrel. *Visual Neuroscience, 15,* 685–91.

Linberg, K. A., Lewis, G. P., Sakai, T., Leitner, W. R., & Fisher, S. K. (2000). A comparison of cellular responses to retinal detachment in cone- and rod-dominant species. *Investigative Ophthalmology and Visual Science, 41,* S570.

Mollon, J. D. (1982). What is odd about the short-wavelength mechanism and why is it disproportionally vulnerable to acquired damage? In G. Verriest (Ed.), *Colour Vision Deficiencies VI* (pp. 145–9). The Hague: W. Junk Publishers.

Nork, T. M., Millecchia, L. L., Strickland, B. D., Linberg, J. V., & Chao, G. M. (1995). Selective loss of blue cones and rods in human retinal detachment. *Archives of Ophthalmology, 113,* 1066–73.

Pokorny, J., Smith, V. C., Verriest, G., & Pinckers, A. J. L. G. (1979). *Congenital and Acquired Color Vision Defects.* New York: Grune & Stratton.

Rex, T. S., Lewis, G. P., Yokoyama, S., & Fisher, S. K. (2001). Cone opsin and phosducin expression in experimental retinal detachment. *Investigative Ophthalmology and Visual Science, 42,* S446.

CHAPTER 41

COLOUR VISION IN CENTRAL SEROUS CHORIORETINOPATHY

MAIJA MÄNTYJÄRVI AND TARJA MAARANEN

Introduction

Central serous chorioretinopathy (CSC) is an eye disorder where serous fluid causes localized detachment of the sensory retina, most commonly in the macular area. Patients are usually young or middle-aged healthy men who complain of blurred, reduced visual acuity. The etiology of this disease is not known. However, psychological stress, vascular disorders, high adrenocorticotrophic hormone, ACTH, and pregnancy have been associated with CSC (Fastenberg and Ober 1983; Gelber and Schatz 1987; Zamir 1997). Spontaneous recovery of visual acuity usually occurs during 3–6 months. Laser photocoagulation has been used as treatment which could prevent recurrences and shorten the duration of the serous detachment (Yap and Robertson 1996).

In colour vision, an acquired blue colour vision defect and displacement of the Rayleigh match towards red in the anomaloscope (pseudoprotanomaly) have been found at the time of the active disease (Jaeger and Nover 1951; François and Verriest 1968; Smith *et al.* 1978; Serra 1978; Folk *et al.* 1984; van Meel *et al.* 1984; Tilanus *et al.* 1998; Bek and Kandi 2000).

The purpose of the present study was to examine colour vision in 12 patients with active CSC and after a follow-up of 1.5 years.

Patients and methods

This study was reviewed and accepted in the Ethics Committee of the University and University Hospital of Kuopio and has been performed in accordance with the ethical standards of the Declaration of Helsinki, 1994. The patients of the study gave their informed consent.

A thorough eye examination and colour vision examination of both eyes were performed in 12 patients (10 men and 2 women) with active CSC. The age of the patients varied from 37 to 52 years (mean 45.2 ± 5.6, SD). Nine of the patients were examined with the fluorescein-angiography (FAG), and leakage was found at the site of the localized detachment of the sensory retina. Three of them subsequently had argon laser treatment. Three other patients had only slight symptoms of the disease and therefore, no FAG was performed. All patients were invited to a follow-up examination 1.5 years later, but only

6 of them came. As one of these patients also then had active CSC, only 5 patients were examined in the follow-up study.

Colour vision was examined with the Farnsworth–Munsel 100 (FM100) hue test. The error scores were calculated as square roots (Kinnear 1970) and the axis according to Smith *et al.* (1985). The scores of the patients were compared to the normal error scores in different age groups defined by Verriest *et al.* (1982). Scores of >mean $+ 2 \times$ SD (one-tailed level of confidence of 97.5%) were considered abnormal. The result in the FM 100 test was considered abnormal if the error score and/or the axis deviated from normal. The illumination was provided by the Macbeth Easel lamp, 1000 lux. In addition, the Nagel anomaloscope was used. Normal values for the anomalous quotient (AQ) and matching range (MR) were observed according to Birch *et al.* (1979).

In statistical calculations, paired t-test of Stat View 512+ (Abacus Concepts Inc., Berkeley, California, U. S. A.) was used, and p-values <0.05 were considered significant.

Results and discussion

The patients had no other abnormal findings in the eye examination besides CSC, and they had no medications or diseases which could affect colour vision.

At the time of active disease, the visual acuity (VA), red-green AQ and MR as well as the FM100 score and axis in the CSC eyes and contralateral eyes can be seen in Table 41.1. Six CSC eyes and two contralateral eyes showed colour vision defects compared to age-related norms (Verriest *et al.* 1982; Smith *et al.* 1985; Birch *et al.* 1979), mostly blue colour vision defects. This is in accordance with earlier studies where also mostly blue defects has been found (Kitahara 1936; Verriest 1963; François and Verriest 1968; Serra 1978; Folk *et al.* 1984). In addition to the blue defects, pseudoprotanomaly was detected in 2 CSC eyes. There was a significant difference between the CSC and contralateral eyes in the VAs, AQs, and FM100 scores, but not between the MRs or FM100 axes (Table 41.1).

During the follow-up study of the five patients (Table 41.2), the pseudoprotanomaly of two CSC eyes had disappeared and the AQ of all five CSC eyes had changed significantly towards green. The blue defects could still be detected in three of the CSC eyes. There was no significant difference between the onset and follow-up results in the VAs, MRs, and FM100 scores or axes. These blue defects have been shown to persist a long time after the active CSC (Folk *et al.* 1984; Serra *et al.* 1989; Maaranen *et al.* 2000) Moreover, apparently healthy contralateral eyes have shown colour vision defects (Serra *et al.* 1989; Maaranen *et al.* 2000) as did the healthy eyes of 2 of our patients in the present study. However, electrophysiological and circulatory studies have shown that CSC really is a disease of both eyes (Iida *et al.* 1999; Marmor and Tan 1999). So, finding colour vision defects in contralateral eyes is not surprising: an earlier subclinical CSC can well explain it. However, this possibility of a colour vision defect in both eyes after CSC should be remembered in occupations where normal colour vision is required.

Table 41.1 Colour vision test results in the eyes of active central serous chorioretinopathy and in the contralateral eyes of 12 patients

| Patient | | CSC eye | | | | | Contralateral eye | | | | |
| | | VA | Nagel anomaloscope | | FM100 | | VA | Nagel anomaloscope | | FM100 | |
No	Age		AQ	MR	Score	Axis		AQ	MR	Score	Axis
1	37	0.7 (20/30)	0.64*	2	23.2*	3.6*	1.2 (20/16)	1.09	0	11.8	2.8
2	38	0.8 (20/25)	0.84	5	15.7*	5.9*	1.1 (20/18)	1.18	3	10.6	4.2*
3	39	0.4 (20/50)	0.62*	3	19.4*	3.5*	1.5 (20/13)	1.12	1	12.1	−0.3
4	40	1.2 (20/16)	1.06	3	7.2	2.4	1.2 (20/16)	0.94	3	8.7	1.4
5	51	0.5 (20/40)	1.03	0	6.8	2.2	1.2 (20/16)	1.06	1	7.8	4.1
6	42	0.7 (20/30)	0.84	1	9.1	2.1	1.0 (20/20)	1.00	2	7.6	1.2
7	45	1.0 (20/20)	0.97	0	16.8*	6.2*	1.0 (20/20)	1.18	1	8.5	3.5
8	49	0.9 (20/22)	0.79	1	13.0	5.0*	1.2 (20/16)	1.18	1	12.0	3.1
9	49	0.8 (20/25)	0.82	2	13.3	1.2	1.0 (20/20)	1.09	4	11.5	0.4
10	50	0.3 (20/60)	0.79	2	19.1*	1.9	1.5 (20/13)	0.94	3	10.3	3.0
11	50	1.5 (20/13)	1.25	1	10.3	0.4	1.2 (20/16)	1.15	2	14.0	7.1*
12	52	0.8 (20/25)	0.82	2	10.9	3.0	1.0 (20/20)	1.15	4	10.1	3.2
Mean±SD		0.8 ± 0.3	0.87 ± 0.18	2 ± 1	13.7 ± 5.2	3.1 ± 1.8	1.2 ± 0.2	1.09 ± 0.09	2 ± 1	10.4 ± 2.0	2.8 ± 2.0
Paired t-test											

Paired t-test   VA $p = 0.013$ s; AQ $p = 0.003$ s; MR $p = 0.572$ ns; FM100 score $p = 0.034$ s; FM100 axis $p = 0.699$ ns

*Result abnormal: pseudoprotanomaly in anomaloscope; abnormal score and blue axis in FM 100 test.

CSC=central serous chorioretinopathy; VA=visual acuity; AQ=anomalous quotient; MR=matching range; FM100 = Farnsworth–Munsell 100 Hue test.

Table 41.2 Colour vision test results in 5 eyes of active central serous chorioretinopathy (1) and in the same healed eyes after the follow-up of 1.5 years (2)

Patient No.	VA		Nagel anomaloscope AQ		Nagel anomaloscope MR		FM100 score		FM100 axis	
	1	2	1	2	1	2	1	2	1	2
1	0.7 (20/30)	0.6 (20/35)	0.64*	0.92	2	6	23.2*	24.8*	3.6	2.3
2	0.8 (20/25)	1.2 (20/16)	0.84	1.00	5	1	15.7*	13.5*	5.9*	5.3*
3	0.4 (20/50)	0.8 (20/25)	0.62*	0.73	3	4	19.4*	18.5*	3.5*	5.4*
4	1.2 (20/16)	1.2 (20716)	1.06	1.18	3	1	7.2	8.1	2.4	3.1
5	0.5 (20/40)	1.0 (20/20)	1.03	1.30	0	0	6.8	6.2	2.2	2.6
Mean±SD	0.7 ± 0.3	1.0 ± 0.3	0.84 ± 0.21	1.03 ± 0.22	3 ± 2	2 ± 3	14.5 ± 7.3	14.2 ± 7.6	3.5 ± 1.5	3.7 ± 1.5
Paired t-test	VA $p = 0.118$ ns; AQ $p = 0.007$ s; MR $p = 0.740$ ns; FM100 score $p = 0.890$ ns; FM100 axis $p = 0.710$ ns									

*Result abnormal: pseudoprotanomaly in anomaloscope; abnormal score and blue axis in FM 100 test.

VA = visual acuity; AQ = anomalous quotient; MR = matching range; FM100 = Farnsworth Munsell 100 Hue test.

Acknowledgement

This study was supported by the EVO (Erityis Valtion Osuus = Special Goverment Share of money for the University Hospitals in Finland)-grant 5503701 of the University Hospital of Kuopio.

References

Bek, T. & Kandi, M. (2000). Quantitative anomaloscopy and optical coherence tomography scanning in central serous chorioretinopathy. *Acta Ophthalmologica Scandinavica*, 78, 632–7.

Birch, J., Chisholm I. A., Kinnear, P., Pinckers, A. J. L. G., Pokorny, J., Smith, V. C., & Verriest, G. (1979). Clinical testing methods. In: J. Pokorny, V. C. Smith, G. Verriest & A. J. L. G. Pinckers. *Congenital and Acquired Color Vision Defects*, New York: Grune & Stratton (pp. 83–135).

Fastenberg, D. M. & Ober, R. R. (1983). Central serous choroidopathy in pregnancy. *Archives of Ophthalmology*, 101, 1055–58.

Folk, J. C., Thompson, H. S., Han, D. P., & Brown, C. K. (1984). Visual function abnormalities in central serous retinopathy. *Archives of Ophthalmology*, 102, 1299–302.

François, J. & Verriest, G. (1968). Nouvelles observations de déficiences acquises de la discrimination chromatique. *Annales D' Oculistique (Paris)*, 201, 1097–114.

Gelber, G. S. & Schatz, H. (1987). Loss of vision due to central serous chorioretinopathy following psychological stress. *American Journal of Psychiatry*, 144, 46–50.

Iida, T., Kishi, S., Hagimura, N., & Shimizu, K. (1999). Persistent and bilateral choroidal vascular abnormalities in central serous chorioretinopathy. *Retina*, 19, 508–12.

Jaeger, W. & Nover, A. (1951). Störungen des Lichtsinns und Farbensinns bei Chorioretinitis centralis serosa. *Graefes Archiv für Ophthalmologie*, 152, 111–20.

Kinnear, P. R. (1970). Proposals for scoring and assessing the 100-hue test. *Vision Research*, 10, 423–33.

Kitahara, S. (1936). Ueber klinische Beobachtungen bei der Japan häufig vorkommenden Chorioretinitis centralis serosa. *Klinische Monatsblätter für Augenheilkunde*, 97, 345–62.

Maaranen, T. H., Tuppurainen, K. T., & Mäntyjärvi, M. I. (2000). Color vision defects after central serous chorioretinopathy. *Retina*, 20, 633–7.

Marmor, M. F. & Tan, F. (1999). Central serous chorioretinopathy. Bilateral multifocal electroretinographic abnormalities. *Archives of Ophthalmology*, 117, 184–8.

van Meel, G. J., Smith, V. C., Pokorny J., & van Norren D. (1984). Foveal densitometry in central serous choroidopathy. *American Journal of Ophthalmology*, 98: 359–68.

Serra, A. (1978). Color discrimination in 23 cases of monolateral central serous retinopathy. *Atti della Fondazione Ronchi*, 2, 242–8.

Serra, A., Fossarello, M., De Martini, G., D'Atri, M., Zucca, I., & Mulas M. G. (1989). Colour discrimination in long-term idiopathic central serous choroidopathy. In: B. Drum & G. Verriest. Colour Vision Deficiencies IX. Doc. Ophthalmol. Proc. Ser. 52 (pp. 229–32). Dordrecht: Kluwer Academic Publishers.

Smith, V. C., Pokorny, J., & Diddie, K. R. (1978). Color matching and Stiles-Grawford effect in central serous choroidopathy. *Modern Problems in Ophthalmology*, 19, 284–5.

Smith, V. C., Pokorny, J., & Pass, A. S. (1985). Color-axis determination on the Farnsworth-Munsell 100-hue test. *American Journal of Ophthalmology*, 100, 176–82.

Tilanus, M. A. D., Pinckers, A. J. L. G., & Aandekerk, A. L. (1998). Anomaloscope examination in macular gliosis, macular holes and central serous choroidopathy. *Graefe's Archive for Clinical and Experimental Ophthalmology*, 236, 326–32.

Verriest, G. (1963). Further studies on acquired deficiency of color discrimination. *Journal of the Optical Society of America*, 53, 185–95.

Verriest, G., Van Laethem, J., & Uvijls, A. (1982). A new assessment of the normal ranges of the Farnsworth-Munsell 100-hue test scores. *American Journal of Ophthalmology*, 93, 635–42.

Yap, E-Y. & Robertson, D. M. (1996). The long-term outcome of central serous chorioretinopathy. *Archives of Ophthalmology*, 114, 689–92.

Zamir, E. (1997). Central serous retinopathy associated with adrenocorticotrophic hormone therapy. *Graefe's Archive for Clinical and Experimental Ophthalmology*, 235, 339–44.

CHAPTER 42

EARLY VISION LOSS IN DIABETIC PATIENTS ASSESSED BY THE CAMBRIDGE COLOUR TEST

D. F. VENTURA, M. F. COSTA, M. GUALTIERI, M. NISHI,

M. BERNICK, D. BONCI, AND J. M. DE SOUZA

Introduction

Colour vision is one of the visual functions severely affected by Type II *Diabetes mellitus* (DMII). Colour vision loss occurs when there is diabetic retinopathy (Remky *et al.* 2000) and is proportional to the degree of retinopathy (Tregear *et al.* 1994, 1997). Colour contrast sensitivity is affected in peripheral vision in the early stages of retinopathy, whereas central (macular) loss is proportional to the stage of the pathology (Fristrom 1998).

These losses have been attributed to vascular changes related to diabetes and not much attention has been paid to the possibility that they may represent neural changes in addition to circulatory ones (Lieth *et al.* 2000). Recent research with various different methods and situations has confirmed that even before the onset of diabetic retinopathy there is colour vision loss (Deschenes *et al.* 1997; Ismail and Whitaker 1998; Kurtenbach *et al.* 2000; North *et al.* 1997*a*) and reduction in contrast sensitivity (North *et al.* 1997*b*). Colour vision may be assessed by different tests and a battery of tests is recommended (Birch 1993) since they measure different aspects of visual function.

A recently released test (Mollon and Reffin 2000) is the Cambridge Colour Test (CCT), from Cambridge Research Instruments, developed by Mollon and Reffin (1989) and clinically adapted by Regan *et al.* (1994). It is a computerized test that uses a psychophysical procedure to estimate MacAdam ellipses, and thus presents quantifiable results (MacAdam 1943).

There is great interest in testing colour vision with the use of a sensitive instrument that gives quantifiable results, since it may allow detection of losses not identifiable with other tests, both in the initial diagnosis and in the follow up of the condition. In DMII, as in any pathology that affects colour vision, better assessment of the losses may result in a more effective therapeutic action.

We therefore used the Cambridge Colour Test to measure colour vision in diabetic patients with clinically normal fundi and in age-matched controls and compared the results with those obtained with other traditionally used tests.

Methods

Subjects

Colour vision was assessed in 9 type II *Diabetes mellitus* (DM II) patients, age 42–76 years, (mean = 60; SD = 11.3) without retinopathy, referred by the Diabetes unit of the University Hospital of the University of São Paulo. Times since DM II diagnosis ranged from 3 months to 14 years. An age-matched group of 9 non-diabetic subjects aged from 48 to 71 years (mean = 60; SD = 9.8) served as control. These Ss were selected from a group of 17 non-diabetic controls because they exceeded the tritan limit of $150 \times 10^3 \, u'v'$ units in the Trivector test, as was also the case of the diabetic patients. Accordingly, they were tested in the Tritanopic Set, as specified in the test manual.

All patients had received ophthalmologic evaluation within a month of colour vision testing. Diabetic patients and control subjects had VA of 1.0, except for one case, for each group, with VA of 0.9.

Colour vision was assessed monocularly in all patients and binocularly in the controls, with the best corrected visual acuity. The patients and the controls were also submitted to the Farnsworth-Munsell 100-hue test (FM 100), to the Lanthony desaturated test, and to the D15 test. An illumination of 1.49×10^3 lux was provided by two fluorescent lamps (Sylvania Octron 6500K FO32W/65K) placed 60 cm above the work surface.

Cambridge Colour Test

We used the commercial version of the Cambridge Colour Test, CCT v2.0, run on a microcomputer (Dell systems) with the VSG 5 graphics card, and a Sony FD Trinitron colour monitor (Cambridge Research Instruments).

The visual stimuli consisted of a target—the letter "C"—on a background of different chromaticity (for details see Mollon and Reffin 1989, 2000). As in the Ishihara test, both were made up of small disks of variable size and luminance. During each trial, the background chromaticity was fixed while the colour of the target was changed in order to determine a discrimination threshold, according to a psychophysical procedure (see below). The opening of the "C" was presented in four orientations (up, down, left, or right). Subjects indicated the position of the opening by pressing the correspondingly situated key on a button box.

The CCT offered two testing situations: the Trivector test and the Ellipses test, each described in detail in an accompanying manual (Mollon *et al.* 2000) and in previous publications (Mollon and Reffin 1989; Regan *et al.* 1994, 1998). The Trivector is a short test, used for rapid screening, in which discrimination thresholds relative to a background chromaticity (0.1977, 0.4689 in $u'v'$ 1976 CIE colour space) are determined in three axes or vectors in colour space: the protan, the deutan and the tritan axes.

The second testing situation, the Ellipses Test, measures three MacAdam ellipses that can be 8, 12, 16, or 20 equally spaced vectors in the CIE colour space. In our groups the 8 vector ellipses were used because the age group tired very easily. The $u'v'$ coordinates for the background chromaticity of each ellipse were: Field 1: 0.1977, 0.4689; Field 2: 0.1925, 0.5092; Field 3: 0.2044, 0.416. For subjects that exceeded a threshold distance of $150 \times 10^3 \, u'v'$ units in the tritan axis of the Trivector test, the ellipses were determined along a red–green axis, in a Blue–Yellow Deficiency Set—Field 1: 0.1977, 0.4689; Field 2: 0.158, 0.4738; Field 3: 0.2422, 0.4634. The software compiled the subject's responses, automatically plotted the threshold for each vector and fitted an ellipse through the thresholds centred on the background colour.

Tests with the CCT were performed in a darkened room, with the computer monitor screen off or dimmed. The subject was positioned 3 m away from the stimulus monitor. The short test version, the Trivector, was determined first, for screening purposes. Eight-vector ellipses were determined. The results were expressed in $u'v'$ coordinates in CIE colour space.

Psychophysical procedure

The CCT used the staircase psychophysical method for threshold determination, presenting two staircases in random alternation. Each staircase began with a saturated hue and proceeded to a less saturated hue every time the S made a correct response. Conversely, an incorrect response or no response was followed by presentation of hues with higher saturation value. Step size was halved or doubled, following correct or incorrect responses, respectively. After six incorrect responses or six reversals, the staircase was terminated and a threshold was computed. Successively, other pairs of hues were tested.

Results

Consistent results were obtained from all Ss, regardless of the lack of preliminary training or the education level. When patients had difficulty understanding the procedure the tester repeated the instructions and allowed a short period of training.

Compared with control Ss (Table 42.1), all patients presented some degree of colour vision loss in the CCT (Table 42.2), ranging from a slight tritan loss (4/18 eyes) to a large tritan loss (4/18 eyes) and from a small to a major diffuse loss (respectively, 7/18 and 1/18 eyes).

Diabetic patients had differences between the two eyes in Trivector thresholds, with the better eye close to age-matched control thresholds and the worst eye showing elevated thresholds (Fig. 42.1). The protan and deutan thresholds were significantly different from those of the controls ($p < 0.005$) but the tritan thresholds were not.

Average ellipse area and length also had much larger values in the worst eye of diabetic patients than in age-matched controls, whereas the angles were close to those of age-matched controls (Fig. 42.2). The fact that DM II ellipses had a narrow distribution of angles, close to 90°, might reflect a tritanopic trend. However, this was not a general rule.

Table 42.1 Test results for age-matched non-diabetic subjects

ID	Age	Eye	Lanthony	FMH100	Trivector test			Ellipses test		
					P	D	T	F1	F2	F3
P. R. S.	48	Both	Normal	36	82	71	163	(32.4, 3.4) 92	(31.6, 2.1) 87	(22.5, 2.5) 43
C. A. S.	49	Both	Normal	52	68	79	236	(39.9, 2.5) 86	(48.4, 2.0) 99	(42.1, 1.5) 88
M. S. F.	54	Both	—	36	120	87	196	(32, 2.0) 89	(37.2, 1.8) 95	(29.8, 2.2) 88
H. R. J.	55	Both	Normal	36	44	51	167	(18.3, 3.2) 102	(29.9, 2.5) 89	(27.3, 2.6) 77
Z. B. N.	55	Both	Normal	52	62	100	173	(25.6, 4.1) 79	(34.2, 2.5) 105	(26.8, 1.9) 55
M. T. A. S.	63	Both	Normal	20	89	69	183	(17.5, 3.9) 80	(21.2, 3.7) 86	(20.3, 3.8) 87
T. C.	71	Both	Normal	40	67	33	163	(31.3, 3.0) 74	(46.9, 3.4) 77	(47.4, 3.4) 68
N. B. G.	72	Both	Tritan	36	92	84	161	(16.3, 2.6) 65	(19.5, 1.9) 111	(20.5, 2.2) 125
E. G. H.	72	Both	Tetartan	48	94	120	181	(43.4, 2.5) 79	(34.6, 1.5) 94	(42.3, 1.5) 74

Table 42.2 Test results for diabetic subjects

ID	Age	Sex	Eye	VA	Lanthony	FMH100	Trivector test			Ellipses test		
							P	D	T	F1	F2	F3
T.P.S.	42	F	RE	1	Normal	172	70	56	118	(67.3, 27) 94.1	(62.9, 47.7) 53.4	(73.8, 53.5) 101.4
			LE	1	Tritan	152	100	110	140	(23.3, 17.6) 69.5	(37.9, 22.4) 78.3	(46.6, 25.1) 89.8
C.C.	60	F	RE	1	—	88	88	101	127	(39.9, 19.2) 88.1	(43.1, 20.2) 87.0	(29.8, 19.9) 64.1
			LE	1	—	108	108	161	179	(25.5, 16.2) 80.8	(38.2, 14.8) 90.8	(36.8, 23.8) 53.4
S.K.	60	M	RE	1	Tritan difuse	128	128	107	101	(27.7, 7.9) 80.8	(36, 11.1) 94.0	(28.6, 9.8) 90.8
			LE	1	Tritan	140	140	72	46	(38.9, 13.6) 88.7	(45.2, 17.5) 97.0	(39.7, 23.6) 82.0
I.A.M.	61	M	RE	1	Undefined	312	132	144	84	(193.5, 2.1) 78.6	(128.8, 2.4) 77.1	(96.4, 2.4) 87.9
			LE	1	Deutan	132	312	144	128	(115.5, 2.4) 84.6	(81.1, 2.5) 91.8	(108.4, 2.0) 78.0
P.B.A.	63	M	RE	0,9	—	116	124	164	193	(58.2, 22.3) 78.8	(35.6, 20.0) 94.6	(42.1, 22.8) 62.5
			LE	0,7	—	140	105	166	369	(44, 17.4) 94.7	(46.3, 16.4) 107.9	(39.1, 19.2) 75.0
A.K.S.	67	F	RE	0,9	Normal	8	—	—	—	(33.9, 1.1) 86.1	(36.8, 1.2) 95.4	(46.6, 1.5) 80.3
			LE	0,9	Normal	0	42	46	153	(154.3, 1.1) 80.1	(39.4, 1.4) 81.8	(55.9, 1.0) 85.2
J.M.P	43	M	RE	1	—	—	81	65	86	(17.0, 9.0) 102.1	(20.8, 13.0) 124.8	(24.5, 9.3) 95.0
			LE	1	—	—	84	90	111	(15.0, 11.0) 104.6	(16.1, 12.5) 72.8	(23.5, 9.7) 103.3
J.L.F.	70	M	RE	1	Undefined	—	119	102	154	(58, 22.4) 79.4	(50, 28.1) 90.8	(79.5, 23.9) 91.0
			LE	1	Undefined	—	86	86	126	(32.4, 18.4) 81.2	(47.8, 25.3) 85.5	(42.8, 18.9) 97.6
N.L.	76	M	RE	0,9	Normal	80	97	73	294	(110.3, 15.4) 84.1	(75.7, 19.8) 88.0	(83.2, 25.6) 76.0
			LE	0,9	Normal	100	143	245	528	(69, 13.1) 88.5	(56.5, 19.9) 89.7	(76.5, 27.1) 72.2

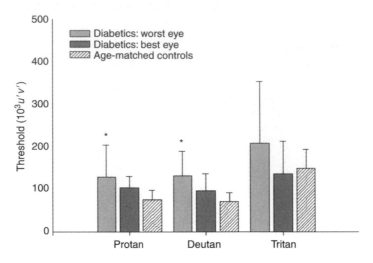

Figure 42.1 Results from the Trivector test showing thresholds in CIE 1976 $10^3\,u'v'$ units obtained along the protan, deutan, and tritan axes for best and worst eyes of diabetic patients and age-matched controls. Asterisks indicate significant differences from the control data.

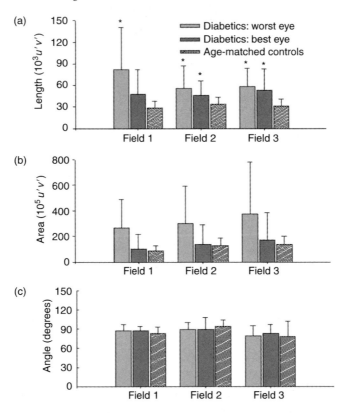

Figure 42.2 Average and standard deviations of CCT ellipse parameters of diabetic patients and age-matched controls. (a) Ellipse length; (b) Ellipse area; (c) Angle of major axis. Asterisks indicate significant differences from the control data.

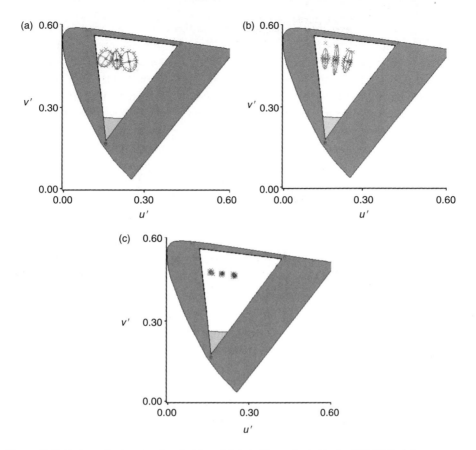

Figure 42.3 Test results showing thresholds and fitted ellipses plotted in the CIE 1976 $u'v'$ chromaticity diagram for: (a) diabetic patient with a diffuse loss; (b) diabetic patient with a tritan loss; (c) normal subject.

Patients were apparently classifiable into two groups: those with clear tritanopic losses and those with diffuse losses (Fig. 42.3).

Duration of DM II

The duration of diabetes was not correlated with the discrimination loss measured by the Trivector test nor with length or area of the CCT ellipses.

Comparison with other tests

The error score in the FM100 hue test was not predictive of CCT loss and showed unspecific losses in 13/16 eyes, a tritan loss in one eye and normal results in 2/16 eyes. The FM score was below 120 for 7/16 eyes, all of which showed losses in the CCT. One of the nine patients was not tested in the FM100.

The diagnosis made with the D15 and with the Lanthony tests coincided with the CCT in only 2/18 cases. Relative to the CCT results, the two tests underestimated losses in 30 per cent of the cases (5/18 eyes in the Lanthony and 6/18 in the D15) or produced a different diagnosis (5/18 eyes in the Lanthony and 4/18 eyes in the D15). The Lanthony desaturated test scores (Bowman 1982) were positively correlated with the protan and deutan axes in the Trivector test, although the correlation was not significant. Comparisons between the CCT and the Lanthony and D15 tests were possible in six patients; measurements were not made in the other three.

Discussion

The finding of colour vision loss in diabetic patients with no retinopathy is consistent with previous reports. Significant lengthening of implicit time and amplitude reduction were detected in the focal electroretinograms of non-retinopathic diabetic patients compared to control subjects (Deschenes *et al.* 1997). Non-retinopathic diabetic patients also had reduced visual acuity and contrast sensitivity and also colour vision loss, compared to normals (Deschenes *et al.* 1997; Ismail *et al.* 1998; Kurtenbach *et al.* 2000; North *et al.* 1997*a*). However, these functions did not distinguish between diabetics without diabetic retinopathy and those in the early stages of retinopathy.

In the present work we found that with one exception, all patients examined with the CCT had some degree of colour vision loss. Although a larger sample would be needed for a stronger claim, it seems that the CCT might be a more sensitive test than the instruments used previously. In fact, in several eyes (5/18) in which FM 100 test scores were relatively low (below 120) for 7/18 the CCT results showed either tritan or diffuse losses. The same happened with the Lanthony and the D15 tests. Of all the comparisons, the best agreement was between the CCT and the Lanthony scores.

The early clinical signs of diabetic retinopathy are mainly related to microvasculopathy represented by microaneurisms. These abnormalities develop after thickening of the capillary basement membrane and pericyte dropout. Since colour vision and other psychophysiological functions seem to be compromised even though clinical signs of diabetic retinopathy were not noticed, a neuropathy may be present. Aldose reductase is found in high concentration in retinal pericyte and Schwann cells and some investigators suggest that diabetic retinopathy and neuropathy may be caused by aldose reductase mediated damage.

We conclude that the CCT has full clinical testability and was the most sensitive of the tests used to detect colour vision loss. It is also evident from the present results that vision should be evaluated in diabetic patients from the earliest stages of the disease. Even though the duration of diabetes was not correlated with the extent of loss in the ellipses data, it was positively correlated with the tritan Trivector results.

Acknowledgements

This work was supported by FAPESP# 99/03013-7, FINEP #66.95.0407.00, CNPq #523303/95-5 and #521640/96-2 grants. Authors D. F. V. and J. M. S. are CNPq research fellows. M. F. C. has a graduate fellowship from CAPES, whilst D. B. O. and M. G. have undergraduate fellowships from CNPq. We thank Claudiel Luiz dos Santos for administrative assistance.

References

Bownan, K. J. (1982). A method for quantitative scoring of the Farnsworth panel D-15. *Acta Ophthalmol. 60*(6), 907–16.

Deschenes, M. C., Coupland, S. G., Ross, S. A., & Fick, G. H. (1997). Early macular dysfunction detected by focal electroretinographic recording in non-insulin-dependent diabetics without retinopathy. *Documenta Ophthalmologica, 94*(3), 223–7.

Fristrom, B. (1998). Peripheral and central colour contrast sensitivity in diabetes. *Acta Ophthalmologica Scandinavica, 76*(5), 541–5.

Ismail, G. M., & Whitaker, D. (1998). Early detection of changes in visual function in diabetes mellitus. *Ophthalmic and Physiological Optics, 18*(1), 3–12.

Kurtenbach, A., Langrova, H., & Zrenner, E. (2000). Multifocal oscillatory potentials in type 1 diabetes without retinopathy. *Investigative Ophthalmology & Visual Science, 41*(10), 3234–41.

Lieth, E., Gardner, T. W., Barber, A. J., & Antonetti, D. A. (2000). Retinal neurodegeneration: early pathology in diabetes. *Clinical and Experimental Ophthalmology, 28*(1), 3–8.

MacAdam, D. L. (1942). Visual sensitivities to color differences in daylight. *Journal of the Optical Society of America, 32*, 247–74.

Mollon, J. D., & Reffin, J. P. (1989). A computer-controlled colour-vision test that combines the principles of Chibret and of Stilling. *Journal of Physiology—London, 414*, 5.

Mollon, J. D., & Reffin, J. P. (2000). *Handbook of the Cambridge Colour Test.* London, UK: Cambridge Research Systems.

North, R. V., Cooney, O., Chambers, D., Dolben, J., & Owens, D. R. (1997a). Does hyperglycaemia have an influence upon colour vision of patients with diabetes mellitus? *Ophthalmic Physiological Optics, 17*(2), 95–101.

North, R. V., Farrell, U., Banford, D., Jones, C., Gregory, J. W., Butler, G., & Owens, D. R. (1997b). Visual function in young IDDM patients over 8 years of age—A 4-year longitudinal study. *Diabetes Care, 20*(11), 1724–30.

Regan, B. C., Freudlander, N., Kolle, R., Mollon, J. D., & Paulus, W. (1998). Colour discrimination thresholds in Parkinson's disease: results obtained with a rapid computer-controlled colour vision test. *Vision Research, 38*, 3427–31.

Regan, B. C., Reffin, J. P., & Mollon, J. D. (1994). Luminance Noise and the Rapid-Determination of Discrimination Ellipses in Color Deficiency. *Vision Research, 34*(10), 1279–99.

Remky, A., Arend, O., & Hendricks, S. (2000). Short-wavelength automated perimetry and capillary density in early diabetic maculopathy. *Investigative Ophthalmology & Visual Science, 41*(1), 274–81.

Tregear, S. J., Knowles, P. J., Ripley, L. G., & Casswell, A. G. (1997). Chromatic-contrast threshold impairment in diabetes. *Eye, 11*, 537–46.

Tregear, S. J., Ripley, L. G., Knowles, P. J., Gilday, R. T., Dealwis, D. V., & Reffin, J. P. (1994). Automated tritan discrimination sensitivity—a new clinical technique for the effective screening of severe diabetic-retinopathy. *International Journal of Psychophysiology, 16*(2–3), 191–8.

CHAPTER 43

COLOUR-VISION DISTURBANCES IN PATIENTS WITH ARTERIAL HYPERTENSION

ANKE SCHRÖDER, CARL ERB, STEFAN FALK,
GABRIELE SCHWARTZE, JÖRG RADERMACHER,
AND ROLF WINTER

Introduction

Arterial hypertension is defined as a diastolic blood pressure > 90 mmHg or systolic blood pressure > 140 mmHg measured several times or as a normotensive blood pressure under antihypertensive medication (Guidelines Subcommittee WHO 1999).

There are different classifications of arterial hypertension based on cause, grade, or course. The most frequently used classification is presented in Table 43.1. Hypertension can result from many causes. But, in most cases, the cause is not known.

The main risk factors are smoking, dyslipoidemia, homocystinemia, diabetes mellitus, age over 60 years, male or postmenopausal female, and cardiovascular diseases in family.

A hypertensive disease increases the risk of severe arteriosclerotic changes in all vessels of the body. These vascular changes have been found in ophthalmic arteries and in the chorioidal vasculature (Meyer and Büchi 1999). Bright (1836) first described a hypertensive retinopathy with clinical manifestations occuring in the retinal vasculature. Since then, our knowledge of the pathophysiology of hypertensive ocular disease has increased. Hypertension affects not only the retinal, but also the chorioidal and optic nerve vasculature. This knowledge has led to a new pathophysiologic approach

Table 43.1 Classification of arterial hypertension based on grade (WHO)

Type	Characteristics
Stage I	No end-organ damage
Stage II	Mild left ventricular disease, retinopathy stage I/II
Stage III	Severe left ventricular disease, retinopathy stage III/IV, cerebral complications, nephropathy

to the classification of hypertensive ocular disease. First and often patients with acute hypertension develop hypertensive chorioidopathy. In this case, unlike the chorioidal vasculature the retinal vasculature is not affected, because it is protected by autoregulatory mechanisms (Bucheli *et al.* 1999; Hareyh *et al.* 1986). These mechanisms stimulate the vascular tone of retinal arteries, which is manifested by focal and diffuse constriction of the arteries. If hypertension is controlled, the retinal vasculature dilates and no permanent damage is inflicted. In uncontrolled conditions the arterioles develop thickening of their walls. Clinical findings of this phase include arterial narrowing, arteriovenous nicking, increased light reflex of the vessels wall, arterial tortuosity and increased angle of branching of the arteries and arterioles. If the autoregulatory mechanisms no longer function there is damage to vascular smooth muscle and disruption of the vascular endothelium with breakdown of the blood-retinal barrier and leakage of fluid and cellular elements. Clinical features of this phase include flame-shaped hemorrhages around the optic nerve head, blot or dot hemorrhages in the deep layers of the retina, hard exudates representing extravasation of lipoproteins and cotton wool spots. As a result of retinal hypertensive arteriosclerosis the patient can develop branch or central retinal artery or vein occlusion and at least a hypertensive optic nerve neuropathy. Consequently this dysfunction of microcirculation, induced by the arteriosclerotic vascular changes, causes ocular dysfunction.

In an earlier study, colour-vision disturbances were found in patients with coronary artery disease (Erb *et al.*, 2001). These patients have a lot of general risk factors and each risk factor should be examined to estimate its influence on the colour-vision. Studies of this kind with smokers and patients with diabetes mellitus have now been published (Erb *et al.* 1999; Fong *et al.* 1999; Kurtenbach *et al.* 1994, 1999).

The purpose of the present study is to examine colour-vision in patients with an early stage of arterial hypertension without end-organ damage.

Methods

Thirty-five patients (14 females, 21 males) with arterial hypertension were included. The mean age ± standard deviation was 51 ± 13 years.

Ophthalmological exclusion criteria were acute or chronic ophthalmological diseases, ophthalmological surgery, congenital colour-vision disturbances, visual acuity <0.6, intraocular pressure >21 mmHg, pathological optic disc, and a hypertensive retinopathy >stage I.

Further end-organ damage by hypertension, for example left ventricular disease, angina pectoris, myocardial infarction, bypass surgery, heart failure, apoplexy, or nephropathy, and risk factors like diabetes mellitus, hyperlipoidemia, smoking or drug abuse, and acute or general diseases and drugs (non-antihypertensive) belong to the general exclusion criteria.

We used a control group of 62 subjects (28 females, 34 males, mean age ± SD = 49 ± 9 years) without any ophthalmological or general diseases.

First visual acuity, refraction, intraocular pressure, slit lamp examination, funduscopy and perimetry (Octopus 1-2-3, Interzeag, Switzerland) were examined.

Next we examined colour-vision with Roth's 28-hue (E) desaturated colour-arrangement test (Roth 1966a,b). This test is a subset of the FM-100, using 28 desaturated color-caps in a circular format. Norms for the test were established by Erb *et al.* (1997). The background used was black cardboard, illuminated with two Osram fluorescent lamps providing 2000 lux at the table (Erb *et al.* 1999). The results are shown in diagrams, which also depict the direction of axes corresponding to several types of colour-vision defects. These axes were calculated by Roth for the 28-hue test from experiments carried out by Verriest (1963) with the FM-100 (Steinschneider 1987). Calculation of global error scores was described by Erb *et al.* (1997), error scores for the red–green (R–G) and the blue–yellow (B–Y) axes were calculated as described by Trick *et al.* [1988].

For statistical comparison of the colour vision test results we used the non-parametric Mann–Whitney-U-test.

Results

The parameters of the ophthalmological examination were within normal ranges in both groups (Table 43.2).

Table 43.2 Results of ophthalmological examinations

	Patients with hypertension		Control group	
	R	*L*	*R*	*L*
Visual acuity	1.0 ± 0.1	0.9 ± 0.1	0.9 ± 0.1	0.9 ± 0.1
Refraction	-0.5 ± 1.5	-0.7 ± 1.6	0.2 ± 2.1	0.1 ± 1.8
IOP	15 ± 2	15 ± 2	15 ± 3	15 ± 3
Cup–disc ratio	0.4 ± 0.1	0.3 ± 0.1	0.3 ± 0.2	0.3 ± 0.2

Table 43.3 Results of Roth's 28-hue (E) desaturated colour-vision arrangement test

	Patients with hypertension ($n = 35$)	Control group ($n = 62$)
Median error score (Median $\pm$ MAD[1])	150 ± 56	72 ± 53.4
Median error score – red/green-axis (Median $\pm$ MAD[1])	81 ± 70	34.5 ± 28.1
Median error score – blue/yellow-axis (Median $\pm$ MAD[1])	99 ± 58	43 ± 26.7
Quotient blue–yellow–green	1.22	1.25

MAD[1] =mean absolute deviation.

In Roth's 28-hue (E) desaturated colour-arrangement test the control group showed an average error score of 72 ± 53.4 (median $\pm$ mean absolute deviation). Patients with arterial hypertension had significantly higher colour-vision disturbances with a median error score of 150 ± 56 ($p < 0.001$, Mann–Whitney-U-test). The qualitative result was a general increase in the error score with no preference for a particular colour-axis (Table 43.3).

Conclusion

Although the ophthalmological examinations were normal we found a significantly higher median error score in Roth's 28-hue (E) desaturated colour-arrangement test for patients with arterial hypertension than for the control group. These results should be taken into account in colour-vision testing to avoid diagnostic interference between specifially ocular diseases (e.g. glaucoma) and arterial hypertension. Similar results were reported recently for smokers and patients with diabetes mellitus (Erb *et al.* 1999; Fong 1999; Kurtenbach *et al.* 1994, 1999).

Indeed, we need to discuss the influence of antihypertensive medication. Furthermore, it would be very interesting if the stage of systemic hypertension and the median error score in Roth's 28-hue (E) desaturated colour-arrangement-test were correlated. We are examining this in a further study.

References

Bright, R. (1836) Cases and observations, illustrative of renal disease accompanied with secretion of albuminous urine. *Guy's Hosp Rep 1*: 338–79.

Bucheli, B., Martina, B., Flammer, J., Hostettler, K., Battegay, E. (1999) Arterielle Hypertonie. In: Erb C, Flammer J (eds) *Risikofaktoren für Augenerkrankungen*. Verlag Hans Huber, Bern: 25–53.

Erb, C., Adler, M., Stübinger, N., Wohlrab, M., Thiel, H. J. (1997) Evaluation of the desaturated Roth 28-hue colour test—preliminary results. In: Cavonius CR (ed.) *Colour Vision Deficiencies XIII*. Kluwer, Dordrecht: 323–29.

Erb, C., Nicaeus, T., Adler, M., Isensee, J., Zrenner, E., Thiel, H. J. (1999a) Colour vision disturbances in chronic smokers. *Graefe's Arch Clin Exp Ophthalmol 237*: 377–80.

Erb, C., Ulrich, A., Adler, M., Isensee, J., Flammer, J., Zrenner, E. (1999b) Influence of illumination on results of the hue-discrimination test, Roth 28-hue desaturated. *Neuro-ophthalmology* 22(1): 33–6.

Erb, C., Voelker, W., Adler M., Wohlrab, M., Zrenner, E. (2001) Color-vision disturbances in patients with coronary artery disease *Col Res Appl 26*: 5288–91.

Fong, D. S., Barton, F. B., Bresnick, G. H. (1999) Impaired Color Vision Associated With Diabetic Retinopathy: Early Treatment Diabetic Retinopathy Study Report No. 15. *Am J Ophthalmol* 128(5): 612–17.

Guidelines Subcommittee World Health Organization-International Society of Hypertension (1999) Guidelines for the Management of Hypertension. *Journal of Hypertension 17*(2): 151–83.

Hareyh, S. S., Servais, G. E., Virdi, P. S. (1986) Fundus lesions in malignant hypertension (VI). Hypertensive chorioidopathy. *Ophthalmology* 93: 1383–1400.

Kurtenbach, A., Schiefer, U., Neu, A., Zrenner, E. (1999) Preretinoptic changes in the colour vision of juvenile diabetics. *British Journal of Ophthalmology*, 83(1) 43–6.

Kurtenbach, A., Wagner, U., Neu, A., Schiefer, U., Ranke, M.B., Zrenner E (1994) Brightness Matching and Colour Discrimination in Young Diabetics without Retinopathy. *Vision Res* 34 (1): 115–22.

Meyer, P, Büchi, E. R. (1999) Arteriosklerose in okulären Gefäßen. In: Erb C, Flammer J (eds) *Risikofaktoren für Augenerkrankungen*. Verlag Hans Huber, Bern: 79–85.

Roth, A. (1966a) Le test 28-hue selon Farnsworth. *Bull Soc Ophtalmol Fr* 66: 231–8.

Roth, A. (1966b) Test 28-hue de Roth selon Farnsworth-Munsell (Manual). Paris, Luneau.

Steinschneider, T. (1987) A new method for presenting the results of the 28-hue desaturated test by means of numerical score. In: Verriest G. (ed.) *Colour Vision Deficiences VIII*. Doc Ophthalmol Proc Ser 46: 151.

Trick, G. L., Burde, R. M., Gordon, M. O., Santiago, J. V., Kilo, C. (1988) The relationship between hue discrimination and contrast sensitivity deficits in patients with diabetes mellitus. *Ophthalmology* 95: 698–8.

Verriest, G. (1963) Further studies on acquired deficiency of color discrimination. *J Opt Soc Am* 53: 185.

CHAPTER 44

VISUAL DYSFUNCTION FOLLOWING MERCURY EXPOSURE BY BREATHING MERCURY VAPOUR OR BY EATING MERCURY-CONTAMINATED FOOD

LUIZ CARLOS L. SILVEIRA, ENIRA TEREZINHA B. DAMIN, MARIA DA CONCEIÇÃO N. PINHEIRO, ANDERSON R. RODRIGUES, ANA LAURA A. MOURA, MARIA IZABEL T. CÔRTES, AND GUILHERME A. MELLO

Introduction

The gold mining activity, in the way that has been done in the Amazon region, has important consequences for several environmental compartments. In the Tapajós river basin, in the heart of the Amazon region, gold mining has been associated with mercury pollution of the environment (Rodrigues *et al.* 1994; Bidone *et al.* 1997; Pinheiro *et al.* 2000*a,b*). Human health can be affected in several steps of this chain of events. Individual pollution occurs in one of the first steps: Amazonian gold miners and other related professionals constitute a group of risk for mercury contamination as a result of exposure to vapours given off during the burning of mercury amalgam (Brown 1990; Palheta 1993). In later steps, the elemental mercury released by the burning of amalgam is converted into organic mercury compounds and transferred to the food chain. These later compounds are also extremely toxic for the nervous system (Hunter and Russell 1954; WHO 1990) and have caused several environmental catastrophes in different countries with serious consequences for human health (McAlpine and Arake 1958; Tsubaki 1968; Harada 1982; Tamashiro *et al.* 1985; Bakir *et al.* 1973; Harada *et al.* 1976). Thus, in the last two decades, the inhabitants of some locations of the Amazon region are at risk of widespread health problems due to environmental mercury pollution (Lebel *et al.* 1996, 1998).

There have been several reports in the literature about the toxic effects of mercury exposure on the visual functions of man and other primates. In the later stages of mercury intoxication there is a severe impairment of peripheral visual field (Iwata and Abe 1986). Notwithstanding this, there are reports of central vision dysfunction, comprising loss of achromatic contrast sensitivity for spatial and temporal modulations (Berlin *et al.* 1975; Merigan 1980; Mukuno *et al.* 1981; Rice and Gilbert 1982, 1990; Lebel 1996, 1998) and loss of colour discrimination (Cavalleri 1995; Cavalleri and Gobba 1998).

The objective of the present work was to evaluate the visual performance of Amazonian gold miners and other workers suffering from mercury poisoning, using chromatic and achromatic spatial tasks. The final goal of this project is to suggest specific and sensible psychophysical protocols that can be used to detect early stages of visual dysfunction due to mercury intoxication.

Methods

We evaluated the visual performance of eighteen subjects who had been exposed to hazardous levels of mercury. Twelve of them were gold miners suffering from mercury poisoning. We have also tested six other patients with different occupational records. Three of them were technicians who had been exposed to high levels of elemental mercury vapour. The other three were inhabitants of communities of the Tapajós river basin, whose hair levels of mercury exceeded the WHO safety level (WHO 1990, 1991). Unlike the other fifteen patients, who were exposed to elemental mercury vapour, the three riverside inhabitants were suspected of having being exposed to organic mercury compounds by eating contaminated fish. The results obtained with the subjects exposed to mercury were compared with those obtained with matched controls with no history of neurological or ophthalmological diseases.

By the time they were tested, the patients had already been removed from mercury exposure by more than six months. Mercury levels were assessed in blood, urine, and hair samples, and were above the accepted WHO safety level (WHO 1990, 1991) in most of patients. However, a dose-response analysis was not performed because of the variable time that the patients were kept away from the mercury exposure before having their sight tested. Routine clinical, neurological, and ophthalmologic examination of all patients was performed prior to psychophysical assessment. The ophthalmologic examination comprised ocular refractometry, fundoscopy, Goldmann perimetry, Humphrey automatic campimetry, Snellen visual acuity, and Ishihara pseudoisochromatic plate test. The exclusion criteria for the present study were the absence of cataract, glaucoma, macular disease or other disorders that could affect contrast sensitivity or colour vision.

The software for psychophysical tests was written using C++ programming language, OFS/Motif 1.1, AIX-Windows R4, and IBM-GL graphic library, all for AIX 3.2.x environment. The software was developed for IBM POWERStation RISC 6000. The stimuli were displayed in IBM 6091 19i colour monitors, 1280 × 1024 pixels, 81.32 kHz horizontal refresh rate, 77 Hz vertical frame rate. They were generated by using IBM GT4-3D graphic adapters, 24 bits/8 bits per gun. We used a dithering routine to obtain 10 bits grey level resolution.

The tests comprised measurements of the achromatic and chromatic contrast sensitivity, colour discrimination ability, and colour discrimination thresholds. All measurements were performed monocularly, both eyes being alternately tested. We measured patient's luminance contrast sensitivity at eleven spatial frequencies, ranging from 0.2 to 30 cycles/deg. The stimuli consisted of stationary, black-and-white, vertical sine-wave gratings, with a mean luminance of 188 cd/m^2, placed at 3 m, subtending 6.5 × 5°. Each measurement was repeated six times and we took the mean value as representative of contrast sensitivity. We have used a modification of the Mullen (1985) paradigm to measure patient's colour contrast sensitivity for red–green and blue–green sine-wave gratings at four different spatial frequencies, ranging from 0.1 to 1 cycle/deg. The stimuli consisted of stationary, isoluminant, vertical sine wave gratings, with mean luminance of 75 cd/m^2, placed at 1.5 m of distance, subtending 13 × 10°. Each measurement was repeated four times and we took the mean value as representative of contrast sensitivity.

We tested the patient ability to perform colour discrimination using a computer version of the Farnsworth–Munsell test. The stimuli consisted of 85 different hues, all with the same mean purity (30 per cent) and luminance (158 cd/m^2), equally spaced on the CIE 1976 chromaticity diagram. They were presented at 1 m and comprised four sets of 21 coloured, 1° square patches. Each measurement was repeated four times, and we took the mean value as representative of patient's score.

We used the Mollon–Reffin test (Mollon and Reffin 1989) to measure patient's MacAdam colour discrimination thresholds. Stimuli were composed of 20 circular patches, with diameter of 0.2–0.6 degrees and random luminance between 7.6 and 17 cd/m^2. The task was to discriminate a Landolt ring against a reference background. The background chromaticity was kept constant while the Landolt ring chromaticity was varied along 20 directions of the CIE diagram, following a staircase and four-alternative forced choice paradigm.

Results and discussion

Two subjects exposed to mercury, one gold miner, and one technician, had performances indistinguishable from control subjects in all tests. All the remaining 16 subjects, 11 gold miners, two technicians, and three riverside inhabitants, had performance lower than control subjects in one or more tests. The subjects exposed to mercury displayed a variable degree of spatial vision dysfunction. Both achromatic and chromatic vision were impaired. They had lower achromatic contrast sensitivity and this effect was more pronounced in the medium spatial frequency range, from 2 to 30 cycles/deg (unpaired t test, $p < 0.05$) (Fig. 44.1(a) and (b)). The mercury exposed subjects also had lower red–green and blue–green chromatic contrast sensitivity than control subjects in all tested spatial frequencies ($p < 0.0001$) (Fig. 44.2(a) and (b)).

The subjects exposed to mercury had poorer chromatic discrimination than the control subjects did. They scored less in the Farnsworth–Munsell test for colour discrimination ($p < 0.05$) and the errors were diffusely distributed in the Farnsworth–Munsell space

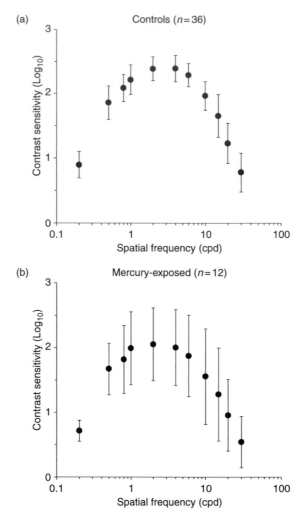

Figure 44.1 (a) Luminance contrast sensitivity for control subjects. (b) Luminance contrast sensitivity for subjects exposed to mercury. Data points and bars represent means and standard deviations, respectively. Seventeen subjects exposed to mercury performed this test. Five subjects were tested following an early version of our psychophysical protocol and were excluded from the means. The subjects exposed to mercury had significantly lower contrast sensitivity than controls for spatial frequencies with between 2 and 30 cycles/deg (unpaired t test, $p < 0.05$).

(Fig. 44.3(a) and (b)). They also performed worse than control subjects in the Mollon–Reffin test (Fig. 44.4(a) and (b)). Their colour discrimination thresholds were higher than normal at all tested directions of the CIE 1976 colour space. The MacAdam ellipses for mercury-exposed subjects had larger area, and both longer major and minor axes than those for control subjects ($p < 0.05$).

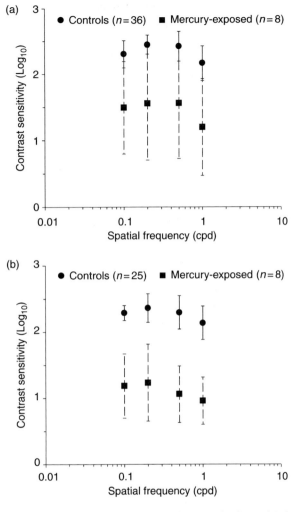

Figure 44.2 (a) Red–green chromatic contrast sensitivity for control subjects (circles) and subjects exposed to mercury (squares). (b) Blue–green chromatic contrast sensitivity for control subjects (circles) and subjects exposed to mercury (squares). Data points and bars represent means and standard deviations, respectively. Only eight subjects exposed to mercury performed this test. The subjects exposed to mercury had significantly lower chromatic contrast sensitivity than controls for all spatial frequencies between 0.1 and 1 cycle/deg (unpaired t test, $p < 0.0001$).

Our results were consistent with those of Lebel *et al.* (1996, 1998) who tested 29 inhabitants of Amazonian communities who had been exposed to high levels of organic mercury compounds by eating contaminated fish. These authors performed a field study in less controlled condition than ours and, as they had a much broader interest, they used a very limited battery of visual tests. They found decreased luminance contrast sensitivity

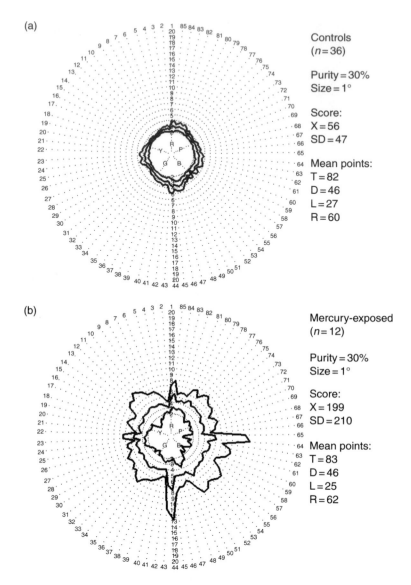

Figure 44.3 Colour discrimination performance of control subjects and subjects exposed to mercury assessed using the Farnsworth–Munsell test. (a) Results for control subjects. (b) Results for subjects exposed to mercury. The contours represent mean values plus and minus one standard deviation for the scores of colour ordering. Twelve subjects exposed to mercury performed this test. The subjects exposed to mercury scored significantly worse than control subjects (unpaired t test, $p < 0.05$). The colour discrimination performance of the subjects exposed to mercury was impaired in all directions of the colour space.

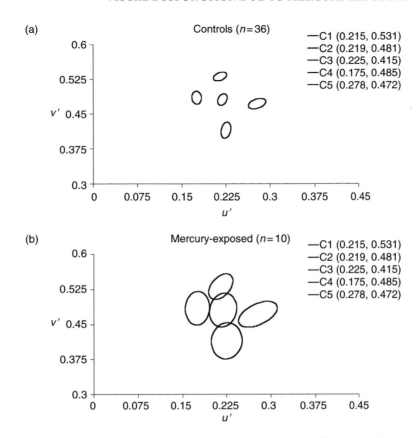

Figure 44.4 Colour discrimination performance of control subjects and subjects exposed to mercury assessed using the Mollon–Reffin test. (a) Colour discrimination thresholds in the CIE 1976 Chromaticity Diagram for control subjects. (b) The same for the subjects exposed to mercury. Ten subjects exposed to mercury performed this test. The subjects exposed to mercury had MacAdam discrimination ellipses significantly larger than those of control subjects (unpaired t test, $p < 0.05$). The colour discrimination performance of the subject exposed to mercury was impaired in all directions of the colour space.

measured using Vistech 6000 printed gratings and decreased colour discrimination using the Lanthony D-15 test. In that study, similar to our own study, there was a large variability of results, which could be explained by different degree of individual exposure. Our findings and those of Lebel *et al.* indicate that psychophysical assessment can be used to quantify the degree of visual impairment of gold miners and other Amazonian population that suffer from mercury intoxication. The functional losses observed in both studies appear to be largely nonselective, and it is not clear that the observed pattern of loss is specific to damage from mercury exposure. Thus, the present protocol must be taken together with clinical story of mercury exposure and confirmatory findings of mercury contamination in tissue samples.

Acknowledgements

This work was supported by PRONEX, FINEP-PNOPG/FADESP #090/00-99, CNPq-PNOPG #550663/2001-0, CAPES-RENOR, CAPES-PROCAD, IBM, and JICA. L.C.L.S. is a CNPq research fellow. E.T.B.D. and A.R.R. had graduate fellowships from CNPq and CAPES, respectively. A.L.A.M. and G.A.M. had undergraduate fellowships from CNPq. We thank Alexandre M. Braga, Antonio T. Silveira, Cleidson R. Botelho de Souza, and Paulo Sérgio S. Rodrigues for software development. We thank Antônio O. Castro, Carolina T. Pinto, and Ruth Mayanna A. dos Santos for helping with the tests.

References

Bakir, F., Damluji, S. F., Amin-Zaki, L., Murthada, M., Khalidi, A., Al-Rawi, N. Y., Tikriti, S., Dhahir, H. L., Clarkson, T. W., Smith, J. C., & Doherty, R. A. (1973). Methylmercury poisoning in Iraq. *Science, 181*, 230–41.

Berlin, M., Grant, C., Hellberg, J., Hellstrom, J., & Schultz, A. (1975). Neurotoxicity of methylmercury in squirrel monkeys. *Archives of Environmental Health, 30*, 340–8.

Bidone, E. D., Castilhos, Z. C., Souza, T. M. C., & Lacerda, L. D. (1997). Fish contamination and human exposure to mercury in the Tapajós river basin, Pará State, Amazon, Brazil? A screening approach. *Bulletin of Environmental Contamination Toxicology, 59*, 194–201.

Brown, N. J. (1990). *Mercury pollution with specific reference to the Amazon basin.* M.Sc. Thesis. London: University of London, Imperial College.

Cavalleri, A. & Gobba, F. (1998). Reversible color vision loss in occupational exposure to metallic mercury. *Environmental Research, 77*, 173–7.

Cavalleri, A., Belotti, L., Gobba, F., Luzzana, G., Rosa, P., & Seghizzi, P. (1995). Colour vision loss in workers exposed to elemental mercury vapour. *Toxicology Letters, 77*, 351–6.

Harada, M. (1982). Minamata disease: organic mercury poisoning caused by ingestion of contaminated fish. In: P. E. F. Jelliffe & D. B. Jelliffe (Eds). *Adverse Effects of Foods* (pp. 135–47). New York: Plenum Publishing.

Harada, M., Fujino, T., Akagi, T., & Nishigaki, S. (1976). Epidemiological and clinical study and historical background of mercury pollution on Indian reservations in Northwestern Ontario, Canada. *Bulletin of the Institute of Constitutional Medicine, 26*, 169–84.

Hunter, D. & Russell, D. S. (1954). Focal cerebral and cerebellar atrophy in a human subject due to organic mercury compounds. *Neurology, Neurosurgery and Psychiatry, 17*, 235–41.

Iwata, K. & Abe, H. (1986). Neuroophthalmological and pathological studies of organic mercury poisoning, "Minamata Disease" in Japan. In: T. Tsubaki & H. Takahashi (Eds). *Recent Advances in Minamata Disease Studies. Methylmercury poisoning in Minamata and Niigata, Japan* (pp. 58–74). Tokyo: Kodansha.

Lebel, J., Mergler, D., Lucotte, M., Amorim, M., Dolbec, J., Miranda, D., Mello, G. A., Rheault, T., & Pichet, P. (1996). Evidence of early nervous system dysfunction in Amazonian populations exposed to low-levels of methylmercury. *Neurotoxicology, 17*, 157–68.

Lebel, J., Mergler, D., Branches, F., Lucotte, M., Amorim, M., Larribe, F., & Dolbec, J. (1998). Neurotoxic effects of low-level methylmercury contamination in the Amazonian Basin. *Environmental Research A, 79,* 20–82.

McAlpine, D. & Arake, S. (1958). Minamata disease. An usual neurological disorder caused by contaminated fish. *Lancet,* 629–31.

Merigan, W. H. (1980). Visual fields and flicker thresholds in methylmercury-poisoned monkeys. In: W. H. Merigan & B. Weiss. *Neurotoxicity of the Visual System* (pp. 149–63). New York: Raven Press.

Mollon, J. D. & Reffin, J. P. (1989). A computer-controlled colour vision test that combines the principles of Chibret and of Stilling. *Journal of Physiology (London), 414,* 5P.

Mukuno, K., Ishikawa, S., & Okamura, R. (1981). Grating test of contrast sensitivity in patients with Minamata disease. *British Journal of Ophthalmology, 65,* 284–90.

Mullen, K. T. (1985). The contrast sensitivity of human colour vision to red–green and blue–yellow chromatic gratings. *Journal of Physiology (London), 359,* 381–409.

Palheta, D. C. (1993). *Investigations of the content of total and inorganic mercury in environmental and biological samples from a gold mining area in the Amazon region of Brazil.* M.Sc. Thesis. Surrey: University of Surrey, School of Biological Science.

Pinheiro, M. C. N., Nakanishi, J., Oikawa, T., Guimarães, G., Quaresma, M., Cardoso, B., Amoras, W. W., Harada, M., Magno, C., Vieira, J. L. F., Xavier, M. B., & Bacelar, D. R. (2000*a*). Exposição humana ao metilmercúrio em comunidades ribeirinhas da Região do Tapajós, Pará, Brasil. *Revista da Sociedade Brasileira de Medicina Tropical, 33,* 265–9.

Pinheiro, M. C. N., Guimarães, G. A., Nakanishi, J., Oikawa, T., Vieira, J. L. F., Quaresma, M., Cardoso, B., & Amoras, W. (2000*b*). Avaliação da contaminação mercurial mediante análise do teor de Hg total em amostras de cabelo em comunidades ribeirinhas do Tapajós, Pará, Brasil. *Revista da Sociedade Brasileira de Medicina Tropical, 33,* 181–4.

Rice, D. C. & Gilbert, S. G. (1982). Early chronic low-level methylmercury poisoning in monkeys impairs spatial vision. *Science, 216,* 759–61.

Rice, D. B. & Gilbert, S. G. (1990). Effects of developmental exposure to methyl mercury on spatial and temporal visual function in monkeys. *Toxicology and Applied Pharmacology, 102,* 151–63.

Rodrigues, R. M., Mascarenhas, A. F. S., Ichiara, A. H., Souza, T. M. C., Bidone, E. D., Bella, V., Hacon, S., Silva, A. R. B., Braga, Y. B. P., & Stilianidi, F. B. (1994). *Estudos dos impactos ambientais decorrentes do extrativismo mineral e poluição mercurial no Tapajós: pré-diagnóstico.* Rio de Janeiro: CNPq–CETEM.

Tamashiro, H., Arakaki, M., & Akagi, H. (1985). Mortality and survival for Minamata disease. *International Journal of Epidemiology, 14,* 582–8.

Tsubaki, T. (1968). Organic mercury intoxication along Agano-river. *Clinical Neurology, 8,* 511–20.

WHO. (1990). *Environmental Health Criteria 101. Methylmercury.* Geneva: WHO.

WHO. (1991). *Environmental Health Criteria 118. Inorganic Mercury.* Geneva: WHO.

INDEX

Achromatopsia 370–377

Adaptation 199, 204, 273–274 (see also Contrast adaptation)

Age, and colour discrimination 337–338; and arterial hypertension 404

Allen, Grant 22

Alouatta, see Howler monkey

Amacrine cell 73–76

Amblyopia 154–158

American Optical Test, see Hardy-Rand-Rittler plates

Anchoring problem 205, 208

Anomaloscope, see Rayleigh equation

Anomalous trichromacy 202–203, 227, 269–270, 274–275, 307, 309, 311–316, 318–325, 343; and lantern tests 356–361; extreme anomalous trichromacy 364–368

Aotus, see Owl monkey

Apes 21, 27, 46, 53–57

Arterial hypertension 404–407

Assimilation 114–120, 231–232, 236–238

Ateles, see Spider monkey

Atherurus, see Porcupine

Baboon 46, 52–57

Benham subjective colours 145–152

Bipolar cell, retinal 63, 71, 73–76, 91

Blue-yellow defect, see tritanopia

Bonobo 53–57

Boundary colours 252, 261

Brougham, Henry *xix–xx, xxii, xxix*

Bushbaby 32, 34

Callithrix, see Marmoset

Cambridge colour test (CCT) 331–338, 370, 373, 376, 395–402; in cases of mercury poisoning 411–12, 415

Camera 269–270

Camouflage 24, 135

Cardinal axes of colour space 123–128, 138–143, 198, 242, 279–287, 374

Catarrhine primates 40, 46, 51–58 (see also Baboon, Bonobo, Colobine monkey, Diana monkey, Green monkey, Macaque, Talapoin monkey)

Central serous chorioretinopathy 389–392

Cercopithecus aethiops, see Green monkey

Cercopithecus diana, see Diana monkey

Cercopitchecus talapoin, see Talapoin monkey

Children 340–341

Chorioidopathy 403

Chromatic aberration 135

Chromatic discrimination, see colour discrimination

Chromatic induction, see colour contrast

Chromatic opponency 191, 195

Circadian rhythm 35

Co-evolution 22

Colobine monkey 27

Colour blindness, see Achromatopsia, Dichromacy, Anomalous Trichromacy, Protanopia, Deuteranopia, Tritanopia

Colour coding 348–353

Colour constancy *xxvii–xxviii*, 204–212, 218–223, 225–229, 239–240, 245, 265

Colour contrast 114–120, 231, 239–245

Colour deficiency, see Achromatopsia, Dichromacy, Anomalous Trichromacy, Protanopia, Deuteranopia, Tritanopia

Colour difference formulae 199

Colour discrimination 98–102, 104, 138–143, 189–212, 289–293, 331–338; relationship to opsin sensitivities 300, 304, 308–316; effect of age 337–338; in incomplete achromatopsia 370; in central serous chorioretinopathy 389–392; in diabetes 395–402; after mercury poisoning 410–415

Colour matching *xxi, xxvii–xxx*, 256–257

Colour naming 174–177, 356–359; in incomplete achromatopsia 371–374 (see also Hue scaling)

Coloured shadows *xxviii*

Colour space 189, 220, 251–265, 266–271, 279–287, 288

Colour vision test, see Cambridge Colour Test, 'Colour Vision Testing Made Easy', D15 test, Farnsworth-Munsell 100-hue test, Hardy-Rand-Rittler plates, Holmes-Wright lantern, Ishihara test, Lantern test, Lanthony test, Pseudoisochromatic plates, Rayleigh equation, Roth's 28-hue test

'Colour Vision Testing Made Easy' 340–346

Colours of thin plates *xxii–xxiv, xxvi*

Complementary colours 253, 261–262

Cones *xxx–xxxii*, 3, 15, 23–24, 31, 35, 39–48, 63–68, 307, 324; microspectrophotometry of *xxx*, 41–48; after retinal detachment 381–387
Cone ratio 39–40 42–48, 51–58, 74
Cone trolands 95
Contrast adaptation 138–143, 203; in Incomplete achromatopsia 371–372, 374–376
Contrast discrimination 94–105, 109–112, 200
Contrast gain 93–94, 201
Contrast sensitivity function, spatial 108, 111–112; in mercury poisoning 411–412
Contrast sensitivity function, temporal 138, 142–143
Contrast response function 92–94, 199, 201
Convergence 160–168
Cryptochrome 35

D15 test 344, 347, 365–367; in incomplete achromatopsia 376; in diabetes mellitus 402
Defective colour vision, see Achromatopsia, Dichromacy, Anomalous Trichromacy, Extreme Anomalous Trichromacy, Protanopia, Deuteranopia, Tritanopia
Depth perception 160–168
Deuteranomaly 202–203, 274–275
Deuteranopia 225–229, 290–291, 300–304, 307, 318
Diabetes mellitus 395–402, 404–405
Diana monkey 53–57
Dichromacy 225–229, 299–304, 307–316, 342
Diet 22–28
Displacement laws 94
Dolphin 32, 34
Dyslipoidemia 404

Edges 79–86, 105, 198
Electroretinogram 15–17, 39–40, 381–387, 402
Emmanuel College *xxii–xxiv*
ERG, see electroretinogram
Evolution of opsins 14–19, 21–28, 31–36
Extreme anomalous trichromacy 364–369
Eye movements 105, 198

Farnsworth-Munsell 110-hue test 331–332, 335, 365–366, 406; in incomplete achromatopsia 376; in central serous chorioretinopathy 390–392; in diabetes mellitus 396, 398–399, 401; computerised version of 411; in mercury poisoning 414
Farnsworth-Munsell D15 test, see D15 test
Fechner-Benham colours 145–152
Fire-fighting 347–353
Flicker photometry 47, 124, 131, 149, 162

Folivory 22–28
Fovea 42–43
Frugivory 22–28, 196, 274

Ganglion cells, retinal *xxxi*, 17, 21, 47–48, 63–68, 71–76, 79–86, 91, 105, 127
Gene expression 299–304, 314, 318–325, 318–325
Gene promoter, see promoter
Goethe *xxviii*, 189, 251–254, 256, 260–262, 265
Gold mining 409–410
Green monkey 54–56
Ground squirrel 382–387
Grouping 242, 245

Habituation, see contrast adaptation
Hardy-Rand-Rittler plates 365–368
Hedgehog 33
Helmholtz, H. von 190, 204, 253, 255–256, 258, 265, 288
Hering, E. *xxxii*, 254
Heterozygote 14, 28, 47, 369
Heterozygous advantage 28
Hippopotamus 32
Holmes-Wright lantern 355, 360
Homocystinemia 404
Howler monkey 19, 21–23, 27–28, 325
HRR test, see Hardy-Rand-Rittler test
Hue scaling 180–185
Hybrid genes 299–301, 304, 307–316

Incomplete achromatopsia 370–376
Interference, Principle of *xix, xxii–xxvi*
International Colour Vision Society, *v–vi*
Ishihara plates 281, 331, 342, 344–345, 347, 365–367; in incomplete achromatopsia 376
Isoluminant stimuli 85, 114, 122–128, 130–135, 148–152, 160–168, 197

Judd (1951) Observer 95, 286

Köllner's rule 381
Koniocellular system xxxi 21, 91, 127
Krauskopf, J. 138–139, 142, 198, 278 (see also Cardinal axes)

Lantern test 354–362
Lanthony test 394–397, 400
Lateral geniculate nucleus (LGN) 21, 91
Leaves, see folivory
LCR, see locus control region

Le Grand, Y. 191, 199
Lemur 14–19, 21–22, 27, 33
LGN, see lateral geniculate nucleus
Lichtenberg, J. C. *xx–xxi*
Lightness contrast 231–238, 242
Line element 288
Locus control region 46, 51–52, 299, 303–304,
    324–325
Luminance noise 281, 286

MacAdam ellipse 199, 271, 288, 292–294, 332, 338,
    395–397, 411–412; effect of intensity on 293
Macaque 40, 46, 51–57, 72, 80–82
MacLeod-Boynton diagram 139, 241, 267, 274,
    280–284 (see also Cardinal directions of
    colour space)
Macular pigment 135, 273–277, 279–281, 286
Magnocellular system 66–68, 79, 82–86, 91–107,
    108, 127–128, 135, 145, 152, 167, 201
Manatee 32
Marmoset 40–41, 44–45, 47
Maxwell, J. C. *xxx*, 189, 256, 258, 265
Mayer, T. *xx–xxi*
MC, see magnocellular system
Mercury poisoning 409–415
Metamers 267–271
Microspectrophotometry 40–48
Minimally distinct border 108, 279
Motion 154–158
Mouse 34

Nagel anomaloscope, see Rayleigh equation
Natural scene statistics 138, 189–212
Newton, I. *xix, xxi, xxvi,* 252–254, 258, 265
Nocturnality 18–19, 32

Object colours 259–260
Opponent colours 254
Opsin *xxxi,* 3–11, 32–36, 39–40, 299
Opsin genes 28, 39–40, 46, 51–58, 299–306; in
    prosimians 14–15, 17–19; exon 2 of 309,
    313–316; in achromatopsia 370 (see also
    Gene expression)
Optical blur 63–65, 68
Optical density 308
Optimal colours 259, 261
Ora serrata 39–40, 44
Ostwald, W. 251, 254, 261–263, 265–266
Owl monkey 32, 34

Palmer, G. *xxii*
Pan paniscus, see Bonobo

Papio, see Baboon
Parvocellular system, *xxxi,* 21, 63–68, 71–76, 79,
    82–86, 91–107, 108, 127, 135, 145, 152, 201;
    in prosimians 17
PC, see Parvocellular system
PCR, see Polymerase chain reaction
Pelage 28
Peripheral retina and peripheral vision 39, 64, 66,
    71, 74, 75, 173–177, 325; in diabetes mellitus
    395; in mercury poisoning 410
Photopigments *xxxi,* 3–11, 14–19, 22–27, 31–36,
    39–48
Platyrrhine primates, see Howler monkey,
    Marmoset, Owl monkey, Squirrel monkey
Pleistochrome 193–198
Polyak, S. 22, 30
Polymerase chain reaction (PCR) 300–301, 309,
    321–322
Polymorphism of opsins 14–19, 21–23, 27–28,
    307–316
Porcupine 31–34
Primate 14–19, 21–28, 33–34, 40, 46–47, 51–58, 72,
    80–83, 325
Promoter 51–58, 324–325
Protanomaly 269–270, 274–275, 368
Protanopia 225–229, 291–292, 299–302, 307; and
    fire-fighting requirements 347
Prosimian 14–19, 21–22, 27, 33
Pseudoisochromatic plates 331, 340–346, 354
Pseudoprotanomaly 389–392
Pupillary reflex 35

Rabbit 32–33
Rayleigh equation 47, 307–308, 313, 315, 331;
    matching range 313, 315–316, 364–369; and
    extreme anomalous trichromacy 364–369;
    in central serous chorioretinopathy 389–392
Reaction time 122–128
Retina *xxxi,* 39–48 See also, Cones, Bipolar cells,
    Ganglion cells, Electroretinogram, Arterial
    Hypertension, Central serous
    chorioretinopathy, Diabetes
Retinal detachment 381–387, 389
Retinitis pigmentosa 105–106
Rhodopsin 3–11, 41–42
Ripeness 23–24, 26–27
Rodents 31, 34–36
Rods *xxx,* 3, 32, 173–186, 267–269 (see also
    Achromatopsia)
Roth's 28-hue test 406–407
Royal Institution *xxiv–xxv, xxvii–xxviii, xxix*
Runge, O. 260, 266

Saimiri, see Squirrel monkey
Schmidt's sign 369
Schopenhauer, A. 251–266
Short-wave (S) photopigment 10–11, 21, 23–26,
    31–36, 42
Short-wave (S) cones 91, 123–128, 130, 142, 148,
    150, 152, 162, 185, 197, 220–223, 240–241,
    279; in incomplete achromatopsia 370; after
    retinal detachment 381–387 (see also
    Cardinal directions of colour space,
    Transient tritanopia)
Sifaka, Coquerel's 17
Simultaneous lightness contrast 231–238 (see also
    Colour contrast)
Single strand conformation polymorphism (SSCP)
    300
Smoking 404–405
Spatial frequency 65, 109–112, 197, 412
Spider monkey 22
Squirrel monkey 47
SSCP, see Single strand conformation polymorphism
Stiles, W. S. 94
Suprachiasmatic nucleus 35

Talapoin monkey 46, 52
Temporal frequency, and contrast adaptation
    138–143
Temporal modulation 145–152
Temporal summation 105
Transient tritanopia 279–287
Trichromatic theory *xx–xxxii*

Trichromacy of colour mixture *xx–xxii, xxvii*
Tritan line, see Cardinal directions of colour space
Tritanopia 32, 218, 220–22, 291–292, 332, 381, 387,
    396, 401
Trivector test 332–325, 396–402

Unequal crossing-over 307, 318–319
Unilateral colour deficiency 204
Unique hues *xxvi, xxxii*, 47, 203–204
Univariance, Principle of *xxx*

Varecia variegata, see lemur
Vergence 160–168
Vernier threshold 79–86
Verriest, G. *v*, 202
Visual evoked potential (VEP) 130–135, 368
Von Kries transformation 205, 274–276

Wave theory of light *xix, xxiv*
Wavelength discrimination 290–294 (see also
    Colour discrimination)
Weber's law 200
White 196, 200, 260

X-chromosome inactivation 40, 47, 369

Young, Thomas *xix–xxxii*, 189, 218